INNOVATION
IN THE
PHARMACEUTICAL
INDUSTRY

D1569800

DAVID
SCHWARTZMAN

Innovation

IN THE

Pharmaceutical Industry

THE JOHNS HOPKINS UNIVERSITY PRESS

Baltimore and London

Manufactured in the United States of America

The Johns Hopkins University Press, Baltimore, Maryland 21218
The Johns Hopkins Press Ltd., London

Library of Congress Catalog Card Number 76-7055
ISBN 0-8018-1844-3 (hardcover)
ISBN 0-8018-1922-9 (paperback)

Library of Congress Cataloging in Publication data will be
found on the last printed page of this book.

For my sons

MICHAEL, JASON, AND PAUL

CONTENTS

TABLES

ACKNOWLEDGMENTS

Whatever merit this book may have as a scholarly contribution depends largely on the novelty and range of data it uncovers and analyzes for the first time. Rarely do students of industry have access to the proprietary data of market research services or the opportunity for detailed technical discussions with operating executives of an industry. In these respects I have been unusually fortunate in obtaining the cooperation of many individuals associated with the pharmaceutical industry and also of Pfizer, Inc., which provided financial assistance.

My creditors in the industry and outside are too numerous to mention, but I should like to acknowledge the comments on early drafts by Yale Brozen, by the late Joseph Cooper, by Harold Demsetz, Solomon Fabricant, Robert Lipsey, John McGowan, John Owen, Merton J. Peck, Jack Taylor, and Fred Weston. Many footnotes acknowledge my debt to IMS America, Ltd., for permission to use their market data; Joan Strauss of IMS was particularly helpful. I also want to thank Thomas Spavins of Yale University for his assistance.

Almost all of Chapter 7 and parts of Chapters 3 and 4 have been taken from my monograph *The Expected Return from Pharmaceutical Research* (Washington, D.C.: American Enterprise Institute for Public Policy Research, 1975) and are reprinted here by kind permission.

Thanks are also due to the American University for permitting me to base Chapter 5 on materials from my article "Research Activity and Size of Firm," in *Regulation, Economics, and Pharmaceutical Innovation: The Proceedings of the Second Seminar on Pharmaceutical Public Policy Issues,* edited by Joseph D. Cooper (Washington, D.C.: The American University, 1976).

My wife, Gertrude, bore the experience of this enterprise with her usual fortitude and good cheer.

INNOVATION
IN THE
PHARMACEUTICAL
INDUSTRY

CHAPTER 1

SUMMARY, METHODOLOGY, AND BACKGROUND

SUMMARY

Pharmaceutical manufacturers compete for sales chiefly by seeking to discover and develop new drugs, and unless this is kept in mind the behavior of the industry is likely to be misunderstood. Competition by innovation in this industry has many consequences, as we will see. To discover new drugs, laboratories must synthesize thousands of new compounds and test them in animals. Few compounds survive these tests and go on to clinical (human) tests, and only a tiny fraction become medically successful marketed drugs. Few prospective drugs satisfy the demands for proof of efficacy in the treatment of a disease and of safety against serious side effects. Adding to the uncertainty, very few of the marketed drugs win large sales. Manufacturers cannot predict the sales of new drugs before doctors have had time to learn about their properties, and very few drugs become popular and financially successful. It is difficult to predict the winners of this game. A few popular drugs which are often the targets of attack have earned large profits, but, as we will see, these are the exceptional successes which have provided the resources for financing the major companies' activities and the incentive for the continued search for new drugs. What is forgotten frequently is that most drugs have small sales. The return from the large investment in research and development (R & D) is highly uncertain.

The failure to recognize that competition by innovation in this industry yields few large-selling new products has contributed to the misunderstanding of the sources and the significance for monopoly power of high concentration of sales among a few firms in many therapeutic classes. (A therapeutic class includes those drugs which doctors prescribe for the treatment of a disease or group of related diseases—for instance, drugs in the therapeutic class of antibiotics are used to treat infections. Market research analysts have devised this classification to be able to record sales by groups of related drugs. For some diseases not all of the drugs in a class are appropriate; for others, drugs from different classes compete—barbiturates, for example, compete against tranquilizers. The classification is only a crude guide as to which drugs are appropriate for particular diseases. Nevertheless, since therapeutic classes include drugs which are substitutes—they are alternative methods of treatment of the same disease—they are taken to demarcate markets. Roughly, then, we can speak of the market for antibiotics in much the same way as we speak of the market for bread or for cereal preparations.) Some economists measure the degree of monopoly power in a market with the concentration ratio, which is the share of total sales accounted for by some small number of leading firms. In a highly concentrated industry, the leaders, according to the theory, face little competition, and they can maintain high prices without inviting entry. Although the validity of the concentration ratio as a measure of monopoly power is dubious,[1] some economists have interpreted the high concentration ratios observed in therapeutic classes to signify monopoly power.[2] But, as we will see, new drugs displace the leaders. Firms therefore constantly search for safer, more efficacious, and more convenient drugs. Patents bar duplicates, but duplicates include only chemically similar drugs, and patents cannot prohibit competition from drugs which are chemically different but offer the same therapy. And patents do expire. The major pharmaceutical manufacturers therefore seek new drugs desperately, the high concentration of sales within therapeutic classes notwithstanding.

The concentration of sales among firms reflects the concentration of sales among drugs, which is the result of the infrequency of effective and safe drugs appropriate for any disease. New therapeutically superior drugs displace older drugs, however popular these older drugs may be.

Without patents, the return from investment in pharmaceutical R & D would fall to zero and private companies would no longer engage in R & D. Because many laboratories can duplicate drugs, patents in this industry have greater value than in other research-oriented industries. Laboratories can analyze the chemical composition of a drug and then proceed to manufacture it without great difficulty. Large resources are required to achieve precisely the desired chemical composition and to ensure quality control, but the technical problems of manufacturing do not prevent imitation. Such duplication is a much smaller threat to the manufacturers of aircraft, computers, and communication equipment, since purely technical manufacturing problems remain difficult even after the designs and processes are well understood. Patent expiration in these industries does not attract a flood of new competitors, in contrast to the expiration of a patent covering a large-selling drug.

Competition by innovation also increases expenditures on promotion. Before they can prescribe a new drug, doctors need information about its numerous potential effects which depend on form of administration, dosage, and patent characteristics. To sell large quantities of a drug, a manufacturer must inform many doctors by promoting it. If companies produced only familiar standard drugs, they would not have to promote them as heavily.

Competition by innovation reduces the extent of price competition. Suppose firms did not innovate. Then as patents expired, duplicates of the original drugs would enter and in time every large-selling original drug would face the competition of several duplicates. Each producer would have little claim to therapeutic superiority for its own product over other products. Some companies would control the quality better than their competitors, and physical differences which are not represented by the chemical formula may cause therapeutic differences. But when the chemical formulas are identical, quality claims have less to stand on and companies therefore tend to resort to price cuts. Thus innovation reduces the incentive to cut prices.

Innovational competition reduces price competition in another way. Despite large research expenditures, companies introduce few large-selling drugs, so usually no more than three or four account for a major part of the sales of each of the major manufacturers as well as of the total sales of therapeutic classes. A given percentage reduction in price will be profitable only if it is less than the resulting percentage increase in sales. A 10 percent price cut will increase profits only if the resulting gain in sales exceeds 10 percent, to say nothing of the increase required to compensate for the additional costs resulting from the growth in output. So large an increase in sales is unlikely for a leading drug with a large share of the sales of a therapeutic group. A cut in the price of a brand will increase its market share rather than the total sales of the group. But an increase in a share which compensates for a cut in the price of a product which already has a large share will provoke retaliation from competitors. Thus, in order to be worthwhile, a 10 percent cut in the price of a product which has 50 percent of total quantity sold must result in an increase of at least five percentage points. This represents a substantial reduction in the market share of competitors, who are bound to retaliate with their own price cuts. When a firm sells only 5 percent of the total, it is more likely to be able to increase by 10 percent the number of units sold, to 5.5 percent of the total, without provoking retaliation. A loss of a half of one percent of the market distributed among several sellers is small for any one of them. A large percentage gain for a small-selling drug is not a significant loss in sales for its competitors.

We must also bear in mind that a leading brand usually represents a large share of its manufacturer's total sales as well as of its therapeutic class. A cut in price which only invites retaliation will therefore reduce profits significantly. Substantial losses in revenue from a single large-selling drug may sharply reduce the margin for overhead and R & D. Not surprisingly, manufacturers of leading brands hesitate to cut their prices. This consideration does not inhibit cuts in the prices of small-selling imitation products, since any resulting loss of revenue from the retaliation of competitors, should it occur, will be small. The manufacturer has other products to fall back on for overhead costs. The share of overhead costs covered by each imitation product can be much smaller than its share of total sales. A company cannot as readily risk a leading brand's contribution to overhead.

In addition, the most compelling appeal of an imitation product, especially of a duplicate, is the price appeal. The manufacturer cannot convincingly claim therapeutic superiority in behalf of a new imitation of an old proven drug. Prices of imitation products are therefore routinely cut in contrast to those of leading brands.

One source of innovative competition has been patents, which have had their intended benefit of encouraging investment in R & D. Since patents have protected most popular drugs, manufacturers have had to develop new drugs in order to grow, and they have in turn had some assurance that duplicates would not wipe out their return on investment. Another souce has been the expectations of continued success created by the successes of the 1940s and 1950s—the sulfonamides, antibiotics, and major and minor tranquilizers, among others—which also set the pattern of competition. This rate of innovation, however, has not been maintained, and the increased cost of research owing to the greater restrictiveness of regulations of the FDA following the 1962 Drug Amendments has reduced the expected rate of return from R & D investment, thus threatening to reduce the number of research projects (if indeed this has not already happened).

A slackening in the search for new drugs would be unfortunate, for they are a more appropriate therapy for a wide range of diseases than are other medical technologies, such as surgery. New drugs have reduced mortality and morbidity rates more than other scientific advances in this century, and future new drugs can be expected to bring further benefits.

Additional new drugs will also diminish medical costs by reducing the frequency of visits to doctors and the number of days spent in hospitals. This view of drugs as an effective and cost-reducing medical technology dominates our study. As we will see, new drugs are likely to yield large savings. This view is in contrast to previous studies' emphasis on monopoly power, which has blinded such studies to the threat which antimonopoly public policies pose to drug innovation and the resulting medical and economic benefits.[3]

The next section of this chapter argues that these studies are representative of many industry studies which view monopoly power as a major problem and as a source of large economic losses.[4] We agree with the view that monopoly power is not pervasive in the U.S. and that the resulting economic losses are small.[5] In particular, the present study demonstrates that drug manufacturers have competed vigorously. Nevertheless, because of the great public clamor the question of monopoly power in the drug industry consumes many pages of this book.

One may question whether the major drug discoveries of the 1940s and 1950s exhausted the promise of drug research; there may be no undiscovered potential drugs for the remaining unconquered diseases. At the end of this chapter we will consider this question, along with questions relating to public policy.

Some people minimize the threat to privately financed research from legislation designed to defeat monopoly power, pointing out that we can rely instead on academic and government laboratories to perform drug research. Although society has left the task of drug research to industrial laboratories, government and academic laboratories may be able to take their place if the measures should discourage industrial research. One's judgment of the seriousness of this threat depends greatly on one's view of the performance of industrial laboratories. If they have done well, then they should be encouraged to continue, for it will be difficult to establish the necessary organizations and develop adequate incentives to perform the research as efficiently. Much of the discussion on this subject represents basic research as being more productive than applied research[6] and thus hinges its arguments on the distinction between the two types of research (the very words "basic" and "applied" suggest where the superiority lies). As we see in chapter 2, this ranking is one of the reasons for many people's distrust of industrial laboratories, which do the applied research, and for their confidence in academic and government laboratories, which do much basic research. So influential is this view that the industry itself is shy about its applied research and boasts of spending a larger proportion of its research budget on basic research than do other industries.[7] The goal-oriented classification applies the term *basic* to exploratory research which is intended to add to knowledge; research which is directed to the discovery and development of new products is designated as *applied.* Some students shrug at the possibility of harmful effects of reductions in the size of the industry's effort, because by definition it is largely applied. For them the ultimate source of new drugs is the basic research which is done outside the industry. It may be a waste of time to deal with a largely definitional argument, but its prominence compels its consideration. In addition, the issues are not wholly definitional, for the evaluation of the work of industrial laboratories requires some discussion of the need for exploratory research in the discovery of new drugs and the extent to which industrial laboratories do such work.

Exploratory research is part of drug research. Scientists cannot simply develop new drugs from findings of earlier exploratory research but must themselves investigate biological processes in order to develop fruitful hypotheses. Usually drug researchers know too little about the related biological processes to permit useful inferences. Use is made of whatever is known, but there is no direct path from biological observations to drugs, as is suggested by the writers who regard basic research as the true source of new drugs. As our description of pharmaceutical research in chapter 3 shows, besides investigating biological processes, the scientists must test hypotheses by synthesizing new compounds which represent potential drugs. Drug research scientists cannot limit themselves to studies which do not utilize such tests in the hope of forming a theory

implying a cure for a disease. The research strategy must include the investigation of numerous hypotheses and testing of these hypotheses with actual
compounds. Drug research thus must be applied as well as basic. Indeed, the
distinction is not very useful for the description of drug research.

The confusion is traceable to the identification of all scientific research with
physics-related research where the distinction between basic and applied research
is useful. Basic research in this field develops a theory which is sufficiently
complete to permit the prediction of practical products and processes given
adequate resources for their development. The original developers of a theory
may not need to test it by manufacturing prototypes of products or processes
(although they may in fact do so). Drug research is different, because the
knowledge of disease mechanisms is incomplete. The scientist can never be sure
that he has the solution to a problem before he tests it with a compound
representing the potential drug. Drug research is therefore constantly seeking
new knowledge about the actions of substances and developing new hypotheses.

One can still dismiss the industry's research effort as trivial, even after the
role of basic research is understood. For this analysis does not preclude the
industry from devoting its efforts to the discovery of trivially new products. A
worse condemnation of the industry's research activities, then, assigns such
research, along with promotion, to the collection of efforts to differentiate
products; "differentiation" connotes insignificant changes.[8] The argument is
that the fear of retaliation to price reductions leads oligopolistic firms to make
minor product alterations which can be expensively promoted as superior to the
original versions. New drugs, according to this view, frequently are simply
molecular modifications of basic agents which the industry owes to basic
research performed by outside laboratories. The molecular modifications, then,
have the same therapeutic effects as the original drugs. In order to support its
assertion about the emphasis on product differentiation, this view leans as well
on the apparently heavy promotional expenditures of drug companies. The
theory views doctors as susceptible to the persuasion of drug manufacturers'
promotional efforts.

The criticism suggests that industrial research differs from the research which
led to the important drugs. Industrial laboratories, however, follow standard
pharmaceutical research procedures. Leads to hypotheses come from a wide
variety of sources, including the observed biological actions of marketed drugs,
and scientists systematically investigate the properties of chemically related
groups of compounds by modifying molecular structures and observing the
resulting differences in biological effects which show up in animal tests.

Chapter 3 includes a description of the work and organization of industrial
laboratories. Certain conclusions emerge. The work requires the close cooperation of a multidisciplinary group of scientists who follow up numerous leads
and, using specially devised animal models of diseases, test the many hypotheses
represented by newly synthesized compounds. The laboratories must have the

facilities for performing massive animal tests and must be able to organize and evaluate clinical tests. In addition, the inconclusiveness of animal tests of efficacy and safety requires the coordination of tasks of different specialists. Final judgments must await a late stage of clinical testing after many different kinds of specialists have participated. Since some potential drugs return for further modification to the chemists who synthesized the original compound, these chemists must retain their interest in the compound until a late stage. This is one reason why it is difficult for scientists who perform some initial animal tests for a compound to "discover" a drug and sell the rights to its development and manufacture to a pharmaceutical company. The high degree of uncertainty prohibits the division of work between laboratories which do only exploratory research and those which continue the research to a later stage of discovery and development. Indeed, a drug cannot be said to have been discovered until the completion of human tests, even though discovery usually is credited to the person or laboratory first observing the desired biological activity in a compound.

The high cost of R & D has also contributed to increasing the dominance of large companies in drug research. Chapter 3 estimates the average cost of R & D per New Chemical Entity (NCE) in 1973 to have been as high as $24 million. The cost is much higher than it was in 1960, owing to the greater restrictiveness of FDA regulations governing the approval of drugs for marketing and to the larger investment of resources in the search for new drugs to deal with such difficult diseases as arthritis and atherosclerosis. Consequently, as chapter 4 shows, the industry discovers the vast majority of new drugs. We estimate that the industry discovered 91 percent of all NCE's introduced between 1960 and 1969.

Related questions concern the relationship between size of firm and number of innovations. Chapter 5 shows that large firms discover and develop proportionally more new drugs than do small firms. This is so because they devote proportionally more resources to research and also because, in this field, large laboratories employ resources more productively.

Chapter 6 shows that competition by innovation has led to a few drugs and therefore a few companies obtaining a large proportion of the sales in each therapeutic class. Many companies conduct substantial research programs, especially in the search for new drugs in therapeutic classes serving many patients. Nevertheless, the new products are few, and even fewer gain large sales. We also will see that competition by innovation has led to a high rate of turnover among leading drugs.

For the industry's R & D investment to continue, its profitability, which is measured by the expected rate of return, must be at least equal to the profitability of alternative investments.[9] Chapter 7 estimates the current expected rate to be 3.3 percent, which is much less than expected rates from other investments. Another reason for anticipating a decline in the level of investment is the fall in the expected rate of return, which in 1960 was 11.4 percent. These estimates are of central importance for this study of innovation in the pharmaceutical industry, for they lead us to expect a continued decline in the rate of innovation.

The expected rate of return from investment is a good index of monopoly power as well as a useful predictor of investment, for monopolistic firms are unlikely to expect a low rate of return. The relevant theory points to the expected rate as the appropriate criterion of monopoly power: this is what economists are estimating, without explicitly acknowledging it, when they use the realized rate of profit as their criterion. The realized rate, however, is a poor estimator of the expected rate, for it is the ratio of earnings to book value of assets, which may be inflated to reflect expected monopoly returns. In addition, the costs of capital equipment are likely to be above book values. Further, since realized rates of profit are estimated for companies, arbitrary accounting procedures which risk large errors are required to make corresponding estimates for groups of products. Finally, a correct estimate of profitability must capitalize R & D expenditures rather than treat them as a current expense, as is usually done with R & D expenditures in arriving at estimates of realized rates of profit.

The other popular index of monopoly power, the concentration ratio, has weak theoretical and empirical support, and its reliability suffers from uncertainty about the location of market boundaries.

The expected rate of return is much more easily defended. The estimate assumes current input and output prices, the best current technology, and average operating efficiency, and it is computed for a specific product or range of products. A high expected rate of return provides a good prima facie case for the exercise of monopoly power. As we have mentioned, the expected rate of return from investment in R & D in the drug industry is low, and the major part of total investment by far is devoted to R & D. It follows that the expected rate of return on total investment is low, and consequently monopoly power is absent.

The evidence of monopoly power provided by the high realized rate of return earned by drug manufacturers, however, cannot be rejected out of hand. The average rate of return on stockholders' equity in the period 1968–72 was 18.1 percent, or 7.5 percentage points more than the average rate in all manufacturing industries, which was 10.6 percent. Large as it is, the difference is accounted for by factors other than monopoly power. We will see in chapter 7 that the largest single component is the result of the accounting practice of charging R & D expenditures as a current expense rather than as an investment. The appropriate procedure of capitalization would reduce the difference by 3.5 percentage points. Investment in the drug industry is more risky than that in other industries, owing to the importance of investment in R & D and the riskiness of drug R & D in particular. Adjustment for relative riskiness reduces the difference by an additional 2.8 percentage points. The third element is the growth of demand. Profits in the drug industry have been high because demand has increased more than in other industries. An adjustment for this component reduces the difference by 1.1 percentage points, leaving a final residual of only 0.1 percentage point. Monopoly power evidently does not explain the relatively high realized profit rate in the drug industry.

The expected rate of return from investment in R & D would be much smaller than it is were it not for patent protection. The Nelson Bill, which aims to diminish monopoly power in the drug industry by reducing patent life, presumably assumes that the present protection is unnecessary to produce the desired level of investment, thus raising the question of the actual length of life of drug patents. The nominal length of life, which is measured from the date of issue of a patent to its expiration, is seventeen years. But drugs are marketed only after extensive animal and clinical tests, and the effective life therefore begins usually much later than the issue of the patent. Chapter 8 estimates that the average effective patent life of drugs introduced in the period 1970–73 is 12.4 years, or 4.6 years less than the nominal life. Short as this period is, it must include the period of introduction in which sales are small and the cost of marketing is high. The companies thus have considerably less time in which to earn a return on their investment in R & D than is generally believed. This short average effective patent life is partly the result of the increased stringency of regulatory demands by the Food and Drug Administration (FDA) for evidence of efficacy and safety following the 1962 Drug Amendments. Regulatory procedures have delayed and therefore reduced the effective patent life of recently approved drugs more than that of earlier ones. Our study demonstrates that the effective length of life declined by 1.5 years from 1966–69 to 1970–73. It took longer in the more recent period to perform the tests and otherwise meet the requirements of the FDA regulations.

A prominent issue concerns the magnitude of promotional expenditures. Excessive promotional expenditures allegedly raise prices. Those who support this view observe that there is a higher ratio of promotion expenditures to sales in pharmaceuticals than in other industries; they also point to doctors' complaints about the large number of visits by detail men and the large volume of promotional mail. Some writers infer not only that costs are excessive but also that the promotional effort persuades doctors to prescribe the wrong drugs and to overmedicate patients.[10]

We have referred to the explanation of apparently high promotional expenditures offered by the model of differentiated oligopoly. Our alternative view is that doctors need information to prescribe correctly, and firms therefore must promote their drugs to sell them. The data, which are reported in chapter 9, fail to indicate excessive influence on doctors. Detail calls, which account for a large proportion of total promotional costs, must be frequent for detail men to have excessive influence, but the detail men of each of the eight leading firms call on each doctor an average of only 3.4 times per year. Nor is the volume of mail as large as the complaints suggest, for each of the same firms mails only an average of 34 pieces annually to each doctor, despite the large number of drugs marketed.

The potential savings to consumers from the reduction of promotional expenditures would be small. Our best estimate of total promotional expenditures is 12.4 percent of manufacturers' sales, which is equivalent to 6.2 percent of consumer drug expenditures, retailers absorbing the difference. For consumers to save this amount, manufacturers must spend nothing at all on promotion, and both they and retailers must pass the resulting savings on completely to consumers. Retailers will pass on about half of any resulting savings, thus leaving 3.1 percent as the potential savings to consumers. This is a maximum estimate, because companies would, of course, have to supply some information about their products.

The estimate that the cost of promotion represents 12.4 percent of manufacturers' sales may rest on shaky data, albeit the best available. If, following the same line of analysis, we accept the frequently proposed high estimate of 20 percent, the potential savings to consumers would be less than 5 percent, or not much more than our best estimate. This small saving can only come at the cost of a drastic cut in the flow of information to doctors, and any resulting deterioration in the quality of prescribing would raise the cost of medical care. Although the companies are not the sole source of information, a severe cut in their promotional efforts would be unfortunate. Busy doctors cannot be expected to increase their reading of the published literature on drugs sufficiently to offset the loss in information resulting from decreased promotion. Not only must they learn about the many properties of new drugs, but they also must relearn some of the things they've forgotten, and the amount of knowledge to be disseminated about a drug increases with its use. Information concerning drugs also speeds up the adoption of new drugs by doctors and thus results in better therapy. Doctors do not prescribe new drugs immediately after they are introduced, partly out of caution but also because of ignorance. As we see in Chapter 9, more rapid adoption of tuberculosis drugs would have reduced the mortality rate from tuberculosis more rapidly. Heavier promotion would also have reduced the costs of hospitalization due to tuberculosis more rapidly. Public policy designed to limit promotional expenditures and so reduce the cost of drugs is likely to result in a deterioration in therapy and in a larger increase in the cost of hospitalization.

Promotion also has certain important indirect benefits. The manufacturers of well-known brand-name drugs value their reputations for high quality, particularly since reports of any harmful effects of these drugs attract a great deal of attention. Promotional expenditures, then, create an incentive to guard against defective products, and they thus indirectly assure the public of high quality.

The condemnation of the apparently high level of promotional expenditures ignores the influence of the large numbers of companies, of doctors to be informed, and of drugs, as well as the special importance of information in this industry. The average sales per doctor of each of the eight leading firms is only $1,500. Modest promotional expenditures per doctor per product quickly add up to a substantial amount.

Promotion is also blamed for the high prices of brand-name products compared to those of generic versions, which raises the question of the relative quality of the two groups of products—a matter which we consider in chapters 10 and 11. The FDA's assurance of the good quality of all marketed drugs may render unnecessary the special claims made in behalf of promoted drugs. However, studies of the FDA's surveillance of manufacturing practices deny the validity of the agency's guarantee. Studies have also demonstrated that the large manufacturers meet higher standards of quality than small manufacturers. The user of a generic product thus risks poor quality, particularly when he is ignorant of the source.

Generic prescribing, nevertheless, has increased as the patents of the leading drugs have expired and the rate of innovation has declined. One consequence has been sharp price cuts, especially in antibiotics. We see in chapter 12 that the large sales of popular drugs have exposed their manufacturers to price competition from imitations produced by rivals. As we have already suggested, the attraction of price competition is increased by the imitations' small share of total sales of their therapeutic class and of their manufacturer's sales as well as by the high ratio of overhead to total costs, so that even large firms have not hesitated to cut prices.

The popular belief that their indifference to drug prices encourages doctors to prescribe high-price brand-name products makes a mystery of the observed price competition. For, in that case, a price cut would induce only a small increase in the quantity sold, one which would be insufficient to offset the direct loss in revenue resulting from the price cut. But manufacturers know the effects of price cuts on their sales. When they cut their prices, they increase their market shares, reducing those of manufacturers which maintain their prices. In recent years doctors have written more generic prescriptions, and pharmacists fill generic prescriptions with low-price generic and brand-name products. Generic prescribing, however, cannot account for the price competition of the early 1960s, so we must look elsewhere for the explanation. A large part of the responsiveness of market shares to prices may be due to the substitution of low-price drugs for high-price drugs which are specified in prescriptions. Such substitution is generally illegal without the prescribing doctor's express permission, which is both a nuisance for pharmacists to request and for doctors to give. Our study indicates that many pharmacists substitute low-price drugs for prescribed drugs without first obtaining a doctor's consent. Thus, the apparent indifference of doctors to prices has been of no consequence. As has been observed in other contexts, the market often overrules the law.

Our major conclusion is that public policy toward the industry should seek to encourage innovation. Continued investment in R & D promises to produce beneficial drugs. This study will show that there is little basis for the pre-eminence of the monopoly issue both in the economic literature on the industry and in proposals for public policy.

METHODOLOGY

The structuralist theory of oligopoly provides the framework for most recent studies of industries: it is the prevalent theory of industry behavior. Such studies describe the structure of an industry—structure referring to such characteristics as the concentration ratio, the condition of entry, the availability and impor-tance of the economies of scale of plant and of firm, the number of buyers, and whether the individual firms' products which are essentially similar to competi-tive products can readily be differentiated in the minds of consumers by means of advertising. These structural characteristics are the result of technology or other aspects of the industry which are independent of the behavior of firms. The concentration ratio is seen as the result of difficult entry, which in turn reflects the need for large size of plant in order to minimize the cost of production. The combination of the technological conditions of production and the prices of the various factors which are employed determine the costs of production and thus the concentration ratio. In this model it is not the behavior of firms which determines the concentration ratio. Since concentration is caused by difficult entry, profits can be high in such industries without attracting the competition of new firms, and established firms can continue to maintain prices yielding excessive profits. The leaders in a highly concentrated industry will find it in their interest to maintain high prices, and they will do so. The structuralist theory dismisses as unimportant the problems raised by the practical difficulties of colluding in the face of the Sherman Act and the dissatisfaction of some firms with their small market shares. It also ignores the possibility that the observed high concentration comes from the past successes of leading firms and their ability to maintain their superior efficiency over other producers rather than from difficult entry owing to economies of scale or other barriers.

The authors of structuralist studies hope to be able to classify industries according to the structural characteristics and thus predict firms' behavior. The concentration ratio and the differentiability of the product receive emphasis, since the theory holds that sellers in highly concentrated markets prefer to differentiate their products whenever possible rather than to cut prices.[11] The theory thus suggests that prices in the drug industry, which has been taken to be an example of differentiated oligopoly, are higher than those which would prevail in a many-seller market in which companies did not promote brand names. Each structuralist study seeks to determine whether the structure cor-responds to differentiated oligopoly (i.e., whether the market is concentrated and products are differentiated) or some other market model, such as atomistic competition, in which there are many sellers and products are undifferentiated. The studies then go on to determine whether the indicated model predicts the competitive behavior well. The studies conclude by evaluating the social performance of the industry. They look at profits, the ratio of advertising expenditures to sales, efficiency, and progressiveness. Since the latter two aspects of performance are difficult to judge, profits and advertising attract most of the attention, the other two dimensions receiving only token service. The prediction is that a high degree of concentration leads to excessive profits and promotional expenditures. The popularity of the structuralist model of differentiated oligopoly notwithstanding, the evidence in its favor is inconclusive. Some studies show only weak relationships between the concentration ratio and the profit rate,[12] and the ratio of advertising expenditures to sales,[13] and others show none.[14]

Some economists therefore have suggested that the structuralist models may be inadequate. F. M. Scherer, among others, suggests that competitive behavior may be independent of structure and therefore that studies of structure provide poor predictions of performance.[15]

Others suggest that firms in concentrated industries may compete in price and, indeed, that the concentration ratio may be the result of rather than the source of the competitive behavior.[16] Highly efficient firms can be expected to seek a large share of sales and to succeed. The usual list of structural variables thus may fail to predict industry behavior. In addition, industries differ sufficiently to prohibit good predictions based on answers to a few questions. Acceptance of the model of differentiated oligopoly thus does not save authors the effort of examining the peculiar features of an industry's environment, technology, and experience if they wish to explain persuasively its observed behavior. Inquiries must be "historical" or open-ended; the theory really does not perform the desired service of delimiting the important questions. The peculiarities of the drug industry include the special role of information, the unusual importance of defective quality, the large investments in R & D, the technical and commercial uncertainty of innovation, and the experience of the industry. This experience includes the innovations of the 1940s and 1950s, which led to a high expected rate of return from investment in R & D, which in turn induced a high level of investment. Finally, patients represented by doctors are an unusual group of consumers in their enthusiasm for new products. Firms have recognized the value to doctors of new and potentially helpful therapeutic tools.

The weakness of the evidence does not appear to have reduced significantly the appeal of the structuralist oligopoly theory, which every industry study must honor by reciting the measures of concentration, commenting on the condition of entry, examining promotional expenditures, and so on. The theory has defined the issues even for industry studies which deny the presence of monopoly power. Disagreements generally are confined to such questions as the definition of market boundaries and whether or not the evidence with respect to collusion or other competitive behavior is conclusive—issues which do not challenge the validity of the model itself. Fundamentally, most studies have accepted the unsupported theoretical criteria of monopoly power.

The political appeal of the model of differentiated oligopoly which attacks a few large apparently profitable firms attracts many economists, along with large segments of the general public. The model also has the advantage of supplying a plausible summary answer for many complex questions: it saves work. The model saves industry studies from becoming open-ended, difficult to manage, and requiring a great deal of thought. In addition, it is easier to refute or confirm a few hypotheses which are suggested by a theory than it is to evaluate a free-standing argument. Moreover, the theoretically guided studies win approval by observing the scientific tradition of testing theoretically specified hypotheses. Nevertheless, what matters in the end are the conclusions which evaluate the performance of the industries, and these often are unwarranted. The studies do not usually confine themselves to the scientific task of testing hypotheses. Uncautiously they go on to reach conclusions concerning sources of competitive behavior and to evaluate performance, thereby implicitly assuming that they are applying a hardy model which has withstood the rigors of previous tests. This is not so, and the conclusions therefore are unwarranted. The persistent application of the model of differentiated oligopoly has harmed the study of industrial behavior by "scientifically" justifying the exclusion of important evidence from the examination of competitive behavior and performance and thereby encouraging premature judgments.

Our approach thus has much to recommend it. The peculiarities of industries generally, and of the drug industry in particular, and the weakness of the criteria of monopoly power warrant the skepticism regarding oligopoly theory. We leave the study open to evidence which we might otherwise reject as irrelevant. Our persuasiveness will depend on the quality of the evidence and of the logic. This openness makes a great demand on readers, for it is easier to judge whether or not the data support a well-known and familiar theory than it is to evaluate an independent argument. But such judgment is unavoidable in any case, and it is better to be aware of and advertise the necessity than to ignore or conceal it.

Finally, our approach is not committed to the view that monopoly is the paramount issue. Unfortunately, concern with monopoly power dominates the field of industrial organization to the exclusion of other, more important, problems. Instead of investigating conditions favoring innovation, economists pose the narrower question relating monopoly power to innovation, price rigidity, plant efficiency, and advertising expenditures.[17] They assume without any basis that the effect of the degree of monopoly power on any of these and other aspects of firm behavior is large. The cost of making price changes may have a greater effect on the speed of such changes,[18] and surely the demand for information has much to do with the volume of advertising.[19] The dominance of the monopoly issue over other questions thus has distorted severely the investigation of many problems, blinding economists to the importance of certain variables which would otherwise be obvious.

Since the quality of studies of the drug industry seems especially to have suffered, the present study attempts a broader scope than most others. We do investigate the monopoly issue—in fact, it is difficult for us to avoid making the same assumptions which we have criticized—but our approach stresses the need for new drugs, to which we now turn.

DRUGS AND THE COST OF MEDICAL CARE

Public policy for reducing the surfering and both the indirect and direct costs of disease is a major and increasingly urgent political issue. The indirect costs resulting from the ill health and premature death of members of the labor force exceed the direct costs of medical care, but it is the latter which are at the center of public attention, and society as a whole is assuming an increasing share of these costs. Two factors are causing the direct costs to grow. First, the growth in numbers of the elderly adds to the demand for medical care, and, second, the costs of medical care, notably those of hospital treatment, have been rising rapidly with the development of such costly medical technologies as kidney dialysis, open heart surgery, and coronary bypass implantation. These trends increase the cost-reducing effect of the substitution of drug therapy for other forms of therapy and thus increase the social benefits of drugs.

The cost of medical care absorbs a large and growing fraction of the gross national product. Currently the share is 7.7 percent, and it has risen rapidly since the introduction of Medicare and Medicaid. A national health insurance program would increase the burden by placing massive new demands on the present limited supply of services which can be expanded only slowly. Depending on the assumptions which one makes regarding the extent of a national health plan, estimates for health cost outlays for 1980 range from $174 billion to $199 billion,[20] compared to current health costs in the vicinity of $120 billion.

For some diseases drugs provide relatively inexpensive therapy. The advent of broad-spectrum antibiotics and of tranquilizers had the effect of reducing the demand for hospitalization for the treatment of infectious diseases and mental illness, and were it not for these drugs, medical costs today would be much higher than they are. The work being done to develop drugs as a low-cost substitute for surgery in the treatment of gallstones and other research promises additional economies.

It is in the public interest that this relatively inexpensive form of therapy be developed. Medical practitioners, whose stated objective always is to provide patients with the best available care regardless of cost, are not accustomed to a cost-benefit analysis of choices among alternative therapeutic methods. This tradition of disregarding costs has some advantages: a doctor need not restrict expensive but effective therapeutic programs to rich patients, and he need not consider costs in prescribing treatment for terminal patients. However, we need not resolve any moral issues in order to urge doctors to choose an economical form of therapy when it is as safe as other forms. Moreover, since drug therapy has the advantage of wider applicability than other technologies, including surgery and radiology, the use of drugs permits larger reductions in morbidity and mortality rates[21] and thus reduces cost of disease.

The alternative forms of therapy are much more costly than drug therapy because they rely on the employment of professional skills and costly equipment. A dramatic example of costly treatment is the heart transplant, the expensive technology of which prevents it from coping with heart disease for a large number of patients. Such advances in technology have contributed to the catastrophic costs of certain illnesses for individual families and thus have resulted in public pressure for national health insurance.[22]

There are other factors in the economies from the use of drugs. Patients can usually take drugs without frequent professional or skilled help; and to facilitate self-administration, drugs are made up in oral dosage forms when possible rather than in injectable forms. The modification of an injectable drug to permit oral self-administration is an economic advance, if not a major medical advance.

The mass production of drugs has also reduced costs. Before the 1940s, pharmacists compounded drugs as required for each prescription. This handicraft method became prohibitively expensive as wages increased, and costs of pharmacies fell after pharmaceutical manufacturers took over the manufacture of final-dosage drugs. The same economic forces which promoted self-service groceries and the displacement of custom-made apparel and shoes by mass-produced, ready-to-wear clothing were at work in this industry.[23] It is frequently recognized that the old method became technologically obsolete, for the retail pharmacist simply could not compound the new antibiotics or antihistamines. But the influence of the rise of wages was also important. Thus, pharmaceutical manufacturers took over the production of virtually all of the old drugs, and today the retail pharmacist does virtually no compounding at all.

The economic benefits of drug therapy have grown with the increases in the prices of medical services. Since the prices of drugs have remained virtually stable, their relative cost to the customer has declined. The increase in the utilization of medical services has also increased the potential savings resulting from the substitution of drugs for medical services.

Because the human benefits are more familiar to most people, we have emphasized the economic benefits of the new drugs developed since 1940. These new drugs, especially the antibiotics, were an important factor in the increase in the average life expectancy in the U.S. from 62.9 years in 1940 to 70.8 years in 1970.[24]

It is difficult now to imagine what medicine was like prior to the 1940s. The number of drugs which were then available to the doctor was very limited by modern standards. The work of Koch and Pasteur had produced vaccines against anthrax and against rabies. By the end of the nineteenth century, effective vaccines had been developed for typhoid fever, cholera, and plague. In addition, there were antitoxins against diphtheria and tetanus. Paul Ehrlich had developed drugs which were effective against trypanosomiasis, African sleeping sickness, and syphilis. Banting and Best introduced insulin in the 1920s, and the anticoagulant heparin became available in 1918. In addition, the first sulfa drug was patented in 1932. Other drugs which were available included digitalis, quinine, ipecac, caffeine, some anesthetics, some pain relievers, and certain sedatives. There were, of course, many other drugs available, but most of them have minor therapeutic effects if any at all. The dramatically successful introduction of penicillin in the late 1940s was followed by that of the broad-spectrum antibiotics, the tetracyclines. The period of the late 1940s and early 1950s witnessed the introduction of cortisone and its greatly improved successors, hydrocortisone and prednisolone. The 1950s also saw the first major tranquilizer, chlorpromazine, which is used in the treatment of schizophrenics and psychotics, and the first minor tranquilizer, meprobamate, which is used in the relief of anxiety and tension. This decade also saw the first antihypertensives and the introduction of new anti-inflammatory drugs. This period of prolific drug discovery also introduced oral contraceptives, new diuretic drugs, antidiabetic drugs, and important new penicillins which were effective against bacteria which were resistant to the original penicillin.

The economic discussion of the industry has failed to emphasize the industry's major potential contribution to the public welfare: the development of new drugs. Public attention tends to focus instead on the secondary goals of reducing manufacturers' selling costs and profits, which constitute a small fraction of the nation's total medical expenditures. In 1974 U.S. sales of ethical drugs of pharmaceutical manufacturers accounted for only $6 billion of the nation's total medical expenditures of over $100 billion, and total selling costs and profits accounted for much less. Thus the opportunities for realizing savings by lowering prices in the drug industry are probably less than those which exist in other components of the medical care industry, and any savings from cutting drug prices could well be wiped out by offsetting increases in the cost of medical care resulting from reductions in the rate of innovation of drugs.

Despite the medical contributions of the "wonder" drugs of the last three decades, new drugs are needed for the treatment, prevention, and cure of major diseases, as is detailed below.

INFECTIOUS DISEASES. Although treatment of infectious diseases has seen the greatest pharmaceutical triumphs, much remains to be done. Antibiotics have greatly reduced the debility and mortality from pneumonia, meningitis, tuberculosis, septicemia, and other diseases. Nevertheless, infectious diseases as a group still account for about 7 percent of all deaths[25] and a significant amount of severe disability.

Furthermore, in recent years certain infectious diseases which had been effectively treated with drugs have reemerged. For example, in 1974 gonorrhea was the most prevalent reported infectious disease, with over 870,000 active cases.[26] In part the problem has reemerged because the bacteria have become resistant to penicillin, which is now effective against gonorrhea only in very large doses. A more important factor, which is social rather than medical or bacteriological, is the permissive contemporary attitude toward sex.

Paradoxically, some other currently important bacterial diseases are the by-products of therapeutic successes. Hospital gram-negative infections, for example, have now become a more common terminal disease of patients who are alive because of success in treating their cancers or the injuries and burns they received in major accidents. These bacteria, which do not usually cause disease in humans, do so in these weakened patients. The incidence of gram-negative infections has increased also as a result of the increase in the number of people in the older age groups, who are more susceptible to such infections. Unfortunately, the ability to treat gram-negative infections still is modest, and new drugs are required.

CARDIOVASCULAR DISEASE.   Cardiovascular diseases are the leading cause of death in the U.S., accounting for 53 percent of all deaths in 1968.[27] Part of the reason for this is the increase in size of the most susceptible fraction of the population—those over 45 years of age.

Despite the rise in the proportion of older persons in the population, the annual death rate from cardiovascular disorders fell from 515.1 to 494.0 per 100,000 between 1960 and 1970.[28] Drugs, doubtless, were a factor in this decline. The diuretics and antihypertensives now in use against this disease were first introduced in the late 1950s and early 1960s, but few new ones have been introduced since.

The reduction in the annual death rate from hypertensive heart disease and hypertension has been even more dramatic; from 44.1 per 100,000 in 1960 to 11.0 per 100,000 in 1970.[29] The great improvement is largely due to the use of antihypertensive drugs. Recently there has been a growing use of drug therapy to regulate abnormalities of lipid metabolism, and greater attention is now being given to the identification of the causes of atherosclerosis.

In the 1960s, innovation in the cardiovascular field was slow, in part because the long-term use required of drugs such as these increases the risk of toxicity, which in turn has made FDA licensing especially restrictive. The importance of developing new drugs in this field is demonstrated by the fact that when such drugs have become available, physicians have shifted to them rapidly and academic experts have endorsed them.

ARTHRITIS.   About 50 million persons suffer from arthritis to some degree; approximately 17 million require medical care, and 3.4 million are disabled. [30] Except in the case of gout, the causes of arthritic diseases are unknown. Current treatment provides only symptomatic relief. The available drugs include steroid hormones and nonsteroidal anti-inflammatory compounds such as phenylbuta-zone, indomethacin, and aspirin.

CANCER. Cancer is a major area in which new drugs are needed. In response to federal support, medical research has concentrated heavily on cancer and has succeeded in developing new drugs which have contributed to an increase in survival rates for certain types of cancer. In 1967 fewer than one-fifth of all patients survived for five years or more after beginning treatment; by 1970 the survival rate had risen to one-third.[31] New drugs, however, have been only one of several factors involved in this success; early cancer diagnosis and advances in surgery and radiology probably have been more important factors in the in-creased survival rate.

MENTAL ILLNESS. Mental illness remains a very serious problem, even though important advances in treating it have been made by drug therapy. New tranquilizers and antidepressants have helped reduce the number of patients in mental hospitals from 558,000 in 1955 to 339,000 in 1970. During those years the average stay in a mental hospital dropped from 8 years to 1.4 years. These two factors have had the effect of reducing the American mental hospital population to half of what it otherwise would have been. Further improvement, however, still is desirable.

Other illnesses akin to mental illness, such as alcoholism and narcotics addiction, are susceptible to drug therapy in conjunction with other appropriate therapies. One estimate of the total cost of alcoholism alone to the U.S. economy is $15 billion per year, consisting of $10 billion in lost work time, $2 billion in health and welfare services, and $3 billion in property damage and medical expenses—and this estimate does not include the losses due to reduced life expectancy, traffic fatalities, and arrests.[32] New drugs are needed to help reduce these burdens.

VIRAL INFECTIONS. Antiviral drugs, although not of practical therapeutic use today, are one clearly promising field for further research. Interferon, which is a natural substance induced in mammalian cells by exposure to a virus, inhibits the growth of the virus in the infected cells and prevents its appearance in neighboring cells.[33] The potential economic benefits arising from effective treatment of the common cold alone are enormous.

DRUG RESEARCH AND PUBLIC POLICY

Frequently the suggestion is made that additional R & D efforts are unlikely to be productive because the major discoveries of the 1940s and 1950s have exhausted the available opportunities. It is said that new discoveries must await a major breakthrough of the magnitude of penicillin and that such a prospect is dim. This position does not seem valid. Many of the new drugs introduced since 1960 have proven to be therapeutically significant. Some examples are as follows: ampicillin, which has a wider antibacterial range than either penicillin G or penicillin V and which destroys such penicillin-resistant, gram-negative organisms as Salmonella, Shigella, Haemophilus influenzae, and some species of Proteus, is especially effective against urinary tract infections which typically involve gram-negative organisms. Cephalosporins, a family of relatively new wide-spectrum antibiotics, have the important advantage of efficacy against penicillinase-producing Staphylococci and Streptococci which resist older penicillins. Other important new antibiotics include gentamicin and carbenicillin, which are effective against severe and often life-threatening infections caused by gram-negative organisms resistant to most other antibiotics.

The bulk of discovery research has been located in the pharmaceutical industry because innovation is the focus of competition. Since most significant products are or have been protected by patents, companies must develop new and patentable products to expand their share of the market. In 1973 the U.S. ethical pharmaceutical industry invested over $800 million in research, which is equal to about 14 percent of domestic sales and nearly 9 percent of the world sales of the U.S. industry. By contrast, R & D expenditures in U.S. manufacturing as a whole have been approximately 1.3 percent of total sales.[34]

The expenditures on R & D early in the 1960s resulted in an average of 36.5 new single entities per year. In more recent years the rate of innovation as measured by the number of new single entities has dropped to a level of about 12.3 per year. Despite this sharp decline, which is discussed in later chapters, the focus of competitive efforts within the industry remains innovation; the major firms continue to increase their R & D expenditures. Thus the current level of R & D expenditures is more than three times as large as the expenditures in 1960. In 1961 the industry employed 13,464 individuals in its research activities, compared to 21,725 in 1971.

If we accept these three related conclusions—that drugs are the most important technology of medicine, that new ones are badly needed, and that they come from industrial R & D—then the distribution of total medical research expenditures by types (table 1-1) and the trend in such expenditures are disturbing. We would expect a large part of the total expenditures for medical research to be located in the pharmaceutical industry, but in 1972 its share was only 22 percent. We would expect the trend to be in the direction of an increasing share of total expenditures to be made by the industry, but expenditures outside the industry have been growing at a faster rate than those within the industry. Worse still, federal funding of cancer research promises to result in an even greater allocation of resources to nonindustrial laboratories. HEW plans to increase annual appropriations from the current $500 million to $1.7 billion by 1982,[35] and though the National Cancer Institute will use some of the funds

TABLE 1-1
National Support for Performance of Medical
Health-Related Research by Source of Funds ($ Millions)

	1960	1965	1970	1972
Government	$471	$1,229	$1,740	$2,223
Federal	488	1,174	1,664	2,144
State & Local	23	55	76	79
Private	121	158	193	211
Foundations & health agencies	76	88	108	124
Other private contributions	12	25	32	33
Endowment	19	19	19	19
Institutions' own funds	14	26	34	35
Industry	206	328	566	668
Industry percentage of Total	26	19	23	22
Total	798	1,715	2,499	3,102

Sources: Industry expenditures: Pharmaceutical Manufacturers' Association. Other expenditures: Associate Director for Program Planning and Evaluation, Office of Resources Analysis, National Institutes of Health, March 1973.

Note: 1972 figures for industry represent budget amounts rather than actual expenditures. Other 1972 figures are estimates of actual expenditures.

to screen possible anticancer compounds much as the industry might do, a large part of the funds will be devoted to basic research.

This spending pattern will divert the limited supply of trained research personnel into basic research and will thus reduce the resources available to the industry for drug discovery and development. The diversion will take place through bidding up the costs of research; to retain their present research staffs, the pharmaceutical manufacturers will have to pay higher salaries. Thus, a paradoxical result of the additional government funding of research may be a reduction in the flow of new drugs.

The shift of medical research resources away from industrial laboratories and toward others is also the result of other changes in public policy. Although expenditures by the industry have continued to increase, it is likely that they would have grown at a faster rate were it not for the increase in costs of R & D required for a new drug to reach the market. Since the 1962 Drug Amendments, the FDA has become much more strict in its demands for assurances of efficacy and safety. The costs of R & D have risen accordingly, and it now costs considerably more to develop a new drug than it did before 1962.[36] The resulting decline in the expected rate of return from investment in R & D will reduce such investment and also the rate of innovation. The rate of innovation, in fact, has fallen, even though expenditures for R & D continue to increase as measured in constant as well as in current dollars.

In addition, changes in public policy may very well bring about an actual decline in R & D expenditures. The continuing investigation of the industry by congressional committees, the FTC, and other public agencies has focused on the alleged monopoly power exercised by pharmaceutical firms. The investigations have resulted in the Maximum Allowable Cost (MAC) regulations, under which HEW will pay only the prices of generic products when these are widely available at lower prices than those of the corresponding brands. The Nelson Bill calls for the compulsory licensing of drug patents three years after the drug is marketed. The MAC regulations and the Nelson Bill risk the reduction of the flow of innovations by reducing the expected rate of return from investment in R & D.

Society will suffer a loss from a decline in the rate of innovation. Critics of the industry,[37] who disparage new drugs as being merely minor products, ignore the possibility of such alterations improving therapy significantly or adding to patient convenience and reducing drug costs. The replacement of an injectable by an oral dosage form may not be recognized by medical authorities as a major advance in treatment. But an oral dosage form frees the patient from the need for professional assistance and thus may save a great deal of money. A major economic advance is not to be dismissed as a trivial improvement. In this highly empirical field, moreover, leads to major drugs come in the search for new drugs.

Scientists in industrial laboratories have the same incentives as other scientists to make discoveries, while management has the economic incentive to encourage such discoveries. Such incentives have led laboratories to persist in the face of discouraging tests of compounds; the desired biological activity all too frequently is associated with toxicity, requiring difficult decisions as to the advisability of continuing a line of research. These kinds of judgments are uncertain, but one cannot help feeling that the usual criteria employed in funding academic research and the usual academic incentives would be inadequate to allow the completion of many pharmaceutical research projects. For example, Lederle Laboratories' massive random screening project to discover the antitubercular drug ethambutol lasted fifteen years. Upjohn's large prostaglandin project is now more than fifteen years old and is still continuing, and only one product has been introduced. Examples of lengthy difficult projects which were discontinued and revived later could be also cited. Naturally, major discoveries are few, but this fact should not lead to condemnation of innovational activity.

BACKGROUND INFORMATION

The ethical drugs industry produces prescription drugs which are advertised to physicians rather than to the general public. We are not concerned in this book with proprietary drugs, which are promoted in the popular media.

The industry distributes its products to consumers through three primary channels: retail pharmacies, hospitals, and government agencies. Pharmacies are the most important, accounting for 74.5 percent of sales at the wholesale level. Table 1-2 shows the distribution of sales.

TABLE 1-2
Percentage Distribution of Manufacturers'
Domestic Sales among Retail Pharmacies,
Hospitals, Government Agencies, 1970

	Percentage	($ millions)
Retail	74.5	4296.9
Hospital	14.4	831.8
Government	11.1	639.4[a]
Total	100.	5768.1

Sources: For retail and hospital sales,
IMS America, Ltd., *U.S. Pharmaceutical
Market, Drug Stores and Hospitals* (Ambler,
Pa.: IMS America Ltd., 1970). Data sum-
mary, U.S. Dept. HEW, Social Security
Admin., Office of Research and Statistics,
SS Pub. 59-71 (5-71), 1971.
[a]Prescription drugs only.

In 1972 there were 880 manufacturers of ethical drugs. Of these, the top
twenty firms accounted for 73.5 percent of total sales. These firms conducted a
full range of operations, including research and development. The companies
promote the drugs chiefly through sending detail men to physicians. Many of the
larger companies have their own distribution network. The smaller companies'
sales consist principally of generic products, many of them producing tablets and
capsules from bulk materials supplied by the larger companies; they are essentially prepackagers or finishers. Many of these smaller companies operate only
within regions or even states.

Table 1-3 shows the percentage distribution by number of employees of
establishments in the census classification "pharmaceutical preparations" in
1967. Most of the establishments were very small. A majority had fewer than
nine employees, and together they accounted for only 0.6 percent of sales. The
43 percent of all establishments which were in the smallest size class had average
sales of only $38.8 thousand. We can assume that nearly all of the small
establishments are owned and operated by single-plant companies. Thus, even
though the largest twenty companies account for nearly three-quarters of total
sales, the vast majority of companies in this industry are very small. In fact, the
census figures understate the number of establishments and thus the number of
companies producing drugs. The census data for pharmaceutical preparations
report only the number of establishments which are classified as members of the
industry. Other establishments producing drugs are classified in other industries
because drugs are not their primary product. The government's General Accounting Office has estimated that the FDA must inspect 6,400 plants manufacturing drugs.[38]

TABLE 1-3
Size of Establishment in Pharmaceutical Preparations Industry (SIC 2834),
by Employment

Number of Employees Per Establishment	Establishment		Value of Shipments		Average Value of Shipment ($000)
	Number	% of Total	($ Millions)	% of Total	
1–4	379	43.3	14.7	.3	38.8
5–9	83	9.5	12.8	.3	154.2
10–19	95	10.9	36.7	.8	386.3
20–49	107	12.2	101.8	2.2	951.4
50–99	81	9.3	167.8	3.6	2,071.6
100–249	55	6.3	460.4	9.8	8,370.9
250–499	28	3.2	575.3	12.2	20,546.4
500–999	24	2.7	768.2	16.4	32,008.3
1,000–2,499	14	1.6	1,227.3	26.1	87,664,3
2,500 and over	19	1.0	1,331.5	28.4	147,944.4
Total	875	100.0	4,696.4	100.1	5,367.3

Source: Bureau of the Census, Census of Manufacturers 1967, table 4, pp. 280–89.

Table 1-4 reports a distribution of sales in various years broken down by therapeutic field. The therapeutic fields are used by market analysts to study changes in demand and in shares of individual companies' products of sales within submarkets. The classification which is used in table 1-4 can be broken down further or it can be aggregated more. Chapter 6 discusses the problem of locating the boundaries of drug markets. Table 1-4 is presented here only for the purpose of providing an impression of the relative importance of different classes of drugs and of changes in their importance. Currently antibiotics and ataractics (including both major and minor tranquilizers) are the two leading classes, accounting for 13.2 percent and 11.0 percent, respectively, of total sales of ethical drugs in 1972. Hormonal drugs (including contraceptives) and cardiovascular drugs are the next two therapeutic fields in order of sales, accounting for 8.7 percent and 7.4 percent, respectively. We can also see some marked changes in the distribution of sales among therapeutic fields since 1957. The shares of ataractics, analgesics, antiarthritics, cardiovascular drugs, and diuretics have increased considerably while those of antibiotics, anti-infectives, have declined. None of the classes show an absolute decline in sales. The declines in market shares reflect the introduction of new drugs and rapid expansion of sales in other classes.

The table also reveals a rapid rate of increase in total ethical sales. The increase in current dollar sales was 185 percent between 1957 and 1972. Owing to the fall in the prices of drugs, the growth in constant-dollar sales was even larger, 204 percent. This is equivalent to an average annual rate of growth of 7.7 percent, which can be compared to an average annual rate of growth of constant-dollar GNP of 3.8 percent. A large part of the rapid rate of increase has

TABLE 1-4

U.S. Wholesale Sales of Ethical Drugs, by Therapeutic Category ($ Millions)

	1957		1960		1965		1972	
	$	%	$	%	$	%	$	%
Analgesics	65.2	3.9	76.8	4.0	129.8	4.8	256.3	5.4
Anesthetics	15.8	0.9	16.9	0.9	36.1	1.3	55.1	1.2
Antiarthritics	—	0	15.8	0.8	35.8	1.3	100.0	2.1
Anti-infectives[a] and anthelminthics	42.3	2.5	40.6	2.1	65.0	2.4	108.0	2.3
Antibiotics and sulfonamides	335.2	20.2	335.5	17.4	418.2	15.5	625.2	13.2
Antiobesity	6.8	0.4	63.7	3.3	94.4	3.5	71.8	1.5
Ataraxics	111.1	6.7	144.2	7.5	253.0	9.4	520.2	11.0
Bronchodilators	7.9	0.5	17.1	0.9	40.8	1.5	69.2	1.5
Cardiovasculars[b]	82.9	5.0	103.3	5.3	175.7	6.5	346.3	7.3
Dermatologicals	—	0	49.3	2.5	52.6	1.9	108.7	2.3
Diabetic therapy	28.1	1.7	55.2	2.9	79.8	3.0	126.6	2.7
Diuretics	17.5	1.1	47.6	2.5	79.7	2.9	163.6	3.5
Gastrointestinal drugs[c]	125.5	7.6	147.5	7.6	201.6	7.5	350.8	7.4
Hormones	124.6	7.5	147.0	7.6	237.4	8.8	411.3	8.7
Muscle relaxants[d]	8.6	0.5	21.5	1.1	26.1	1.0	54.6	1.2
Psychostimulants	4.2	0.3	13.4	0.7	42.9	1.6	73.3	1.6
Sedatives	31.1	1.9	36.3	1.9	49.5	1.8	61.0	1.3
All others	651.5	39.3	599.8	31.0	685.1	25.3	1,217.0	25.8
Total Ethical Market	1,658.1	100.0	1,931.5	100.0	2,703.4	100.0	4,718.8	100.0

Source: IMS America, Ltd., U.S. Pharmaceutical Market, Drug Stores and Hospitals, various years.
[a] Antibacterials and antimalarials. Excludes antibiotics and sulfonamides.
[b] Also includes digitalis preparations and vasopressors.
[c] Includes antacids, antidiarrheals, antinauseants, antispasm, and laxatives.
[d] Surgical and nonsurgical.

been due to the development of new drugs. Sales have also grown as a result of the growth of demand for existing drugs. This growth is the result of the increase of demand for medical care generally, which can be traced back to the rise in income per capita, the growth of population, and to changes in public policy as expressed by Medicare and Medicaid.

CHAPTER 2

BASIC RESEARCH
AND INVENTION

INTRODUCTION

Most of today's important and effective drugs were discovered and developed during the past three decades and have played a central role in the revolution in health care witnessed since World War II. During the past ten years, however, something appears to have gone wrong with the productivity of drug research. If we take as our measure of productivity the number of new drug entities that have appeared in the past decade, we must observe that there has been a serious decline in the rate of therapeutic innovation. Some writers have assailed drug research, as it is conducted by the pharmaceutical industry, for this decline, charging that the number of important drugs is small because the pharmaceutical manufacturers engage in "applied" rather than "basic" research.[1] Basic research has been regarded as the ultimate source of advances in science and thus of discoveries. In this context, "basic research" means fundamental research or research which leads to the understanding of natural phenomena, as contrasted with research which merely develops some useful implications of scientific knowledge and the resulting new products or manufacturing processes. Later we will consider the usual definition of basic research, which is similar to this one but is not identical with it. The usual definition, as we will see, has produced some confusion.

Unfortunately the arguments concerning basic and applied research have led to the erroneous suggestion that the rate of new drug discovery is independent of the return on investment in applied research by pharmaceutical manufacturers and therefore that the government can reduce the life of drug patents and otherwise reduce incentives to invest in industrial research without fear of reducing the number of important new drugs introduced annually. However, as we shall go on to see, drug discovery is an intricate and complex process, differing in important ways from other forms of scientific research. The process of discovery often taken as the model for research is the one occurring in

29

physics-related sciencies, and wherein principles discovered by basic research generally find ready application. In the process of pharmaceutical R & D, however, there exists no simple flow-through from basic to applied R & D. Basic research advances relevant to drug discovery, in contrast to the role of basic research in other fields, do not lead in any direct way to new drugs. New drugs cannot be designed by logical deductions from valid general principles; chemical theory alone is not enough and biological theory is woefully inadequate. In some diseases such as rheumatoid arthritis and cancer we are still too ignorant of causes even to know how best to look for therapeutic remedies. As a consequence, the search for new drugs is frequently organized on the basis of provisional hypotheses and empirical tests. These provisional hypotheses are based on bits of chemical and biological knowledge. The hypotheses are constantly being revised in the light of new findings, but they provide a direction to research and serve as a sort of feedback mechanism which generates new hypotheses and sets the stage for fresh experiments.

While it is true that drug research is an applied discipline in that it seeks new drugs as its ultimate goal, it is frequently very fundamental in its approach and long-range in its accomplishments. Indeed, most drug research is characterized by intimate links between basic science and its application; applied research progress typically leads to progress in basic knowledge and vice versa. It is essential to understand this seeming paradox of drug research. While drug research is applied in its objective and able to flourish only if it receives constant nourishment from basic research, such research necessitates a great deal of basic research in the process of trying to achieve the applied result, and thus it contributes to the pool of basic understanding itself. In this context it is a matter of great concern that government regulation, modified and influenced by political pressure, threatens to handicap the applied research component of drug research and may in fact already have done so. Because of the intimate links between basic and applied research in the biomedical field, such interference and the resultant slowdown in applied research reduces the rate of progress in basic research. Regulatory interferences with the ultimate indicator of progress in drug development—namely, testing in humans—has reduced the ability of biomedical scientists to test hypotheses and validate laboratory inferences. Moreover, in the past, leads to new potential applications of drug prototypes were frequently derived from its use on man when a drug designed for one purpose demonstrated unexpected properties. This important source of leads has been reduced by the restrictions on the marketing of new drugs.

If public policy makers are to design optimal policies for the encouragement of new drug discovery and development, the basis of industry's expertise in biomedical research needs to be clearly understood. Accordingly, this chapter deals with the concepts of basic and applied research examining their relative contributions to industry's R & D and the process of drug discovery, and the need for empiricism in drug research.

BASIC VERSUS APPLIED DRUG RESEARCH

New drugs are often pictured as one of the fruits of applying the discoveries of "basic" research. Unfortunately this has resulted in an impression in the minds of some people that most basic research is restricted to academic laboratories and that the really important drug discoveries have emanated from them whereas the industrial laboratories have been mainly concerned with production problems or routine research of a lower grade, disparagingly referred to as "applied" research.

There may have been some truth in this idea, during the pre–World War II era, when drug companies were concerned largely with formulating existing drugs and commercial exploitation of findings of original research in universities. However, such an image of the pharmaceutical industry today must be regarded as completely distorted. Although sometimes it is difficult to assign ultimate credit for discoveries, it can be safely said that the pharmaceutical industry laboratories have made a significant contribution to science, and that they will continue to be a primary source of new medicinals. Indeed, it often comes as a surprise to some people, particularly to the laymen of influence who affect public decisions, that drug research today is concentrated in the laboratories of the drug industry and that these laboratories are the only major institutions where the search for new and better drugs takes place on a large and sophisticated scale.[2] Drug discovery today requires an inordinately expensive and a highly organized multidisciplinary research team effort, well beyond the scope of academic laboratories which have neither the resources nor the facilities or temperament to indulge in the development of new drugs. A case in point is the development of the antibiotic field. An enormous effort was made by industrial laboratories all over the world over a span of more than twenty years in a search for new antibiotics. Yet, the practical outcome of this mammoth effort was the discovery of a mere handful of antibiotics which found clinical application. From the financial point of view alone, such a costly undertaking, resulting in relatively few winners, could only have been possible in the goal-oriented atmosphere of the industrial laboratories.

It is difficult to imagine what the practice of medicine would be like today without the research contributions of the pharmaceutical industry. The list of important medicinals credited to industry is quite long and includes agents such as sulfa drugs, antibiotics, hormones, vitamins, hypoglycemics, diuretics, antihypertensives, tranquilizers and antipsychotics, and analgesics.[3] Nevertheless, claims to the contrary continue to persist.[4] These claims are based on studies of lists of inventions in many industries, of which the drug industry is only one. The results of the frequently cited study by Jewkes, Sawers, and Stillerman,[5] which emphasizes the importance of the individual inventor, have been interpreted by Mansfield to signify that of sixty-one major inventions after 1930, barely 20 percent emerged from laboratories of large corporations.[6] Inventions such as air-conditioning, automatic transmissions, and jet engines, it has been noted, were the work of independent inventors. Such studies, which deal with technologies based on a wealth of known physical and basic principles and concerned with problems of design and engineering development, however, can be exceedingly misleading because they deal largely with advances in technologies quite different from those involved in drug discovery. In all these cases, basic principles were known before the inventions. The inventors perceived the practical implications of these principles. The situation in drug discovery is quite different.

The research and development of new drugs is an intricate and complex scientific process. It differs from other forms of scientific research in its unusually heavy dependence on empirical exploration and inference. Drug research makes much more use of experiment and observation than other fields because the basic knowledge and theories are so incomplete. It is inferential research in that it logically attempts to discover therapeutic agents based on the limited available basic knowledge. The process uses new techniques and theories and combines them with inferences, insights, and experience in a coordinated effort to discover a new drug.

Unlike the fields of modern technology which are essentially based on physics and engineering, pharmaceutical research operates at the borderline of the unknown in basic research. Specific differences between the development of a nuclear device or of an IBM-370 computer system and that of a new drug consist in the degree to which the underlying scientific knowledge can be efficiently mobilized for achieving practical goals. Theoretical physics had been far advanced in the 1930s following the discovery of artificial radioactivity by Enrico Fermi. Development of the atomic bomb became feasible once Lise Meitner's experiments in Copenhagen (inspired by similar, though less precise, experiments done a few months earlier in Berlin by Otto Hahn and F. Strassmann) demonstrated the possibility of nuclear fission. This information, brought to Einstein by Niels Bohr in 1939, led him to urge President Franklin D. Roosevelt to initiate development of the atomic bomb by the United States. Einstein's recommendation marked the beginning of the Manhattan Project and the mammoth effort that culminated in the successful development of the nuclear bomb.[7]

Thus, given an applied goal in engineering, there is often nothing but money that stands in the way of achieving the goal, provided basic science has shown this goal to be achievable. Not so in drug discovery; the basic research necessary to demonstrate the feasibility of any given approach of drug design or discovery is necessarily painfully diffuse, and as Weinberg[8] properly points out, the bulk of biomedical science is in the "prefeasibility" stage. Despite the massive progress that has been made in the last several decades in the understanding of the structure and function of living organisms, huge gaps still exist in our knowledge of the fundamental biology and engineering of normal human cells; much less is known about cancerous ones. Scientists are painfully aware of the futility of any all-out "war on cancer," as is amply attested by the lack of any significant breakthroughs on this front despite the many millions of dollars that have been poured into the battle against cancer.

The first step in the drug discovery process, then, is the development of a working hypothesis based on some shred of molecular and chemical knowledge or biological phenomena. This working hypothesis is an idea which is tentatively advanced to explain how a particular pathology occurs and how it might be affected by a specific kind of compound, taking into account the chemical constitution and pharmacological actions of drugs previously used for treatment. If the working hypothesis seems plausible in light of current knowledge and observations, then the promising compounds are synthesized in the laboratory and are examined in a series of tests in animals. Unfortunately, the scientists involved often lack a theory for assessing the efficacy and entire safety of biologically active compounds. Further, in many instances one cannot produce a meaningful model of a human disease in animals. Assuming that a satisfactory model exists, the biologist determines which of the chemicals are active in the desired way and at the same time are relatively free of toxic effects. Obtaining this balance between efficacy and safety in animal tests is of critical importance and is often a difficult challenge. Often it proves to be an impossible task and the compounds are discarded. On the other hand, although animal tests may fail to yield a useful drug, they often provide a better understanding of how the compound and biological systems interact and precipitate a revision in the working hypothesis and the creation of new drug prototypes. Sometimes, of course, the animal tests reveal a promising compound with acceptable levels of both activity and toxicity.

When the research team finds that its compound is promising in these tests in several animal species, it still is ignorant about many of the compound's features. Some diseases cannot be satisfactorily mimicked in experimental animals. More-over, all animal tests are inherently and severely limited in their scientific and clinical usefulness because of the differences that exist between animal species and humans in metabolism, anatomy, and the detectability of side effects (such as nausea or headache). Thus animal tests, even if extensive in scope and duration, can at best yield only inferences of safety and efficacy and can in no way yield conclusive evidence regarding the effects of compounds in humans.

Thus, drug researchers cannot view successful animal tests as conclusive. Although a compound which is a failure in animals is discarded before testing in man (even though it might have been useful for the human species), successful animal tests do not assure success in man. This helps explain the high rate of preclinical rejection of compounds, the large number of compounds which are rejected during early clinical trials, and the reason why the research team must perform extensive and iterative tests in humans before it can obtain conclusive proof that the compound is in fact efficacious and safe for human use—that is, that a drug has been discovered.[9]

Pharmaceutical research laboratories thus do practical applied research in areas where basic feasibility is yet to be demonstrated; fundamental principles are not known, but are only assumed; alternative assumptions are considered and then tried in a series of tests of working hypotheses. Drug discovery is essentially a feedback process between applied research in therapeutics and fundamental biological knowledge. Inevitably, pharmaceutical research generates a great deal of authentic scientific knowledge and contributes to basic knowledge. Although in its objective pharmaceutical research is applied, its very nature necessitates a great deal of basic research in the process of trying to achieve the applied result. Not surprisingly, then, the history of drug discovery is replete with instances where a finding of applied research has been the touchstone for significant advance in the understanding of biological mechanisms.

We can see that the continuing discussion of the relative merits and demerits of basic versus applied research in drug discovery becomes meaningless, since it is based on a misunderstanding of pharmaceutical research. Much confusion has been created by people who assert that the trouble with pharmaceutical research is that it is applied, not basic, research, and that basic research is limited to academic laboratories. Both academic and industrial research laboratories have made contributions of enormous importance to drug research. Both kinds of approach—the academic and the industrial—are indispensable and complement each other. The association of academic with basic research and of industrial with applied research is involved in this unfortunate dichotomization. No discovery could have been more "applied" in nature than the discovery of penicillin, which originated in an academic laboratory. Similarly, several basic discoveries that originated in industrial laboratories, such as the discovery of histamine and acetylcholine proved to be of immense theoretical and academic consequence.

ECONOMIC THEORY OF R & D

The National Science Foundation defines basic research as "research which is directed toward increase of knowledge in science. It is research where the primary aim of the investigator is a fuller knowledge or understanding of the subject under study, rather than as in the case with applied research, a practical application."[10] This definition stresses the aim of the research rather than the results, but as we have suggested, "applied research" can generate fundamental scientific understanding. The definition's stress on the aims confuses the discussion of research, which is primarily concerned with results. Thus, Edwin Mansfield says that the biologist who investigates why certain cells proliferate without having any particular application in mind performs basic research. He contrasts this type of research with projects which seek ways of increasing the ability of steel to resist stresses, methods of inhibiting the growth of streptococci, and methods of obtaining energy from atomic fission directly as energy. Mansfield's illustration and discussion suggest that basic research is the ultimate source of the advance of science and thus of discoveries.[11] The definition, as Mansfield's examples indicate, emphasizes that basic research seeks general principles, while applied research applies them. The possibility that research may have a specific commercial objective and yet produce important scientific advances is ignored.

Arguments that represent applied research as routine, while conceding that there are many technical difficulties, maintain that industrial laboratories pursue projects the outcome of which is less uncertain than that of basic research. This description is especially true for some types of industrial research concerned with problems of design and engineering development. Thus, Edwin Mansfield and Richard Brandeburg found that in more than three quarters of the projects undertaken by the laboratories of an electrical equipment manufacturing company, the probability of technical success was estimated at about 0.8.[12] Only 44 percent of the projects actually resulted in technical success, but even this percentage suggests that the degree of uncertainty is not very high compared with that in basic research. In short, industrial laboratories limit their activities to the application of known principles discovered elsewhere to practical problems, the solution of which is relatively routine after the basic research is completed.

The argument goes on to say that because profit-maximizing companies are reluctant to undertake risky, innovative R & D projects, individual inventors, as pointed out by Jewkes *et alia*,[13] are prominent in lists of important inventions. It is perhaps not without significance that of the illustrations of important inventions in this list, those that are pharmaceutical products—insulin, penicillin, and streptomycin—all belong to an age prior to the development of the modern pharmaceutical R & D.

Thus, most of the discussion of applied versus basic research in economic literature refers to research other than pharmaceutical research. Pharmaceutical research, which is highly dependent on exploration, does not fit the standard model well; the line between basic and applied research is especially fuzzy in this field. While the very definition of basic research would exclude any deliberate search for specific drugs, pharmaceutical discoveries take the form of new drugs.

Economists have suggested that increased expenditures on research other than basic research would not increase the number of inventions. The inventor draws on his knowledge of previous basic research, but his own efforts usually do not closely correspond to the amount of funds he has at his disposal. The efforts depend more on the prospect of economic reward resulting from the patent on a product and on the natural curiosity of the inventor. The examples given suggest that the inventor does not require the resources of the large firm and that economies of scale are unimportant in the research preceding the invention.[14]

The large firm's advantages, it is suggested, are more likely to be present in the development stage following the invention, including the development of the design of the product and of production processes. The advantages of scale in this stage come from the need for the skills of many specialists in different aspects of the problems of manufacturing a new product. Since small firms have difficulty in raising large amounts of capital, particularly when the investments do not produce any collateral, they may be unable to develop a product because of the large expense of making many designs, the practicality of which must be tested through numerous trials. If the project fails, as many do, the inventor may not be able to recover his funds. In addition, the small firm cannot support the large number of different specialists necessary for the development of a product.

Jacob Schmookler extended the model to analyze the forces influencing the rate of innovation. This extension employed the traditional tools of demand and supply.[15] Schmookler conceived of a supply curve of innovations which shifts to the right with reductions in the cost of innovation. The model identifies the amount of available scientific knowledge in the relevant field as the major influence on the cost of innovation. The contribution of basic research is seen as that of reducing the cost of innovation in the particular field of research by providing the necessary underlying knowledge. As knowledge expands, the cost of innovation is reduced, shifting the supply of innovation to the right.

Nevertheless, Schmookler's own emphasis is on the importance of the demand for innovation rather than on the supply. In his view, innovations respond to increases in demand which are the result of the rise in the level of income, the growth of population, changes in prices of competing products, and changes in factor costs.

Schmookler maintained that accumulated knowledge only influences the rate of innovation by limiting the scope of inventions. He did not accept the idea that scientific discoveries alone stimulated inventions. In other words, a shift in the supply curve of innovations to the right would not result in an increase in the number of innovations. There had to be an increase in demand for this to happen; apparently Schmookler believed that the demand for innovations was inelastic with respect to their price. His evidence consisted of the record of inventions in four industries: petroleum refining, paper making, railroading, and farming. In these industries the demand for innovation determined the number of innovations. According to Schmookler, hundreds of inventions could be traced to the recognition of a problem and the use of available knowledge to solve it. In addition, he showed that in railroading the number of inventions increased historically with the amount of investment.

Schmookler argued that even in more science-based fields, research and development expenditures are not influenced greatly by individual scientific discoveries. He recognized that discoveries in pure science sometimes provide the stimulus for invention, but most of the inventions, even in science-based industries, derive from the same stimuli as in the industries which he examined in detail. He therefore concluded that the number of inventions depends more on the expected sales of products embodying the invention.

Other writers, including W. E. G. Salter,[16] give greater credit to the growth of knowledge. Salter suggested that when a new technology arises, it will bring forth a flow of significant improvements and modifications. Salter also suggested that as a technology matures, significant advances become less frequent.

Both Schmookler and Salter ignore certain other conditions influencing the quantity of resources employed in applied industrial research. Other factors include those affecting the cost of research, such as the prices of resources used in industrial research; regulatory requirements, which in the case of the drug industry are important; and the degree of protection provided by patents. Thus, restrictions by the FDA on clinical testing and regulatory requirements governing proof of the efficacy and the safety of drugs raise the cost of research, delay marketing of drugs, and thus reduce the expected rate of return from investment in R & D. Another important factor affecting the amount of resources devoted to applied research is the amount of protection patents give to manufacturers of new products. Those economists who would require drug companies to grant licenses to all applicants three years after the issue of the patent under certain specified conditions apparently believe that the present amount of protection is unnecessary to provide adequate research incentives.[17]

Clearly, analysis of the sources of innovation has been far too general. In some fields—for example, physics, where practical applications may follow fairly quickly on the growth of basic scientific knowledge—the underlying theory may be sufficiently complete for additions to knowledge to be readily translatable into practical devices. Industrial research, which utilizes the results of such fields, in that case, may not diminish significantly with reductions in the protection provided by patents. In addition, secrecy of production processes may adequately protect innovators against rapid imitation and loss of sales. In fact, one study suggests that in many industries firms would not reduce the extent of their research if patents were not available.[18] The much more important consideration, then, may be the availability of a sufficiently large market at prices which provide some profit. Drugs, like all chemical inventions, however, are too easily imitated by too many firms for patent protection to be ignored. This industry differs from others in that patents almost invariably refer to products rather than to processes, and it is relatively easy to imitate the product once it is available on the market and chemists can analyze its composition.[19]

It is important thus to examine the roles of basic and applied research in drug discovery specifically. We will examine their contributions to the discoveries of the important new drugs which were introduced during the 1940s and 1950s. During this golden age of discovery, as it is frequently called, the rate of innovation in the industry accelerated greatly, and it has since declined. We will consider the contributions of basic and applied research in these important drug discoveries.

Pharmaceutical research is highly empirical. Because of this, basic discoveries have often emerged from applied research efforts in the field. For example, a popular theory of the way drugs exert their effect on bacteria was the product of applied research. Some of the tools of chemical analysis which drug discovery shares with other fields of chemical research and which might be thought to be the result of basic research were actually the results of applied research. On the other hand, the theories of chemical bonding (e.g. the theory of valence), which organized and so facilitated the chemical investigation of classes of compounds were developed by basic research. But it is important to note that this research was performed in a context completely removed from that of pharmaceutical research rather than in an obviously related field. The recognition of this contribution of basic research thus does not indicate that the government or the industry should support basic research in, say, the biological or other drug-related fields with the expectation of encouraging drug discoveries. Moreover, the evidence, as we are about to see, reveals that the contributions of basic research to drug discovery are unpredictable and would be difficult if not impossible to identify in advance of their use in the applied research process.

The confusion concerning the contributions of applied and basic research to pharmaceutical research, it appears, stems partly from the popularity of the model of research described earlier, but which is totally inapplicable to drug discovery. We anticipate our conclusion when we say that to find new drugs one must search for them directly; therefore, the more money that is invested in applied research, the more new drugs will be discovered.

MAJOR BREAKTHROUGHS IN DRUG DISCOVERY

It is generally agreed that the discovery of the sulfonamides, penicillin, and the histamines were crucial breakthroughs which set the stage for the many important later discoveries that marked the golden age of drug discovery. The trail of the sulfonamides, whose discovery launched the modern era of antibacterial chemotherapy, provides an instructive example of the empirical nature of drug discovery.

SULFONAMIDES. The sulfonamide story began in 1935 with the discovery by Domagk in the laboratories of I. G. Farbenindustrie that the deep red dye sulfamidochrysoidine (Prontosil) was effective against lethal streptococcal infections in mice. Interestingly the drug proved to have greater antibacterial activity in vivo than in the test tube (in vitro) suggesting that the animal must be altering (metabolizing) the dye molecule in some way to make it more effective. A French group at the Pasteur Institute soon proved that this indeed was the case, when they discovered that the active drug was the metabolite sulfanilamide, a fragment of the sulfamidochrysoidine molecule. Sulfanilamide provided the structural prototype of a class of compounds which chemists investigated by molecular modification of the prototype and testing the resulting compounds. These investigations led to major breakthroughs in other therapeutic areas and eventually to the discovery of hypotensive, anticonvulsant, diuretic, antidiabetic, and uricosuric drugs.[20]

Because the structure of sulfanilamide is relatively simple, chemists could modify it easily. Initially, derivatives were synthesized in an effort to find drugs which were more effective than the original drug and which would cause fewer adverse effects. Although sulfanilamide was life-saving in many severe human infections, it was prone to cause kidney damage at high doses. It was during the course of these investigations—which culminated in preparation of two of the most successful sulfa drugs, sulfathiazole and sulfadiazine—that chance observations were made which provided the key to the discovery of drugs with effects other than anti-infective effects.[21] In general, it could be said that these discoveries were the result of deliberate investigations through the synthesis and testing of compounds which were derivatives of sulfanilamide and the observation of unanticipated reactions. Scientists had learned from the histories of previous discoveries to be on the alert for effects other than the intended ones. When the discoveries were made, however, it could not be said that they were a direct result of a particular theory or of basic research in the biological sciences.

The empirical nature of drug research is perhaps best illustrated by the discovery of diuretic drugs related to sulfanilamide. Southworth's observation in 1939 that sulfanilamide produced alkaline urine triggered research in several laboratories. Researchers soon discovered that sulfanilamide blocks an enzyme, carbonic anhydrase, found in high concentrations in the kidney, where it is responsible for the normal acidity of urine. Inhibition of this enzyme decreases the formation of hydrogen ions in kidney cells and increases the excretion of sodium, potassium, and bicarbonate ions. The excretion of these ions is accompanied by the excretion of water, and thus sulfanilamides increase the volume of urine.[22] Since there existed a real medical need at that time for better and safer diuretic agents, testing was begun with sulfonamides, examining them either as inhibitors of the isolated enzyme carbonic anhydrase or as diuretic agents in intact animals. A group led by R. H. Roblin at the Lederle Laboratories soon found that the best enzyme inhibitors and diuretics were to be found among the more acidic sulfonamides. This resulted in the synthesis and testing of even more acidic sulfonamides. One of these, acetazolamide, eventually reached the market as the first of a new class of diuretics.

Although Domagk's discovery of Prontosil was the critical one which stimulated a large investigation by numerous research scientists and led to many subsequent discoveries, the seeds of his discovery could be traced to earlier works. In particular, his anti-infective research was guided by Ehrlich's affinity theory, which had been developed much earlier. Ehrlich suggested that certain sites on the surface of bacteria cells have a high affinity for groups of molecules which might be used as drugs, forming with them a tightly bonded complex. He postulated that the toxic portion of the drug might be brought sufficiently close to the cell to produce the desired effect.[23] Thus in this case biological theory apparently made a significant contribution. Nevertheless, it does not follow that the source was basic research, for Ehrlich developed his theory while searching for substances which kill or inhibit the growth of pathogenic protozoa. Ehrlich's work led to Salvarsan, the antisyphilitic agent, and to other drugs, which along with other discoveries in the early 1900s began to make many protozoal infections susceptible to treatment.[24] Ehrlich's methods resembled those used in modern research. He synthesized a large number of compounds and tested them in his search for Neo-Salvarsan, the improvement of the original drug, Salvarsan. His theories were the result of applied rather than of basic research.

The empirical approach of synthesizing and testing a large number of compounds, employed successfully by Ehrlich and Domagk, and which later went on to become the cornerstone of new drug discovery, originated in the experiences of earlier chemists with substances isolated from natural sources. Many of the early plant-derived medicinals were alkaloids, such as morphine, which was obtained from crude opium. The finding of such potent substances from natural sources spawned an intensive but empirical search for medicinals in the plant kingdom and yielded a fascinating array of novel biologically active plant products such as atropine, caffeine, nicotine, quinine, and strychnine.

The isolation of natural drugs was followed by the syntheses of hundreds of compounds in an attempt to empirically devise useful new drugs. Ehrlich is said to have synthesized 605 compounds before preparing his syphillis remedy, arsphenamine, which was relatively effective for that time.

This technique of investigation was used until the advances in understanding of chemical bonding and molecular structure were made in the early part of the twentieth century. These advances, which included A. M. Lewis's theory of valence, permitted chemists to systematize their investigations. They were able to limit their syntheses to classes of compounds sharing those parts of a molecular structure which are observed to cause a particular biological effect.

The theories relating to the molecular structure of substances which came out of basic chemical research have been a pillar of chemical investigations, including those in pharmaceutical research, but they were not developed in anticipation of any utility in pharmaceutical research.[25] Similarly, other chemical concepts (e.g. those of ionization, hydration, and the mechanisms of chemical reactions) which are widely used by pharmaceutical chemists resulted from basic investigations unrelated to pharmaceuticals. It is unlikely that these theories would have been developed earlier had more resources been devoted to basic research aimed at advancing pharmaceutical research.

PENICILLINS. Another path-finding discovery was Sir Alexander Fleming's observation that penicillin prevented the growth of bacteria. Fleming's observation initiated the successful search for many natural and synthetic antibacterial products which now exist. The antibiotics include streptomycin, tetracycline, chloramphenicol, and such semisynthetic penicillins as ampicillin, oxacillin, and the cephalosporins, as well as penicillin itself. Fleming's discovery did not lead immediately to the development of a useful drug. During the late 1930s and early 1940s the work of Sir Howard Florey and Ernest B. Chain at Oxford established the therapeutic properties of penicillin. The problem of producing the required quantities proved to be very difficult, and it was only solved with the stimulus of wartime needs.

Since it is generally agreed that Fleming's work set the stage for the antibiotic research which followed, we must inquire into the nature of his work. Despite the frequent mention of the accidental nature of Fleming's discovery, Fleming was seeking anti-infectives. Thus, in 1922 he detected an enzyme in body fluids which was bactericidal, but the tests were disappointing, for this enzyme killed only harmless bacteria. When he noticed the effect of penicillin, Fleming was studying the influence of changes in environmental factors on the characteristics of microbes. This search for an anti-infective can be classified as applied research.

Like Domagk, Fleming and his successors built on a great deal of previous applied research. Thus Pasteur had empirically recognized the phenomenon of microbial antagonism. The basic methodology for the detection of antibiotics in growth media had been developed much earlier. In addition, according to Lloyd H. Conover, there had even been a commercial antibiotic product produced in Germany as early as 1901 which was effective against bacterial infections.[26]

Fleming's discovery also underlines the importance of unanticipated observations which are made in the search for drugs in stimulating further research; the discovery transformed the investigation of antibiotics from an erratic pursuit to an organized and intensive search.

Conover says that by the time the antibiotics were discovered a great many observations had been made by experimental workers which strongly suggested the possibility of antibiotics, and the actual discovery was long overdue when it occurred. He attributes the delay to the fact that the scientists who were primarily interested in infectious diseases were involved in immunological research, and they had been disillusioned with chemotherapy by the ineffectiveness and toxicity of disinfectants against systemic infections. It was the discovery of penicillin combined with the success of the sulfonamides rather than advances in immunology which led scientists to investigate other metabolites.

ANTIHISTAMINES. The antihistamines were the third important development preceding the stream of discoveries of the 1940s and 1950s. Many important current drugs including the anti-Parkinsonian drugs, sedatives, tranquilizers, antidepressants, and anti-emetics can be traced to the antihistamines.[27]

The initial research which led to the discovery of the antihistamines can be described as exploratory or basic research not directed to the discovery of any specific drug. Soon after histamine was described as a chemical curiosity, Drs. G. Barger and H. H. Dale in 1911 at the Burroughs-Wellcome laboratories isolated it from ergot and intestinal mucosa. Following their discovery, histamine was found to be widely distributed in plants and lower forms of animal life, as well as in all mammals.[28] The interest in histamine which set off the subsequent search for antihistamines was the observation that although normally histamine is bound to certain cellular constituents where it is inert, it is released by a provoking stimulus such as injury or an allergen and causes an inflammatory reaction or the symptoms of allergy such as those of hay fever.[29]

When Bovet at the Pasteur Institute sought a drug to counteract the inflammatory effects of histamine, his work was applied research, since he was looking for a drug with a specific effect. Bovet synthesized as well as collected from other sources numerous compounds for testing. In addition, he devised animal tests to detect the anti-inflammatory effects of compounds. Since the effect of histamine could be shown in animals and in isolated organs, Bovet was able to screen many compounds. The compound which was selected as the lead compound for molecular modification turned out to be one which originally was synthesized by another research scientist in the search for an entirely different drug. In 1937 Bovet observed the antihistamine effects of some compounds synthesized several years previously by his colleague, E. P. Fourneau, who had been searching for a new antimalarial drug. Bovet synthesized an analog which proved to be a more powerful antihistamine than the original compounds, but this new agent was too toxic to be introduced to man.

The chemists at the French pharmaceutical firm Rhone-Poulenc continued Bovet's lead by synthesizing other analogs. Thus, they systematically investigated a class of compounds through the process of molecular modification. They finally succeeded in finding an antihistamine which was sufficiently powerful to treat allergic diseases without being too toxic. This was soon followed both in the United States and in France by the synthesis of other analogs some of which turned out to be therapeutically superior to the original drug.

The greatest achievement derived from this line of research was the discovery of the major tranquilizers typified by chlorpromazine. Scientists at Rhone-Poulenc observed that one of the side effects of the antihistamines they were studying was sedation. They began to search for other effects of the derivatives of the antihistamines on the central nervous system. In 1952 Laborit and his group announced the discovery of chlorpromazine, which they suggested would be useful to enhance the effects of anesthetics during surgery. Later, its unexpected usefulness in the treatment of psychotic states was recognized by the psychiatrist, Dr. J. Delay.[30]

Much of the research which led up to the discovery of chlorpromazine was directed at finding antihistamines. Chlorpromazine, along with other successor drugs, was found through a process of noticing the side-effects and new actions of the antihistamines and modifying compounds to enhance these side effects. The work thus was highly empirical, and again the chemists relied greatly on a research strategy employing the general tools of chemistry, including that of molecular modification.

The above examples of pharmaceutical research suggest some general points about the sources of new drugs as well as about the origins of the high rate of innovations in the 1940s and 1950s.

Most of the work which we have described in connection with these discoveries was applied research. Only the early research which eventually yielded the antihistamines can be called basic research. Curiously, as we noted earlier, this early work on histamine was conducted at a pharmaceutical company rather than an academic institution. The other work was applied research. Thus Fleming was seeking an anti-infective drug, Florey and Chain were attempting to demonstrate that penicillin was an effective antibiotic agent, and Domagk was also looking for an anti-infective agent. We will postpone assessing the implications of these observations for public policy until we have reviewed contributions which research in other disciplines made to the drug discoveries which we have described.

CHEMISTRY, PHYSICS, BIOLOGY, AND DRUG RESEARCH

Important contributions have come from basic research in chemistry and physics. Such research contributed the theories of molecular structure, which, as we have seen, helped to systematize the investigation of classes of compounds. On the other hand, applied research in other industries developed an important technique of chemical analysis. Investigation of the chemistry of the human body required the detection of chemicals present in extremely small quantities in tissues and body fluids. Similarly the search for new antibiotics required methods to detect, isolate, purify, and determine the molecular structures of the metabolities of micro-organisms. By the 1940s such techniques were available. Primary among them was the analytical technique known as chromatography. Chromatography has been one of the basic tools responsible for the success of research in that decade and since. To understand the origins of the basic knowledge on which pharmaceutical chemists have drawn, it is therefore important to know the source of this technique.

The essential work to develop chromatography was done in the petroleum industry in a search for techniques to isolate fractions of crude oil. In 1900 petroleum chemists first utilized chromatographic separation for this purpose. Discovery of the technique, however, is credited to a Russian botanist, Mikhail Tsvet who was attempting to separate the pigments of plants. Unfortunately, chromatography was not widely used until the 1940s. Archer Martin and Richard Synge have been given credit for stimulating the wide use of the method by applying it in an effort to determine the amino acid composition of wool [31] with a view to increasing the usefulness of this fiber. The rediscovery and development of chromatography thus were responses to urgent practical industrial needs.

The attribution of the analytical technique, mass spectrometry, which has been of great value for the identification of the prostaglandins and the determination of their structures, is not quite as simple. The development was the result of an interest in the separation and discovery of isotopes of nonradioactive elements, which can be described as basic research. But this observation is misleading for the development of the technique was a byproduct of this research just as chromatography was the byproduct of the search for techniques for the separation of fractions of crude oil. Mass spectrometry was the result of applied research directed at the specific problem of finding a method of separating isotopes of nonradioactive elements within a general framework of basic research. Both chromatography and mass spectrometry were the results of deliberate searches for methods of analysis within specific contexts, in the one case generally "applied" context and in the other a generally "basic" context. To say that mass spectrometry was discovered by scientists engaged in basic research does not suggest that the discovery would have been made sooner if more funds had been appropriated by the government or by the industry for basic research with a view to accelerating the flow of new drugs.

Before the technique of mass spectrometry could be used in pharmaceutical research, it had to be adapted for the analysis of organic chemicals. The required work was done by petroleum chemists in the petroleum industry who developed this technique because it promised to aid them in analyzing complex mixtures of chemicals. As in the case of chromatography, petroleum industry chemists did the essential work. Apparently, immediate industrial needs provided the necessary stimulus in both cases.

Thus, much of the basic knowledge used in the discovery of drugs was developed in basic research in chemistry and physics by scientists who had no interest in pharmaceutical research. But much of the development of the technique of analysis and measurement resulted from applied research in either academic or industrial laboratories. Pharmaceutical research along with other fields of organic chemical research have benefited from these efforts.

We have so far neglected the contributions of basic biological knowledge, which are much more difficult to trace and assess. Biological research has contributed certain theories including Ehrlich's theory of affinity [32] and derivative theories of drugs fitting target sites in or on cells they affect. These theories are applied in the search for drugs. Basic research in biology and biochemistry has also elaborated theories of cell function on the molecular level which pharmaceutical scientists apply in the formulation of working hypotheses. But it has been very difficult to predict the behavior of even simple, chemically well-understood molecules in cells. The living cell has proved to be far too complex a system. Thus while much progress toward understanding normal and diseased cell function has been made, vast unknown areas remain, including the molecular basis for most of our serious diseases. Because the necessary theories have been missing, pharmaceutical research has had to rely on setting up working hypotheses based on laboratory and clinical observations.

The incompleteness of biological theory is in sharp contrast to knowledge in the field of physics, but it is applied research based on physics that has been commonly though incorrectly thought of as the prototype for applied research in other fields, including pharmaceutical research. Failure to recognize this fundamental difference between the two fields has led to the erroneous belief that the application of knowledge in these two fields proceeds similarly. Application of the principles of physics may be represented as the working out of technological problems. By contrast, applying chemical and biological principles to develop useful drugs requires bridging large gaps in the theoretical framework.

Pharmaceutical research has in the past consistently jumped over theoretical gaps to yield new drugs. For example, pharmaceutical scientists have synthesized analogs of naturally occurring chemicals to yield new drugs in spite of their incomplete knowledge of how these natural substances act biologically. Similarly, chemical modification of steroid hormones has yielded oral contraceptives and anti-inflammatories; alteration of thiazide diuretics has led to antihypertensives; and structural changes of phenothiazine tranquilizers have resulted in psychostimulants. The discovery of the derivative drugs was not a direct follow-through on the understanding of the mechanism of the drug's action on the relevant disease.[33]

Seldom does biochemical or chemical theory predict *de novo* what pharmacologic actions a given compound or chemical change in a compound will have. By intelligent trial and error, pharmaceutical investigators are able in many cases to identify the active parts of molecules and to maximize desired effects. It was empirically observed that some of the antibacterial sulfonamides had hypoglycemic properties. By systematic chemical modification of one of these hypoglycemic sulfonamides, industrial chemists demonstrated that one chemical group which is essential for antibacterial action has no effect on hypoglycemic action. This permitted the development of antidiabetic drugs devoid of antibacterial effects.[34]

The majority of discoveries can be traced to one of three sources: naturally occurring compounds, accidental discoveries, or modifications of previously known drugs. The process of pharmaceutical research thus requires mastery not only of theoretical biology and organic chemistry but also of the pharmacological properties of many tested compounds, only some of which are themselves used as drugs. While drug discovery has benefited from basic research discoveries, the reverse is also true. For example, the discovery of antibiotics, which was initiated by the serendipitous observation of penicillin, was advanced by massive screening programs and selective chemical modification by the industry. The microbiology on which the screening was based came from basic scientific advances. Once the antibiotics were identified, however, and their structure elucidated, basic research laboratories utilized them to selectively affect bacterial cells in ways which have clarified our perception of cell structure. Blocking of protein synthesis by streptomycin, for example, permitted scientists to examine the way proteins are made in the cell. The resulting knowledge of cellular function then became a working part of the search for drugs.[35]

As new types of drugs are discovered, academic and industrial laboratories investigate the mechanisms by which they act and thus expand our basic understanding of cellular function. For example, soldiers exposed to nitrogen mustard gas were observed to have low leukocyte levels in their blood. Since this effect would be desirable in treating leukemia, scientists formulated the working hypothesis that compounds related to the nerve gas might be useful anticancer drugs. In fact, some of the alkylating agents related to nitrogen mustard *were* found to be useful anticancer agents. Subsequently, these drugs were shown to cross-link the strands of DNA, thereby preventing the DNA duplication and cell replication which permit tumors to grow. Thus, elucidation of the theoretical basis for antineoplastic activity of these drugs clarified our understanding of molecular biology.[36]

Pharmaceutical research is highly empirical; trial and error and chance play an important part. Use is made of previous knowledge, theory, and techniques—but the conduct of pharmaceutical research consists primarily of the pursuit of promising leads rather than the search for and discovery of new principles. Even when scientists are familiar with a disease area, they may not know detailed mechanisms of the disease. They may know only that certain molecular structures have been found to have a desired or other specific effect while similar molecular structures may have different therapeutic and toxic effects. Alternatively, the lead may consist of the knowledge that a natural substance that occurs in animals or plants provokes an interesting biological reaction. This information may derive from folk medicine, as in the case of the rauwolfia root, or it may be based on other laboratory observations. To build up a body of knowledge in pharmacology consists of accumulating evidence from one's own experimental work and from that of others.

Basic research in physics, chemistry, and the biological sciences does contribute importantly to formulating hypotheses to direct the search for drugs. Analytical and synthetic techniques from basic research efforts are also of major significance to pharmaceutical research. Historically, however, the important discoveries in drugs have depended to a very large extent on information which was previously obtained in the course of applied pharmaceutical research and on basic techniques obtained from applied research in other fields. Basic research in other fields which are not obviously related to drugs has also turned out to be valuable. In general, however, drug research has progressed primarily on the strength of a vast accumulation of empirical findings of previous drug discovery efforts.

The history of major drug discoveries thus suggests that to yield the most in terms of new drugs, research resources are better devoted to pursuing leads to new drugs than on exploratory basic research in biology and chemistry. Basic research in physics, chemistry, and biology has turned out to be valuable to pharmaceutical research, but expenditures on such research have to be justified on grounds more general than those of benefits to the process of drug discovery. If the past is any guide to sources of new drugs, the optimal fiscal strategy for the development of new drugs would allocate a large fraction of the total resources available for drug research to the synthesis and testing of compounds which are suspected of being able to provoke desired biological activities.

CHAPTER 3

CHARACTERISTICS OF
DRUG RESEARCH

INTRODUCTION

Drug discovery is an intricate and complex process, differing in important ways from many other forms of scientific research. Since new drugs cannot be designed by logical deductions from valid general principles, drug research is a trial-and-error process organized on the basis of a series of provisional hypotheses systematically refined by feedback from empirical tests. In retrospect, the discovery of a drug will be seen to have rested on a few critical findings during the discovery process, although many other observations and false starts will have been made which turn out in the end not to be useful. These cannot be avoided; that they eventually will prove to be of no use can be ascertained only in retrospect. Because of this, the process of discovery of a new drug is long, tedious, and expensive.

Drug discovery requires close intermeshing of chemists, pharmacologists, biochemists, and clinicians, who must be in constant communication with each other. Possible leads must be painstakingly examined, test results must be evaluated, and decisions must be made about further in vitro or animal tests and about the synthesis of additional compounds. This constant exchange permits the use of a great deal of information and the pursuit of leads developed by members of the team or by outside sources.

It is vital to understand how one important characteristic of drug research differs from other chemical research that is undertaken in the typical manner (e.g., the seeking of a new insecticide, dye stuff, or food additive). The drug research scientist is severely limited in assessing the validity of his hypothesis or testing whether any of the chemical structures he synthesized is a lead point in his progress towards a more potent or more selective therapeutic activity. In fact, under the present inadequate state of development of animal models for complex human diseases, the more innovative the therapeutic discovery, the more necessary is its clinical validation before one can say with any certainty that a potentially useful drug has been discovered at all. The drug research scientist cannot really make a discovery in the true sense until he has had recourse to a clinical experiment. In view of this, the process of discovery in drug research is unusually susceptible to government regulations which are apt to cause increasing delays in clinical feedback to the laboratory team. Such regulatory interference bogs down the entire progress of drug discovery because it leaves the scientist without a facile indicator of how his work is measuring up and therefore leaves him unable to identify those critical leads that are demonstrably relevant to clinical therapy.

Many academic laboratories dealing with biochemistry and pharmacology might seek new drugs. One possible advantage of the distribution of efforts among many laboratories is that more hypotheses might be tested than if research were concentrated in a smaller number of laboratories. Indeed, a few drug discoveries have emerged from such academic laboratories, but in practice the structure and goals of academic laboratories are not conducive to the discovery of new drugs. Academic laboratories suffer from serious disadvantages in the search for new drugs. They usually are organized by disciplines rather than as multidisciplinary drug research units. This is understandable because their primary goal is to expand scientific knowledge, which is divided into disciplines, rather than to discover new drugs. When they do undertake drug research, they usually limit it to the testing of compounds previously prepared in industrial laboratories. Some academic laboratories synthesize new compounds in an attempt to identify new drugs, but most do not. Academic laboratories usually would not desire to search for a drug systematically by synthesizing a class of compounds suspected of having a desirable pharmacological property and testing them, because the university functions of education of students and expansion of basic knowledge would not be furthered by such efforts.

When research efforts are dispersed among independent small academic laboratories, there are long delays in following up discoveries. We have seen that Florey and Chain did not investigate penicillin's therapeutic efficacy until ten years after Fleming's initial discovery, and further development would probably have been delayed much longer were it not for the wartime demand for anti-infectives. Some discoveries were lost because they were not followed up, and they had to be made again independently by other scientists before they resulted in new drugs. Thus, in Romania, Dr. Nicholas C. Paulesco discovered insulin before Drs. Banting and Best did so independently in Canada.[1] The later discovery did result in a drug but only after Eli Lilly and Company made possible its development by devising a suitable purification procedure. The company also instituted control procedures to ensure potency and safety and arranged for clinical trials.

As this chapter will show, industrial laboratories have organized their research so as to systematize and accelerate the pursuit of leads, and they have had adequate incentives for the development of drugs which can be manufactured in commercial quantities. This chapter also describes several recent major academic discoveries, noting that they were the result of large-scale programs resembling industrial efforts rather than the usual scattered, independent, small-scale efforts of academic laboratories.

The sequence of research conducted in pharmaceutical laboratories is also examined in this chapter. The description indicates the high degree of specialization of research workers and the numerous disciplines involved, the need for close coordination of the members of a research group representing different disciplines, and the resulting need for large resources. We see that research programs take a long time to complete. Finally, we report on the degree of uncertainty associated with pharmaceutical R & D. This discussion is followed by estimates of the cost of pharmaceutical research.

EXAMPLES OF INDUSTRIAL PHARMACEUTICAL RESEARCH

Several examples of industrial pharmaceutical research will serve to illustrate the advantages of industrial laboratories in this type of research. Such laboratories usually are organized in multidisciplinary teams which can sustain integrated programs over long periods of time. They even promote basic research in academic laboratories and can efficiently exploit leads that may emerge from such sources. The important conclusion which emerges is that they have converted pharmaceutical research from an erratic pursuit into a sustained systematic effort in which much if not all of the available evidence is considered and applied.

The primary approaches to drug discovery are examination of natural sources, screening, and molecular modification. More than one of these approaches may be employed in any one research project. In the first of these methods, naturally occurring compounds are examined for pharmacological activity. Opium, morphine, digitalis, and reserpine are examples of drugs occurring in nature. In the screening approach, hundreds or thousands of compounds are collected from many sources, natural and synthetic, and are examined for desired activity. The molecular modification method begins with a compound with known pharmacologic activity which is chemically altered in an attempt to change its properties. Often these synthetic modifications are guided by a working hypothesis based on previous experience of what pharmacologic changes should be produced by a given chemical alteration.

PENICILLINS. The use of molecular modification as a discovery technique is perhaps best illustrated by the development of some of the earlier "biosynthetic" penicillins.[2] It had been observed that the chemical nature of penicillins produced by fermentation could be altered at will by the presence of certain compounds in the growth medium. As a result, in 1948 a process was developed for synthesis of a variety of biosynthetic penicillins, modified in the acyl moiety, by systematically adding variants of phenylacetic acid to penicillin fermentations. The discovery of penicillin V was made in 1954 by such a process.

In 1958 Sheehan at M.I.T. announced the synthesis of 6-amino penicillanic acid (6-APA), which could be converted to penicillin by acylation. Independently, workers at Beecham laboratories discovered 6-APA and developed a practical fermentation method which yielded large quantities of 6-APA. By varying the chemical groups attached to this nucleus, new semisynthetic penicillins could be synthesized at will. Among these were new drugs which had improved oral absorption (methacillin and ampicillin), penicillinase resistance (oxacillin), and activity against some gram negative bacteria (carbenicillin).

ETHAMBUTOL. The development of the antitubercular agent ethambutol (Myambutol), at Lederle Laboratories illustrates the successful application of random screening. The search extended over twenty-four years.[3] The research was devoted initially to increasing the capacity of the test system. The early screening was slow, requiring ten grams of the compound and ten guinea pigs for each new test. At the end of each test, the guinea pigs were autopsied and eight organs of each animal were weighed, examined, and graded for pathology. The extent of anti-TB activity was measured by comparing treated guinea pigs with those which were untreated. Only five hundred new compounds per year could be tested with this original screen. The new screen, however, required only one tenth of a gram of each new compound to be used in two mice. The test permitted five compounds to be tested at the same time in each animal. Survival of at least one of the mice indicated some anti-TB activity and follow-up study determined which of the five compounds was active. The system was capable of finding compounds with only a small amount of anti-TB activity with a high degree of reliability. The capacity of the new system was 20,000 compounds annually.

Following the development of this screen, Lederle Laboratories systematically tested a file of chemical compounds accumulated by the American Cyanamid Company, its parent company. The file contained 103,000 chemical compounds (to which 5,000 were added annually) which had been developed in the company's other divisions for a variety of purposes. In 1965, after thousands of compounds had been tested, one which had originally been developed as an antioxidant additive for rubber and which had failed in its original purpose was found to be potent against tuberculosis. The structure of this chemical is relatively simple and very different from that of other anti-TB drugs. As research was continued on analogs, six hundred new structures were synthesized, one of which was found to be more active and less toxic than the lead compound. Additional work revealed that the activity was limited to the dextro isomer, while the toxic effects accompanied both isomers. Further work led to isolation of the dextro isomer and elimination of the toxic but ineffective levo isomer. The research program which led up to ethambutol thus was a combination of large-scale random screening of thousands of compounds and a program of molecular modification to uncover the best analog.

In the work leading to ethambutol, the ingenuity of research workers was expressed in the development of an economical and reliable screening system which could process many compounds. Much of the other work was of a highly routine character. Random screening is becoming less common. But even when there are leads, hundreds and sometimes thousands of compounds must be screened. The development of reliable screens which can handle many compounds economically is therefore a recurrent problem.

TETRACYCLINE. Tetracycline was first obtained by synthetic modification of a fermentation product, chlortetracycline. Tetracycline proved to be both more stable and better tolerated than its fermentation-produced progenitor. The complexity of the tetracyclines made further synthetic modification difficult,[4] and during the 1950s new tetracyclines were fermentation products, such as demeclocycline, rather than products of synthetic modification.

Eventually the chemistry of the C_6 hydroxyl function was found to hold the key to new drug discovery. In 1958 Pfizer scientists reported the successful removal of the C_6 hydroxyl, paving the way for synthesis of several new tetracyclines. Similar work was reported later by Lederle Laboratories. Methacycline, doxycycline, and minocycline were the result of this increased synthetic ability. Studies of the effects on potency of different molecular structures and electronic properties have both guided drug discovery efforts and explained the unique properties of new tetracyclines, such as the efficient absorption of doxycycline.

PROSTAGLANDINS. The search for active substances in animals or plants is best illustrated by prostaglandin research.[5] The prostaglandin story began in 1930 when these lipide-like acidic substances were first detected in human semen and were shown to contract or relax strips of human uterus. Believing that the active substances came from the prostate gland, Von Euler named them prostaglandins. (The name turned out to be misleading, since prostaglandins are produced throughout the body).

At the time of their discovery and in the nearly three decades that followed, research with prostaglandins moved at a slow pace, partly due to wartime pressures and partly as a result of the scarcity of the naturally occurring materials and a lack of suitable methods for their isolation, purification, and analysis. Finally, in 1956, Bergstrom of the Karolinska Institute in Sweden tackled the problem of the structure of these "curiosities." Aided by a grant from the Upjohn Company, and using some of the sophisticated techniques of isolation and purification that had just then become available to organic chemists, Bergstrom was successful in obtaining a pure crystalline sample of the first prostaglandin. By 1966 he had isolated and elucidated structures of the whole family of new prostaglandin substances.

Prostaglandin total synthesis studies began in several laboratories long before clear evidence of therapeutic potential was established. Early successes, particularly in the area of biosynthetic techniques, enabled the Upjohn Company, in particular, to assist work in the field by freely supplying synthetic prostaglandins to scientists wishing to study their effects in physiological systems. This greatly stimulated the accumulation of a vast body of basic knowledge in this area. The elegant work of Corey and his associates at Harvard, who successfully executed the synthesis of all naturally occurring prostaglandins in pure optically active form, is an outstanding example of the application of organic synthesis to solve the problem of a limited supply of a natural product. These and other syntheses provided technology for the preparation of analogs, several hundred of which have been synthesized since then, in the ongoing effort to produce prostaglandins which eventually can play an important role in therapy.[6] The clinical phase of prostaglandin research is already well advanced throughout the world. The clinical efficacy of prostaglandins in abortion and induction of labor is well established, and synthetic $PGF_{2\alpha}$ has recently been introduced for use in these indications. Successful clinical studies with a variety of prostaglandins and related analogs as gastric antisecretory agents, bronchodilators, and agents for the treatment of cardiovascular diseases are appearing with increasing frequency, leading to the expectation that perhaps several will find their place in therapy during the next decade.

These descriptions indicate that the search for a drug with the desired characteristics requires a continual awareness of the literature, new patents, and symposia in order to track down worthwhile clues. Many groups throughout the world may be doing related work. What is more, the elusive nature of the problems and their solutions means that it is unlikely that any single group can hit on a solution completely on its own. Frequently, therefore, pharmaceutical manufacturers with a special interest in an area support related work done elsewhere through the supply of materials, technical assistance, and financing. A large firm which has a considerable investment of its own in a certain area will encourage academic research in the same area even at the risk of its competitors sharing the benefits. Because its own research puts it in the lead, the firm can expect to gain from the work done elsewhere. This is the reason Upjohn supported Bergstrom's research on prostaglandins and Merck supported Waksman's group at Rutgers.

The advantages of an industrial laboratory are also apparent when we examine the descriptions of drug discoveries in academic laboratories. The Salk vaccine, the birth control pill, and cortisone were supported by large and unusually well funded organizations. Without such support, these discoveries might not have been made or would have been greatly delayed.

SOME ACADEMIC DISCOVERIES

SALK VACCINE. Salk's virus laboratory at the University of Pittsburgh was very unusual for it benefited from a well-financed crash program, and Salk may have been the most lavishly supported biologist in history.[7] Carter quotes an anonymous critic to the effect that Salk's laboratory was the "smoothest, biggest, damnedest thing you ever saw, like a big, damned industrial plant except it was in a medical school." The National Foundation for Infantile Paralysis, headed by Basil O'Connor, supplied the large funds.

Before the foundation became active, polio research had stagnated because of erroneous theory and the costliness and difficulty of research. In 1935 virologists agreed that the cause of polio was a virus, which they incorrectly concluded grew only in living nerve cells, entered the body through the nose, and spread to the brain and spine through the nervous tissue.

Dr. Harry M. Weaver, the foundation's director of research, organized a virus-typing program which required large resources and included a great deal of mechanical drudgery. Salk was one of the small handful of scientists willing to undertake this work. Weaver was the much-needed organizer of the various research efforts supported by the foundation. He anticipated trends in research and organized among the foundation's grantees discussions which served to provide a forum for ideas and a means of communication among the workers. In attempting to direct research, he contradicted previous practice; traditional practice had been for scientists to act independently. Weaver coaxed the grantees to develop new areas of research, encouraging them to investigate the possibility of vaccination at a time when the prevailing view was to rule it out.

Salk was unusual among academics in being ready to use large resources for biological research. According to Weaver,

> His [Salk's] approach was entirely different from that which had dominated the field. The older workers had all been brought up in days when you didn't accept a grant of more than $400 or $500 from an outside source without having a long conference with the dean. Everything was on a small scale. You made do with one or two laboratory animals because you couldn't afford to pay for the twelve which were needed. Jonas had no such psychology. He thought big. He wanted lots of space and was perfectly comfortable with the idea of using hundreds of monkeys, and running dozens of experiments at a time. He always wanted to expand his program so that it would encompass as much of a subject as possible. He was out of phase with the tradition of narrowing his search down to one or two details, making progress inch by inch. He wanted to leap, not crawl. His willingness to shoot the works was made to order for us. Furthermore, he was entirely without fear of the concept of vaccination.

Much of Salk's time was spent dealing with administrative problems. Many of them arose out of the shortage of monkeys which had to be obtained for tests.

The shortage led the foundation to develop new methods of trapping, transporting, and feeding monkeys. It acquired the Okatie farm in South Carolina, where the monkeys were conditioned for laboratory use.

Certain critical discoveries preceded the development of the vaccine. Dr. John Enders at Harvard proved that the virus would grow in non-nervous tissue. Dr. Isabel M. Mountain reported experiments with monkeys in which the virus, inactivated with formalin, produced antibody levels and immunity similar to that achieved with live viruses. Although the discovery commonly is attributed to Salk, the contributions of other scientists also were important.

Not only did the foundation organize and finance the research done by different scientists, but it also stimulated competition among them by organizing conferences at which the grantees presented reports. The conferences served to accelerate the rate of progress, for the scientists were no longer isolated and dependent solely on reports in journals published long after the actual experiments. In effect, the foundation simulated the competitive environment which a market provides for the industry. The competition did not focus on economic rewards but on the recognition of a peer group. This difference is not of critical importance. What is crucial is the observation that the foundation provided an exceptional set of circumstances for the development of a new drug. In certain important respects, this organization resembled that provided by industry.

This history of the polio research program indicates the importance of large resources, large-scale effort, effective organization of this effort, the active leadership provided by the foundation, and speed in following leads.

CORTISONE. The discovery of cortisone as a clinically useful drug involved a large-scale research program employing different groups of investigators, substantial financing, and leadership by one or two individuals.[8]

In 1942 the National Research Council authorized an extensive investigation to develop a chemical technology for the synthesis of corticosteroids. The investigation involved teams from Yale, the University of Chicago, the Mayo Clinic, Northwestern University, Princeton, and two pharmaceutical companies, Merck and Squibb. Sarett of Merck and Kendall of the Mayo Clinic were the principal leaders. The main problem was to prepare a large enough supply of cortisone to study its activity. By 1946 both Kendall's Compound A and cortisone had been prepared on a small scale in the laboratory.

Compound A was tested in man but showed no promising activity. Sarett's group at Merck persevered in an attempt to synthesize sufficient cortisone to conduct a clinical test. By May 1948 Sarett had enough cortisone to allow Kendall and Hench of the Mayo Clinic to test the compound in arthritic patients. The dramatic relief provided by the drug put a high priority on an efficient way to make large quantities of cortisone. However, the synthetic technique developed by Sarett and Kendall was a complex and difficult one. A great deal of ingenuity went into Merck's development of a feasible commercial process for cortisone, which was completed by late 1949. In 1951 Schering (U.S.A.) developed a similar process.

It is interesting to note that, despite the large effort and investment by Merck in the discovery and development of cortisone, it was soon displaced by prednisone and prednisolone. The undesirable effects of cortisone included the retention of water and salt, which was associated with an increased burden on the heart and increased blood pressure. In addition, stomach ulcers were aggravated and long-term treatment sometimes was associated with loss of calcium and spontaneous bone fractures. In 1954 scientists at Schering were able to modify the structure of cortisone to produce prednisone and prednisolone. These minor alterations in the molecular structure increased the potency three to five times and reduced the side effect of salt and water retention which had limited the use of cortisone.

THE BIRTH CONTROL PILL.   Another important discovery associated with an academic institution is that of the birth control pill.[9] Again there was leadership by a foundation, large financing, and the coordination of effort in different institutions.

In 1950 Abraham Stone, medical director of the Planned Parenthood Foundation, persuaded Gregory Pincus, co-director of the Worcester Foundation for Biological Research, to undertake development of a contraceptive agent. Pincus knew from the work of Makepeace, Weinstein, and Friedman that progesterone injected into rabbits inhibited ovulation. He therefore *fed* rabbits large doses of progesterone and observed that whereas they mated, they did not ovulate. The experiment suggested that pregnancy might be prevented by an oral agent. Pincus obtained the assistance of Dr. John Rock, of Harvard University, and tests were carried out on a group of women. These experiments demonstrated that chemical contraception in the human was possible.

The high oral dosages required to inhibit ovulation, and the imperfect control of menstruation with progesterone, however, made it essential to look for better progestational agents. Pincus then asked Searle, which had been supporting efforts of the foundation, to help in the search for an acceptable oral contraceptive. Dr. Frank Colton at Searle made several steroidal compounds and tested them for progestational activity in animals. He sent samples of the more promising compounds to Pincus for further study. In this manner norethynodrel was prepared and was found to be at least ten times more potent orally than progesterone. Rock's clinical trial using fifty women demonstrated that the compound was effective as a contraceptive and of low toxicity. Later it was discovered that a small amount of a powerful estrogen, mestranol, is required along with the progestational agent for optimum activity. Searle then conducted extensive field trials in Puerto Rico in which more than 1,600 women participated over a period of four years. Upon successful completion of these tests, Searle was granted approval to market its contraceptive in 1960. Since that time, further research by several pharmaceutical firms has contributed to development of even more effective oral contraceptives, and has eliminated most side-effects, such as nausea and weight gain experienced by some users of earlier forms of the pill.

The work which led up to the discovery and development of the birth control pill involved the active efforts of a foundation, heavy financing, the cooperation of several institutions, and the synthesis of new steroids and the organization of large-scale clinical tests by the pharmaceutical industry. Thus, although much of the research leading to oral contraceptives was conducted in a nonprofit private laboratory, it was done on an industrial scale and industrial methods were applied.

The foregoing descriptions of the research on polio vaccine, the cortico-steroids, and the pill all underline the fact that important academic drug discoveries came about as a result of large coordinated campaigns financed by government or other agencies. Without considerable outside support and the organization which is associated with it, it is unlikely that academic laboratories will muster sufficient resources to achieve drug discovery. This is especially true now when the average new single entity requires, as we shall see, approximately $24 million in funds invested in research.

Unless there is a national campaign against a disease, academic research is unlikely deliberately to pursue the discovery of a new drug. The costs of research and development are usually too great, and academic departments are not organized for the purpose of finding drugs.

A DESCRIPTION OF PHARMACEUTICAL RESEARCH

A description of pharmaceutical research will shed additional light on the advantages of industrial pharmaceutical laboratories. In particular, the description provides a background for the later discussion of the economies of scale in pharmaceutical research.

The basic decision for a drug company is whether to undertake research in a particular therapeutic field, for this decision involves a commitment to build up expertise in the area over a ten-year period without any assurance of developing a single new drug, let alone one that will have enough sales to provide an adequate investment return. Having committed itself, a company will examine the drugs which are available in the field to determine the possibilities for developing drugs which are more effective and less toxic or which exhibit new properties.

In chapter 2 we saw how the first step in the drug discovery process is the development of a working hypothesis which takes into account both the nature of the disease against which the drug is to be effective and also the chemical constitution and pharmacological activity of drugs previously shown to be useful for treatment of that disease. We also saw how feedback from "screening" of compounds synthesized in the laboratory leads to the synthesis of yet more compounds until the scientists obtain a promising agent with a satisfactory balance of efficacy to safety in animal tests. Counts of discoveries for the purpose of estimating the importance of industrial or of academic laboratories as a source of drug discoveries, such as are reported in chapter 5, usually give credit for the discovery of a drug to the scientists involved in the initial synthesis and testing of the compound. But the synthesis and the early animal tests are very early in the process of the discovery and development of a drug, as we will see. The drug is not really discovered until the much later clinical tests which establish efficacy and safety. Many compounds which demonstrate desirable biological activity in the initial tests do not go much further, and few reach the stage of clinical tests, to say nothing of marketing. The scientists only have a working hypothesis to go on and too much depends on the later tests to be able to have confidence that a discovery has been made following initial animal tests. This is the consequence of working on the edge of the unknown with only bits of information on which to base hypotheses which are revised as experiments continue.

Thus, compounds surviving the primary screen go into secondary, more detailed screens, where they are extensively studied. They are also examined in other primary screens, in particular the cardiovascular, pulmonary, renal, and central nervous system screens. Occasionally a drug originating in one field is discovered to have therapeutic effects in another field; but the major purpose of the screens in other fields is the detection of undesirable side effects, which are frequent. The requirement that a compound go through tests in other therapeutic areas is important for our later discussion of the economies of scale, since it gives a laboratory which spans many therapeutic fields an advantage over others which are limited to one or few fields. Only a large laboratory will be able to support significant research projects in many therapeutic fields.

The early animal tests can at best yield only inferences of safety and efficacy and can in no way yield conclusive evidence regarding the effects of a compound in humans. It is at this stage that a medical review committee evaluates the animal test results and makes the decision to proceed to the first clinical (human) tests. Before this can be done, however, the compound must be subjected to intensive and rigorous animal toxicology and pharmacological tests. The toxicologist does not join the drug design team, but instead independently conducts animal tests of compounds reaching him from all fields in that organization. These tests determine (a) the highest dose range—that is, that which causes obvious side effects but does not kill the animal before the end of the test; (b) the second dose range—that which causes borderline side effects; and (c) the low dose range—that which is the maximum dose that shows no side effects at all. The initial clinical dose will be some fraction of this smallest dose. FDA regulations require at least thirty days of animal toxicology testing to accumulate data before making initial human tests. The animal toxicology testing continues after initial human trials in order to determine effects over the lifetime of the animal.

If the results of the thirty-day animal tests are satisfactory, an Investigational New Drug Application (IND) is sent to the FDA, and phase I of clinical research, or initial trials with normal subjects, begins after permission. Clinical testing is divided into phases I, II, and III. Although these phases are in sequence, they overlap in time to some extent, and tests on normal subjects are called phase I studies whenever they are performed. It is perhaps unnecessary to point out that the only purpose of tests with normal subjects is to determine safety rather than efficacy. Tests for efficacy must await phase II tests with patients who are suffering from the disease. So it is not before this late stage that scientists know whether or not a drug will be effective.

Returning to the animal toxicology tests, the ninety-day subacute toxicity tests are conducted on two species. The latter part of these tests is conducted concurrently with phase I human trials. A New Drug Application (NDA) requires eighteen months of chronic toxicology tests on rodents and twelve months of such tests on other animals.

Preparation for clinical research begins early in the history of a compound, when it is scheduled for toxicology. The physician who then joins the team usually knows the therapeutic field from work with previous compounds in that area. He supervises phase I clinical studies which are usually limited to healthy volunteers in a prison or special hospital unit. Potential subjects of these tests must be given full information about the studies and must demonstrate willingness to participate by their informed consent. Phase I determines the maximum dose of drug which is free from unacceptable side effects, and is usually conducted with a small number (10–20) of volunteers. Although many observers seem to perceive great risks to the subjects of these early human trials, they are in fact conducted under close medical supervision and in practice have proven to be extremely safe. An article published by the Food and Drug Administration states: "the safety record of such research is excellent. FDA knows of no volunteer patient who has been permanently harmed as a result of Phase I (early clinical) testing of hundreds of new compounds under the FDA procedures established in 1962."[10]

If the compound successfully passes these early clinical trials, it is now considered an active drug candidate. It is ready to be tested for long periods of time (often two or two and a half years), in animals with metabolic pathways similar to those in man, to derive an indication of its long-term safety characteristics. At the same time it is also ready to be tested in human subjects with the target disease in order to determine the extent of its efficacy. These human tests (Phase II) are usually conducted by independent clinical investigators who are both physicians with responsibility for their own patients and at the same time trained scientists who work closely with the drug research team. They perform careful, controlled studies with the drug candidate in order to demonstrate efficacy and to help determine proper dosage and profiles of use.

Even if the drug candidate proves promising in these clinical trials, it still must undergo a series of wider scale studies (phase III), usually under outpatient conditions and in larger groups of people (500–1500 patients) in a search for low-incidence side effects and proof of efficacy in a large patient population. In both phase II and phase III the independent clinical investigator uses sophisticated technology (including the double blind design in which neither he nor the patient knows if the drug or a different compound is being administered) to validate efficacy, safety, and eliminate the effects of psychological suggestion and random chance.

If these tests prove successful, the new drug candidate will have completed a rigorous, time-consuming, and costly research and development program from the working hypothesis through synthesis and preclinical and clinical trials. It is now ready for governmental review and approval for public use. Nevertheless, companies continue to test features of their new drug even after the FDA's acceptance of the NDA and the beginning of marketing. Application for additional dosage forms or for new uses of the drug require additional clinical trials.[11]

Typically, for every new product thousands of compounds are synthesized. In 1970 PMA members prepared, extracted, or isolated for medical research purpose 126,060 substances, and pharmacologically tested 703,900 substances. The number that reached the stage of clinical testing in that year was only 1,013. That same year only 16 new compounds (from previous years) were successful in passing all clinical tests, obtaining approval from the FDA, and reaching the market.[12] The vast majority of experimental compounds are eliminated by the primary and secondary screens; very few reach even the animal toxicology stage.

There are many factors which can halt the progress of a compound. A recent study by Drs. Louis Lasagna and William Wardell, based on a survey of the fifteen major American-owned companies, reports the total number of new chemical entities which were clinically tested world-wide from 1963 through 1973, the number of IND's (filed in the U.S.) for new chemical entities, the number of such IND's which are still active, the number discontinued prior to NDA approval, and the number of NDA's approved (table 3-1). The results indicate that only a small percent of the IND's become new chemical entities approved for marketing. By April 1974 only 7.1 percent of all such IND's filed from 1963 through 1967 had resulted in approved NDA's. Were a later cutoff date than 1967 used, the percentage would be even lower. These data indicate that there is only a .07 probability of a clinically tested new chemical entity being marketed.

There are many factors which can halt the progress of a compound. Clinical side-effects must be balanced with activity, and the acceptability of the side-

TABLE 3-1

Analysis of IND's for New Chemical Entities Filed by Fifteen Companies
between 1963 and 1973 (as of April 1974)

	Number of IND's				Percentage of IND's			
	Filed	Discontinued prior to NDA approval	Approved as NDAs	Still active	Filed	Discontinued prior to NDA approval	Approved as NDAs	Still active
1963	63	59	2	2	100	94	3	3
1964	87	76	10	1	100	87	12	1
1965	73	60	5	8	100	82	7	11
1966	58	53	0	5	100	91	0	9
1967	43	32	6	6	100	74	14	12
1968	48	31	4	11	100	65	8	27
1969	55	36	1	18	100	66	2	32
1970	51	30	0	21	100	59	0	41
1971	42	21	1	22	100	50	2	48
1972	28	6	0	22	100	21	0	79
1973	41	4	0	37	100	10	0	90

Source: Louis Lasagna and William Wardell, "An Analysis of Drug Development Involving New Chemical Entities Sponsored by U.S.–Owned Companies, 1962–1974," paper presented at the Conference on Drug Development and Marketing, American Enterprise Institute for Public Policy Research, Washington, D.C., July 25–26, 1974.

effects depends not only on their severity but also on the effectiveness of the drug and the suffering caused by the disease. Another factor is the efficacy of the drug relative to that of other drugs already on the market. Only rarely is there no activity at all or extremely serious side effects; the preceding animal tests are usually reasonable predictors in these respects.

The comment may be made that a small number of successes out of many attempts does not signify a high degree of risk, if a given investment in R & D can be counted on to generate a specific number of successes with a high degree of certainty. Such certainty clearly is not characteristic of pharmaceutical R & D investment. As we will see in chapter 6, some of the largest firms have introduced very few new drugs over an extended period.[13] This is evident already in table 3-1, in the data on the number of NDA's for which the fifteen companies surveyed by Drs. Lasagna and Wardell were able to obtain approval in the period 1963–73. We also know that large pharmaceutical research projects have had to continue for many years before they have been able to yield new products such as ethambutol, the prostaglandins, and doxycycline.

Thus pharmaceutical research entails the synthesis and testing of numerous compounds by a variety of specialists. Only a small number of compounds out of the thousands tested in laboratories in the discovery stage of research survive to be clinically tested. The clinical tests, which are broken down into three phases, are carried on simultaneously with continued intensive animal toxicology tests. Large R & D expenditures and a highly organized research effort are required if research is to be conducted on a sufficiently large scale to ensure a reasonable probability of success. And even when the yearly expenditures run into ten millions of dollars, the companies cannot be assured of success.

ADVANTAGES OF LARGE FIRMS IN PHARMACEUTICAL RESEARCH

As we have seen, some economists have suggested that a large size of firm does not confer any advantages on an inventor. According to these economists, the chief ingredients of major inventions are imagination and familiarity with recent scientific advances—ingredients which come cheaply—rather than a variety of skills and much specialized equipment. Further, the large corporation is described as conducting relatively routine research and as declining projects having a high probability of technical failure. The large corporation's only advantages are argued to be in developmental research, which is costly because it requires the cooperative efforts of many different individuals.[14]

According to this model, the inventor can dispose of the burden of the developmental work by selling the patent to a large corporation. Once he has formulated the basic idea, the inventor's job is done, and the developer can design the products and production processes. The developer does not take much technical risk because the company can recognize a feasible idea. The developer's major risk is the commercial risk of manufacturing and selling a new product at a profitable price. A large company, in fact, must take over the patent, for a bank or other financial institution is unlikely to invest in the development of a new product.

Little systematic empirical work has been done to test this model, particularly in relation to pharmaceutical research. The discussion of pharmaceutical research frequently cites the accidental discovery of penicillin by Fleming to make the point that the important innovations in this industry have also come from individuals and small laboratories. But while the accidental nature of this discovery is mentioned, little use is made of it.

The model in fact does not apply to pharmaceutical research. Pharmaceutical research has not become bureaucratic. Few administrative layers intervene between the directors of laboratories and the highest policy-making level, and laboratories usually have considerable independence. Management, recognizing that research scientists have to be given considerable independence, intervenes minimally, perhaps only to replace a director who has obviously failed. Within the laboratory the discovery research is carried on by independent small teams of chemists and pharmacologists, each of which has a mandate to seek a certain kind of drug. They periodically report their progress to the director, who does not attempt to provide detailed direction.

Also contrary to the model, the firms take great risks. Some have been disappointed after large funds have been spent on research in particular fields over long periods. This has been especially true in recent years, when successfully marketed products have been few. The high profits which firms have continued to earn from previous innovations have concealed but not eliminated the risks.

The model is also incorrect in its characterization of discovery as applied to the drug industry. In this industry products are usually discovered after systematic effort and much trial and error rather than by an insightful individual. In contrast to the model which sees the inventor as combining in his own head the results of basic research in different disciplines, drug discoveries require the cooperation of many different specialists. Moreover, a team usually will have tried many compounds and will not be certain of its success until a late stage of the research. At the time they are made, the critical observations may not appear to be any more significant than other observations. Only the process of trial and error finally reveals which compound possesses the desired properties. The frequent attribution of a discovery to an individual reflects the erroneous standard assumption that one person was responsible for discovering a key to the problem, rather than the usual case in which an accumulation of information leads to a discovery.

Nor is the distinction between the discovery and the developmental stages very useful in describing pharmaceutical research, for the two stages are not clearly separate. The interest and involvement of the chemists who synthesize a compound do not end with its discovery. At any time in its life, a drug may be returned to the chemist's laboratory for additional molecular modification in an attempt to remove unwanted effects or to enhance efficacy. So the chemists and the associated pharmacologists keep a close watch over compounds late into clinical testing. They observe the toxicology testing, even though it is not their primary responsibility, in order to learn more about the toxic as well as the therapeutic effects of a given chemical structure. The chemists and pharmacologists also assist in planning the clinical tests and in designing the dosage forms and the manufacturing processes. The converse is also true: from their discussions with the discovery team, the development scientists learn what to look for in their tests.

Drug companies do not purchase lead compounds from academic laboratories or from other companies' laboratories because pharmacological theory provides little guidance for identifying promising compounds. Moreover, few compounds demonstrating desirable biological activity eventually become safe, effective drugs which physicians can use routinely. Even in the same firm, clinicians who are responsible for the human tests behave like an internal FDA, skeptical of the claims of chemists and pharmacologists, especially in relatively undeveloped therapeutic fields in which reliable animal tests are difficult to devise. But because they are in the same laboratory as the discovery team and in frequent communication with them, they may be willing to test molecular modifications of compounds which have failed the tests in their original forms. Clinicians in other firms will be even more severe in their judgments of compounds offered to them for sale.

The uncertainty concerning the safety of a drug until late in its clinical testing, the resulting disagreement between physicians who test it clinically and chemists and pharmacologists who develop it, and the interdependence of the different parts of the research program make the negotiation of sales of patent rights very difficult. R. H. Coase has said that under these conditions firms prefer to do their own work rather than purchase finished products: firms will not purchase when costs of negotiation exceed the costs of supervision.[15] Thus most drugs are discovered by the firms which introduce them. Between 1960 and 1970, 75 percent of the new single entities were discovered by the same firms which manufactured them.[16] Most of the other new single entities were discovered and developed by foreign-based companies whose marketing and distribution organizations in this country were inadequate and which therefore licensed the new drug to a large U.S.-based firm. The developmental research for these drugs was essentially complete before the transfer.

The different activities of pharmaceutical laboratories require the employment of specialists from many different disciplines. List 3-1 shows that Pfizer's research laboratories employ nine different classes of specialists, which are further broken down into thirty-five subspecialties. The table reveals interesting differences in the degree of specialization between chemists and biologists. The chemists are broken down into only two broad subspecialties: chemotherapy

List 3-1
Types of Professional Specialists
Employed in Pfizer Laboratories, 1972

1. Medicinal Chemists
   a. Chemotherapy (antibiotics or other anti-infective agents)
   b. Noninfectious diseases
2. Research Biologists
   a. Psychopharmacologists
      1) Behavioral psychologists
      2) CNS biochemists
      3) Neurophysiologists
   b. Cardiopulmonary pharmacologists (o physiologists)
      1) Cardiovascular pharmacologists
      2) Bronchopulmonary pharmacologists
   c. Gastrointestinal pharmacologists
   d. Biochemists, biochemical pharmacologists
      1) Intermediary metabolism specialists
      2) Lipids specialists
      3) Enzymologists
      4) Fermentation specialists
   e. Immunologists
   f. Microbiologists
      1) Bacteriologists
      2) Parasitologists
      3) Virologists
   g. Specialists in drug metabolism
   h. Toxicologists
      1) Teratologists
      2) Genetic toxicologists
      3) Hematologists
   i. Pathologists
3. Pharmaceutical chemists, pharmacists
   a. Physical pharmacists
   b. Formulation development—solid forms specialists
   c. Formulation development—liquid forms specialists
   d. Pharmacists (clinical supplies)
4. Analytical chemists
5. Process chemists
6. Clinical researchers
   a. Medical monitors (M.D.'s)
   b. Statisticians
   c. Data processors
   d. FDA liaisons
7. Data coordinators
8. Technical literature specialists
   a. Librarians
   b. Literature retrieval/search specialists
9. Research administrators (research planning, budgeting)

Source: Pfizer, Inc.

and noninfectious diseases. Apparently chemists can shift around easily with little loss of skill from one disease area to another within the two broad areas. Their skills consist of a familiarity with widely applicable techniques of analysis and synthesis rather than information pertaining to particular chemical substances, individual classes of bacteria, or actions of compounds which were developed in the past. The numerous subspecialties of research biologists, by contrast, indicate that they are much less easily moved around between different disease areas. The commitment by a company to investigate a therapeutic field signifies the commitment to develop a group of biologists with the required knowledge of the field. The large number of subspecialties also confirms the characterization of biological research as largely empirical. Biologists apparently specialize very narrowly in order to be able to absorb a significant body of literature. This is one of the sources of the advantages of large scale in pharmaceutical research.

THE COSTS AND TIME REQUIRED FOR R & D

Another element in the importance of the industry as a source of new drugs and more particularly of the large firm is the large investment in R & D required to discover and develop a basic new agent. True, the federal government has the financial resources and has appropriated funds for drug research, but most of the drug research funded by the federal government has been confined to the cancer field. No large research projects directed to discovering drugs in other areas have been supported by the government.

Currently the costs of drug research are so large, as we shall see, that they exclude small firms from engaging in R & D on a sufficiently large scale to expect success. The cost of R & D per new drug has reached a level of $24 million; this estimate includes the costs of research on drugs which do not reach the market. Not all of the funds are invested at one time, since the R & D period is long. But the firm has to have sufficient financial resources to invest in several projects in order to be able to expect that one of them will result in a new drug.

We must also consider the effect of the expected sales per drug on the inclination and the ability of firms to engage in drug research. However, a full discussion is postponed until chapter 6, where we discuss the consequences of innovational competition. Here we will note some of the effects of the uncertainty of drug research on incentives to undertake such research. The sales of most drugs are too small to result in profits that pay for the research which led up to them; were it not for the relatively few exceptionally large-selling drugs, the investment in R & D by the industry would yield a loss. Much of the investment by individual firms does not result even in technical success, as we have seen, to say nothing of financial success. Under these conditions firms which have no large accumulation of retained earnings and which have no current large revenues against which to charge the costs of research are unlikely to contemplate undertaking R & D directed at the discovery and development of new drugs (i.e., basic new agents, as opposed to new dosage forms or new combination drugs, the components of which are established drugs.) The large firm which can charge the costs of R & D as current expenses against income is investing after taxes approximately half of the amount actually spent on R & D. This opportunity for deducting the cost of R & D from income and thus reducing the after-tax cost is not open to a new entrant not already established in some other industry. Nor is the securities market likely to be a good source for funds for R & D, given the uncertainty of pharmaceutical research. Unlike investment in plant and equipment, investment in R & D does not result in physical collateral which can be sold in the event that the investment does not result in additional revenue. The importance of the availability of internally generated funds is emphasized by the consideration that the investment in R & D is tied up for a long time. The research period itself is long, and the income which is produced by a successful drug does not become available immediately after the completion of the research.

We will estimate the average cost of a new drug for the industry as a whole. The average, it should be noted, is computed as a weighted average, with the large firms given a greater weight than the smaller ones. We compute the average cost of R & D per new single chemical entity (NCE), using industrial aggregates. Since large firms contribute most of the total R & D expenditures and discover most of the NCE's, the average reflects their experience more heavily than that of small firms.

In order to limit the list of drugs to important discoveries, we eliminated certain minor items from Paul de Haen's list of NCE's.[17] The amended list also excludes drugs discovered and developed by companies which are not members of PMA. The reason for the exclusion is that the estimate of the cost of R & D is based on PMA's estimate of R & D expenditures, which is limited to those of its members.

The estimation of the current cost of R & D requires certain assumptions. Specifically we shall assume that the discovery and development of a new drug in the future will require as much effort as was required for the drugs introduced in the recent past, which for the purpose of the estimate is represented by the period 1966–72.

As we have indicated, PMA estimates of R & D expenditures are the measure of research effort. These estimates appropriately include total world expenditures of U.S.-based member companies, but they include only expenditures in the U.S. of foreign-based member companies; expenditures in their home countries or elsewhere thus are not included. Since the NCE's of these foreign-based companies are included in the number, the estimate of the average total R & D cost per NCE will be understated.

The R & D period for an NCE is estimated to be ten years. This estimate is based on previous ones made by Dr. Lewis Sarett and by Mr. Harold Clymer. According to Dr. Sarett, the time required to develop a product after it completes the discovery stage (in the period of 1968–72) is 5½ to 8 years, exclusive of the average two-year period which he estimates is required for a company to obtain FDA approval. The total development period thus is 7½ to 10 years. Dr. Sarett does not estimate the length of the discovery period; nor has anyone else in the industry done so explicitly, probably because the beginning of research directed to a particular compound is difficult to identify. The exploratory research in a disease area that eventually leads to a drug may have begun many years before identification of the compound which leads directly to the final drug, and over the years many compounds which turn out to be false leads may have been synthesized.[18]

Harold Clymer estimated the development period inclusive of FDA approval to be 5 to 7 years.[19] Clymer's estimate of the average time required for development and regulatory approval agrees with that of Drs. Lasagna and Wardell. They found that the mean time from IND submission to NDA approval for NCE's approved in 1973 was 6.6 years (table 3-2). Clymer's estimate of the entire R & D period is 10 years, which implies a discovery research period of 3 to 5 years. If we were to add this estimate to Sarett's more recent estimate of the development research period of 7½ to 10 years, the total R & D period

TABLE 3-2
NDA's Approved for NCE's by Fifteen Companies, by Year
of Approval, and Mean Number of Years Required for
Development and Approval

	Number of NDA's approved	Mean Number of Years for Development and Approval
1963	0	
1964	0	
1965	0	
1966	3	2.7
1967	2	3.0
1968	2	4.0
1969	2	3.0
1970	5	5.0
1971	3	5.7
1972	5	5.2
1973	5	6.6

Source: See table 3-1.

would be estimated at 10½ to 15 years. Our assumption that the entire R & D period lasts ten years is less than the lower limit of the range derived from the Sarett and Clymer estimates and thus is conservative.

We will estimate the R & D cost per NCE in 1973. Since we have estimated the research period to be ten years, we are estimating the cost of R & D for a ten-year period represented by 1973. We will assume that the effort required to discover and develop a drug, the research for which is being done in 1973, is the same as that required for drugs introduced in the period 1966–72. The research period for the drugs appearing in 1966 was 1956–66, of which 1961 is the middle year. Similar reasoning for each of the other years of the period 1966–72 results in the selection of the years 1961–67 as the period on which we base the estimate of R & D cost. The average annual expenditures during these years, according to PMA, was $281.4 million.

To obtain the current cost of R & D per NCE, we must adjust this figure for the increase in prices since 1961–67. For this purpose we use 1964, the middle year of this period, as the point of reference, and we estimate that the change in the cost of R & D due to price changes between 1964 and 1973 was 48 percent.[20] During the 1960s the FDA increased its demands for evidence of efficacy and safety, resulting in higher costs of development, as Clymer and Sarett show. We should therefore include an estimate of the additional cost of R & D due to increasing stringency in these regulatory demands. But as it is difficult to estimate this cost increase, we will deliberately bias the estimated increase on the low side by making no correction for the increase due to the greater demands of the FDA for evidence of efficacy and safety. The total current cost of industry research which would result in the same average number of NCE's, new combinations, and new dosage forms per year as appeared in 1966–1972 would equal 148 percent of $281.4 million, or $416.5 million.

We must now estimate the part of this R & D total that is allocable only to NCE's. Since the industry's discovery effort is devoted wholly to the search for NCE's, its cost must be allocated entirely to these drugs. Our estimate of discovery research's share of total R & D cost is 50 percent,[21] yielding an estimated annual cost of a contemporary discovery research program of the same size as that which resulted in the NCE's discovered in 1966–72 to be equal to 50 percent of $416.5 million, or $208.2 million. Since the average number of NCE's produced each year by the industry was 12.3, the average discovery cost per NCE would be $16.9 million in 1973.

Developmental, as opposed to discovery, costs of R & D must be distributed between NCE's and other new products, including combination and dosage forms.[22] The resulting estimate of the developmental cost adds $7.5 million to each NCE, for a total of $24.4 million. Although a company's total R & D cost per NCE before taxes is $24.4 million, a company in fact invests only the after-tax costs, which is approximately half or $12.2 million.[23]

THE INCREASE IN COST OF R & D

According to Martin Baily and Sam Peltzman, the increase in the regulatory requirements of the FDA for drug approval following the 1962 drug amendments, increased the cost of R & D per NCE.[24] This would have the effect of reducing the expected rate of return from investments in R & D and therefore the level of investment.

We will estimate the cost of R & D per NCE in 1960. The estimate is based on the number of new single entities appearing during the years 1955–58. Over this period the average annual number of new single entities was 36.5. We group derivatives with the original products and, since the R & D period was much shorter than it is now, we assume it to have been five years. Hence the period in which the research was done for the products emerging in 1955–58 can be estimated from the average expenditures per year in 1952–55, which was $74.8 million. Following the same procedure as in our previous estimate, we are using the middle years of the research periods resulting in the drugs introduced in the period 1955–58. Since this was a period of price stability, it is reasonable to suppose that in 1960 it cost no more to do the required R & D for an NCE than it did in 1952–55. As before, we estimate that discovery research accounted for 50 percent of total R & D costs, and all of this amount is assigned to NCE's. The discovery cost per NCE was thus $37.4 million divided by 36.5 NCE's, or $1.02 million per NCE.

The cost of developing an NCE was $285,000. To arrive at this estimate, we distributed total developmental expenditures (estimated at 50 percent of total R & D expenditures) among NCE's, new combination drugs, and new dosage forms as described for the 1973 estimate. We added this amount to the discovery cost to obtain a total R & D cost per NCE of $1.30 million before taxes. We then distributed the after-tax cost, $.65 million, equally over the R & D period of five years.[25] (Thus, $.13 million was the annual cost of R & D for an NCE.) The increase in prices of goods and services used by research laboratories between 1960 and 1973 was about 68 percent.[26] Thus, the increase in costs of R & D due to sources other than price increases is 1,015 percent. Not all of this increase can be attributed to greater severity of the regulatory requirements. Some of it is the result of the increased difficulty of discovering and developing new drugs in therapeutic fields where many good drugs exist, and some is due to the fact that more effort and resources are currently being devoted to the discovery of drugs for diseases about which relatively little is known and which are intrinsically more difficult to deal with, such as arthritis and diseases of the cardiovascular system.

Other studies also indicate large increases in the cost of R & D per NCE. Thus, Dr. Sarett estimates that the development cost of a new drug (as opposed to discovery research) rose from $1.2 million in 1962 to $11.5 million in 1973.[27]

Developmental research only begins when the laboratory has decided, on the basis of animal tests, that a compound is sufficiently promising to warrant clinical tests in humans. Our own estimate of the share of total R & D costs devoted to development—an estimate which is based on industry sources—is 50 percent. The closeness of Dr. Sarett's estimate of developmental costs per NCE in 1972 to our own provides some assurance of the validity of these estimates and so thus also supports the conclusion that the costs have increased greatly.

Other studies by Baily and by Peltzman provide estimates of the effect of increased regulatory stringency on R & D costs. Baily estimates that the drug amendments increased the cost of R & D required for a given number of new single entities by 136 percent. Peltzman estimates that they doubled the cost.

As a consequence, the industry has not been able to maintain its pre-1962 rate of innovation, despite a large increase in spending. The rate of increase in the cost of producing innovations has outstripped the rate of increase in spending. Another consequence of the increase in cost has been, as we will see in chapter 7, a sharp reduction in the expected rate of return from R & D investment. If this expected rate of return declines still further, we can anticipate that investment in R & D will decline and the rate of drug innovation fall even more.[28]

CONCLUSIONS

Industrial laboratories have systematized and accelerated the process of discovery and of evaluation of new drugs. They have transformed drug research from a casual and erratic search to a large-scale, intensive, and sustained pursuit.

The methods are basically the same as those used in the research which led up to the major discoveries of the 1940s. Industrial laboratories still depend largely on empirical leads, synthesis, molecular modification, animal screening, and clinical tests. But the organization of multidisciplinary teams within laboratories permits them to exchange information developed within different disciplines, to use and to test numerous leads, and to systematically investigate large numbers of related groups of compounds.

The large industrial laboratory benefits from the integration of discovery and development stages of pharmaceutical research. A compound may be developed into a marketable drug even after it has failed animal toxicology or clinical trials. The chemist in the discovery team may be able to further modify the compound so that it does pass the tests. Such modifications are made much more difficult by the physical separation of discovery from developmental research. Members of the discovery team are more likely to maintain their interest in a compound after it has failed certain tests when they are part of the same laboratory which conducts these tests and when they can communicate easily with the scientists conducting the further tests than when the discovery and development efforts are physically separated. Similarly the physicians in charge of clinical trials are more willing to test subsequent modifications of compounds which have failed earlier tests when they have been in regular communication with members of the discovery team. This willingness to postpone final judgment on a class of compounds is important in drug research, where predictions of the results of clinical trials based on animal tests are uncertain, the early clinical tests may not reveal effects of low incidence, and apparently minor modifications of compounds may result in significant therapeutic improvements. The separation of discovery research from developmental research thus is likely to result in the loss of potentially valuable drugs.

Economies of scale in pharmaceutical research can be expected to result from the employment by industrial laboratories of many different kinds of specialists, especially in the biological sciences. We have also seen that research tends to be limited to large firms by the high costs of research per new chemical entity. The estimate of this cost for 1973 is $24.4 million. A firm must have large sales or other sources of revenue to finance such expenditures. The expenditures are not concentrated in a single year but are spread over an estimated period of ten years. On the other hand, a firm must carry on research in several areas to maintain the necessary employment of specialists in different fields and to have some reasonable probability of success. Few drugs are successfully marketed from the thousands of compounds tested. The uncertainty contributes to the problem of outside financing of research. Firms depend, therefore, on retained earnings to finance their research.

These conditions have encouraged the concentration of pharmaceutical research in larger industrial laboratories. That this is the case is confirmed by the histories of important nonindustrial drug discoveries, which resulted from unusually large financing by foundations and other sources. The research, moreover, benefited from sustained leadership, industrial methods of research, and rapid and close communication between scientists in different laboratories. The laboratories were also unusual in their dedication to the pursuit of specific drugs rather than in exploratory research. The research which led to the drug discoveries by nonindustrial laboratories was not representative of the research usually done in such laboratories.

The next chapter shows that industrial laboratories account for a large majority of drugs discovered and that this share has been increasing; the subsequent chapter tests the hypothesis that large firms enjoy economies of scale in pharmaceutical research. Another closely related question also will be investigated: Does research effort increase more than proportionally with firm size among pharmaceutical firms? The argument that society gains from large firm size in this industry depends not only on the demonstration of economies of scale but also on whether such firms devote relatively more resources to R & D than do smaller firms. Finally, we shall examine the relationship between size of firm and the number of innovations. If there are economies of scale in R & D and if large firms devote more resources to R & D than small firms, then large firms should produce relatively more new drugs.

CHAPTER 4

THE IMPORTANCE
OF INDUSTRIAL SOURCES
OF NEW DRUGS

INTRODUCTION

A public policy designed to encourage the discovery and development of new drugs must be based on a consideration of the likely sources of their discovery. The description of pharmaceutical R & D in the preceding chapter suggested that industrial laboratories would be the primary source of new drugs. Illustrations of both industrial and academic drug discoveries pointed in the same direction. The argument, however, remains incomplete without an analysis of sources of a comprehensive list of drug discoveries, for the few descriptions presented earlier are open to the criticism that they are selected. An estimate of the likely sources thus can only come from knowledge of the sources of past discoveries. In the Kefauver hearings the question was asked more than once how large a share of all drug discoveries came from the pharmaceutical industry. The industry claimed credit for having discovered most drugs. Critics maintained that most of the drugs discovered by the industry were in fact derived from discoveries which had been made by academic and other nonindustrial scientists. In other words, the industry and the critics disagreed about the relative importance of different discoveries rather than about the origins of the discoveries.[1]

In the following discussion there are four estimates of the industry's share of drug discoveries. Jerome Schnee's estimate is based on one selection of important discoveries. A second estimate is based on another selection of important drugs, made in 1972 by Dr. Marvin Seife, Office of Scientific Evaluation, Bureau of Drugs, FDA. The third estimate is based on a more recent FDA list. A fourth estimate is based on our own study. Since the primary question is the importance of the industrial sources of new drugs for the future, what follows looks at changes in the industry's share of discoveries over time, with a view toward determining the historical trend. In addition, we will discuss the results of a

TABLE 4-1
Percentage of New Chemical Entities
Discovered and Introduced by the
Pharmaceutical Industry 1950–59, 1960–69,
and 1950–69

	Periods in which Drugs Were Introduced		
	1950–59	1960–69	1950–69
Industry	86	91	88
Other	14	9	12
Total	100	100	100

Source: List of NCE's, selected from Paul de
Haen, *New Product Survey* and *Nonproprietary
Name Index*.
Note: See chapter 5 for basis of selection.
Discoveries attributed on basis of the *Merck
Index* and Paul de Haen *Nonproprietary Name
Index*. Codiscoverers are each given half credit;
where the source of discovery could not be
determined, it was assigned to other.

survey of private nonprofit and industrial laboratories concerning the nature of
their drug research and will also consider the work at the National Institutes of
Health.

THE PRESENT STUDY'S ESTIMATES

In order to limit the list to important discoveries, we eliminated certain minor
items from Paul de Haen's list of NCE's. The *Merck Index* and the de Haen *New
Product Survey* and *Nonproprietary Name Index* were used to identify the
source of each NCE classified as "industrial" or "other."

The estimates of the present study are reported in table 4-1. They show that
in the 1960s, the drug industry was the most important source of drug discoveries,
accounting for 91 percent of the total number of new drugs introduced. The
industry's share was slightly smaller in the 1950s: over the years the industry has
become an increasingly important source of new drugs.

Both foreign and domestic discoveries are included in the list of discoveries
tabulated. Companies based in the United States accounted for 49 percent of all
drugs introduced in the United States in 1950–59 and 54 percent in 1960–69,
but the share of all discoveries accounted for by U.S. laboratories is larger than
these percentages indicate. Although U.S. companies conduct some research
abroad, most of their research is done in the United States. The share of new
drugs accounted for by the discoveries of foreign laboratories is smaller than the
share of introductions by foreign-based companies (37 percent of all NCE's in

both periods). This is not surprising, since much of the research of Hoffmann-LaRoche, Ciba-Geigy, and Burroughs-Wellcome is conducted within the United States. Schnee provides an estimate of the share of all new drug introductions in the United States that are based on discoveries in foreign laboratories as distinguished from foreign companies. His estimate will be taken up later on.

It must be pointed out that the attention given in the Kefauver hearings to the foreign share of all discoveries had its origins in a misunderstanding of the relation between the number of discoveries and the degree of patent protection in different countries. The conclusion reached in the hearings that strong patent protection did not encourage discovery was based on the fact that a large number of drugs were discovered in Western Europe, especially in Switzerland, where inventions were less generously protected by patents than in the United States. But U.S. patents protect these products of foreign-based companies sold in the United States as much as they do the products of domestic companies, and the United States is by far the largest single national market for drugs.

Similar conclusions come from an appraisal of the impact of foreign regulation of prices on drug R & D. British companies find it worthwhile to spend large sums on R & D despite the low prices paid by the National Health Service in the United Kingdom, because they have significant sales in other countries where prices are higher; in fact, of the four largest firms, three—and some others—made a major portion of their sales outside the United Kingdom. Table 4-2 shows foreign pharmaceutical sales as part of the world sales of major British companies in 1968–69. The United Kingdom accounted for less than half of the pharmaceutical sales of Glaxo and Beecham. Wellcome's United Kingdom share was only slightly larger than half. ICI is the single exception to the general pattern, with U.K. sales accounting for 82 percent of its world sales.

TABLE 4-2
Foreign and Domestic Sales of Selected
U.K.–Based Pharmaceutical Manufacturers,
1968–69

Company	Sales (£ millions)		Percent Distribution	
	U.K.	World	U.K.	Other
Glaxo	53.8	112.0	48	52
Wellcome	36.1	63.7	57	43
ICI	25.0	30.4	82	18
Beecham	21.6	62.8	34	66

Source: Estimates based on M. H. Cooper and A. J. Culyer, *The Pharmaceutical Industry* (London: Economists Advisory Group and Dun and Bradstreet, Ltd., 1973), p. 14.

The policies of other governments toward the drug industry can be seen as restricting returns to R & D. As a result, foreign R & D would decline were it not for the returns available in the United States. This may seem to impose an unduly large share of the costs of R & D on U.S. consumers and taxpayers. The remedy, however, is not to reduce the profitability of research. In fact, as we shall see, the current expected rate of return on investment in R & D is already well below the level required to attract continued investment. If this were generally known, other governments might be more cautious in adopting policies which tend to reduce the industry's investment in R & D, even though the United States currently is bearing more than its due share of total R & D costs.

SCHNEE'S ESTIMATES

Schnee undertook separate studies of the sources of important new drugs in two periods: 1938–1962 (which was further broken down into two subperiods, 1935–1949 and 1950–1962) and 1963–1970. His selection of drug discoveries for the period before 1963 was obtained from a study of significant discoveries by the Commission on the Cost of Medical Care of the American Medical Association.[2] In 1963 the Commission had asked 400 physicians and pharmacologists to select the most important advances from a preselected list of eighty-nine drugs introduced after 1934. His selection of important drug introductions in the 1963–1970 period was largely based on a survey by *The Medical Letter* of 170 physicians at medical schools.[3]

Schnee defined discovery as the first identification of a drug's biological activity. He located the discoverers of two-thirds of the drugs introduced between 1935 and 1962 from a study of medical journal articles; the others were identified on the basis of reports in secondary sources, which he listed. De Haen's *New Product Survey* and *Nonproprietary Name Index* identified the sources of drugs introduced after 1962. Schnee checked the validity of de Haen's attributions by an independent investigation of medical journal articles and found only one minor discrepancy.

Schnee's results show that the drug industry has consistently been the major source of new drug discoveries (table 4-3). Even in the first period, when nonindustrial discoveries were numerous, industry accounted for more than half of all significant discoveries. In the second period, 1950–1962, the industry accounted for 69 percent of all significant discoveries, and in 1963–1970, the industry's share of important discoveries rose to 82 percent.

Strictly speaking, the judgment of the industry's importance should be based on a comparison of its share of discoveries with that of universities, hospitals, and research institutions, rather than on a comparison of its share of all introductions with the remainder, which includes the unassigned "other" category. This category includes previously known drugs, those whose discoverers are difficult to identify, and those discovered by a domestic company which was

TABLE 4-3
Schnee's Distribution of Drug Discoveries, 1935–70

Source	1935–49	1950–62	1963–70
Industry	52	69	82
Universities, hospitals, or research institutions	34	16	9
Other	14	15	9
Total	100	100	100

Source: Based on Jerome Schnee, "The Changing Pattern of Pharmaceutical Innovation and Discovery," mimeographed (New York: Columbia University, Graduate School of Business, 1973).

Note: In Schnee's table the classes include "innovator and discoverer" and "foreign firm" as well as "universities, hospitals, or research institutions" and "other." We have grouped "innovator and discoverer" and "foreign firm" under "industry." "Other" includes a few cases where the discoverer was a domestic company which was not the innovator.

not the innovator. (Schnee's "other" includes foreign firms which were the discoverers but not the innovators; these have been assigned to "industry" in table 4-3). Thus by focusing on that share of *all* introductions which are represented by industry's discoveries, we tend to understate industry's true importance.

Schnee also measured the industry's share of discoveries weighted by their medical importance as evaluated by the ratings of physicians responding to the AMA survey for the period 1935–1962 (table 4-4). Hence the industry's share of medically weighted innovations in the early period also represents a majority.[4]

Schnee also estimated the distribution of innovations weighted by economic importance as measured by sales of all three periods (table 4-5). The table reveals a marked increase in the industry's share of economically weighted discoveries

TABLE 4-4
Schnee's Distribution of Drug
Discoveries, Weighted by Medical
Importance, 1935–62

Industry	52
Universities, hospitals, and research institutions	37
Other	11
All sources	100

Source: See table 4-3.
Note: See note to table 4-3 and text.

TABLE 4-5
Schnee's Distribution of Drug Discoveries,
Weighted by Sales, 1935–70

	Percent Distribution		
	1935–49	1950–62	1963–70
Industry	33	82	85
Universities, hospitals, and research institutions	66	8	8
Other	1	10	7
Total	100	100	100

Source: See table 4-3.
Note: See note to table 4-3.

between 1935–1949 and 1960–1962. In the 1960s the percentage was about the same as in the previous period. Thus, universities, hospitals, and research institutions discovered the majority of economically weighted drugs introduced in the 1935–1949 period, but their importance declined sharply in the succeeding period and has remained low since. The discrepancy between Schnee's results and the results of this study reflects different lists of "important" drugs, difference in periods, and Schnee's inclusion in the "other" category of some discoveries by firms other than the innovator.

Schnee's results show a trend toward the growing importance of the industry as a source of new drugs. An analysis based on Seife's selection of important drug innovations also corroborates the industry's major role in the discovery and development of significant compounds.

ESTIMATES BASED ON SEIFE SELECTION AND RECENT FDA LIST

Dr. Marvin Seife selected, from among all of the new drugs introduced in the 1960–1969 period, those that he considered to be the most important therapeutic advances. In his judgment, 109 important new drugs came into the market.[5]

When the *Merck Index* and the *Nonproprietary Name Index* are used to identify the discoverer, Seife's list produces an estimate of the industry's share of important discoveries close to the estimates based on the two other lists. As table 4-6 reports, 86 percent of the drugs on the Seife list were discovered in industry laboratories.

In August 1974, in testimony before the Kennedy Subcommittee, FDA Commissioner Schmidt presented a list of the drugs which represented important gains in medicine in the judgment of the FDA. An analysis of this list is presented in table 4-7. According to the FDA list, the pharmaceutical industry accounted for more than two-thirds of the important discoveries in 1950–1962 and for more than four-fifths of those in the period 1963–1970.

TABLE 4-6
Sources of Discoveries of Important New
Drugs Introduced in 1960–69, Selected
by Seife

Source	Percent Distribution
Industry	86
Other	14
Total	100

Source: "Selection of Drugs by Dr. Marvin
A. Seife of the Office of Scientific Evaluation,
Bureau of Drugs, Food and Drug Administration," reported in William McVicker, "New
Drug Development Study," mimeographed
(Washington, D.C.: Food and Drug Administration, 1972).
Note: Attributions according to the *Merck
Index* and Paul de Haen, *Nonproprietary Name
Index.* Where source could not be determined,
drug was assigned to "other." Codiscoverers are
each given half credit.

Both the Seife and the FDA studies conclude that the pharmaceutical industry discovered the majority of all new drugs discovered and that the contribution of the industry increased in importance in recent years. Nevertheless, though these findings are not entirely new, many of those in policymaking positions still do not believe that the industry is society's principal instrument for the dis-

TABLE 4-7
Percentage Distribution of Discoveries of
Important New Drugs Introduced in 1950–62
and 1963–70, Selected by FDA

Source	1950–62	1963–70
Industry	69	82
Other	31	18
Total	100	100

Source: Commissioner Schmidt's statement
to the Subcommittee on Health of the Senate
Committee on Labor and Public Welfare,
August 16, 1974, appearing in August 26,
1974, FDC Reports. Discoveries assigned by
Paul de Haen, *Nonproprietary Name Index,* and
the *Merck Index.*
Note: The sources of five of the eighty-one
drugs introduced in the period 1950–62 could
not be identified. They were counted as nonindustry discoveries. The total number of important gains in 1963–1970 was forty-three.
Codiscoverers are each given half credit.

covery and development of new drugs. In fact, the literature on drug innovations is confused on the importance of industrial sources.

For example, a recent report of the President's Science Advisory Committee states that "external sources [such as universities, hospitals, and research institutes] have played a major role in the technological program of the ethical pharmaceutical industry in the United States.[6] The committee cites the Schnee study, and the critical word in the quotation is "external." The report obviously interprets "external" as defining discoveries made by laboratories external to the industry. But in the original study "external" defines any source other than the innovator, including other firms as well as universities, hospitals, and research institutes. This distinction is important in the analysis for 1935–1949, when nonindustry sources allegedly accounted for the majority of drug discoveries. A reanalysis of Schnee's data for these years shows that non-industry sources accounted for 46 percent (rather than 62 percent) and industry sources for 54 percent of all drug discoveries. A similar analysis for 1950–1962 shows that non-industry sources accounted for 38 percent for those years.

A SURVEY OF ACADEMIC LABORATORIES

Because a large organization with large resources is required to conduct effective pharmaceutical research, such research is unlikely to be conducted in nonprofit and university laboratories. An informal survey which we conducted of nonprofit laboratories engaged in research in the life sciences obtained seventeen responses; sixteen of the respondents claimed to be engaged in research on drugs; thirteen of them reported that they performed animal tests of drugs; and thirteen stated that they were engaged in clinical testing. On the other hand, only five reported that they were attempting to discover new drugs. Most of the laboratories were small: ten of the seventeen employed fewer than twenty scientists, and only two of the laboratories employed twenty or more chemists. The largest laboratories were engaged in cancer research. Roswell Park Memorial Institute was the largest laboratory to respond to the questionnaire. This laboratory employs 300 scientists, 150 of whom are chemists. Its animal facilities contained 100,000 mice. The reason for the large number of scientists and the apparently lavish facilities is that the institute's work is in the field of cancer research, which currently is well financed and is the focus of a national campaign.

Four of the laboratories reported having discovered drugs. Those listed were all anticancer agents, except for the oral contraceptive pill listed as discovered by the Worcester Foundation. In general, then, we can conclude that academic and other nonprofit laboratories are unlikely to be an important source of new drugs for the treatment of diseases other than cancer.

THE NATIONAL INSTITUTES OF HEALTH

The National Institutes of Health have the required resources to undertake drug research, and such research is performed at the NIH, particularly in the area of cancer drugs. Their research is, however, limited primarily to basic biological research and to testing the effects of drugs. For the most part, the NIH leaves the synthesis of drugs to the industry.[7] Over 95 percent of the compounds which have been studied by the NIH have come from the pharmaceutical industry. Very few compounds come from nonindustry grantees of the NIH.

The laboratories of the National Heart Institute have conducted investigations into the interaction of drugs with hormonal and metabolic processes of the body; the penetration of drugs into biological membranes; the distribution of drugs in body tissues; the compounds resulting from the metabolism of drugs by the body, and the mechanisms which are involved in the inactivation of drugs.[8] The National Heart Institute laboratories cooperate with the pharmaceutical firms, which have placed their store of chemical compounds at the disposal of the institute. The firms have also made available to the institute their organic chemists. The collaboration has resulted in new enzyme inhibitors, antimetabolites, and pharmacological agents.[9] In particular, the institute carries on studies of the efficacy of available drugs, as for example in the cooperative coronary drug study. This study, which was scheduled to terminate in 1974, was budgeted for $43 million and was intended to examine the effects of available drugs.[10]

The NIH has carried on research directed at the development of vaccines for influenza, venereal disease, and hepatitis, and it has contracted research for the investigation of cancer drugs and carried out screening for anticancer in house. However, most of the work that is carried on at the institute itself appears to have consisted of investigations of drugs which are discovered elsewhere.

Recent testimony of the NIH before the Committee On Appropriations of the House of Representatives indicates that aside from efforts to develop vaccines and to find anticancer agents, the institute was not significantly involved in efforts to identify new drugs.[11]

CONCLUSIONS

The discussion of the descriptions of pharmaceutical research in the preceding chapters concluded that the industrial laboratories are likely to be the primary source of drug discoveries. We saw there that these laboratories have systematized drug research and have mobilized and organized the necessary resources. This chapter confirms our expectation. The analysis of the discoveries by sources indicates that the pharmaceutical industry has been the major source by far and that its importance has increased since the 1940s. The same conclusions are reached regardless of which list of important discoveries is used.

We can expect the drug industry to continue to be the major source of new drugs. Academic laboratories are unlikely to devote themselves in a routine and systematic manner to drug discovery. Except under unusual circumstances such laboratories have neither the required interest in drug discovery nor the required resources. The NIH has the resources, but it has not used them systematically to search for new drugs except in the area of cancer. The fact that the NIH has not done so appears to reflect the recognition that to undertake such research effectively requires an organization of skills which is difficult to develop and that the industry's laboratories have achieved the necessary expertise and organization.

Firms in the industry, however, will have to invest in R & D in order to supply new drugs. As we have noted, the rate of innovation has declined since the late 1950s, owing to both the increased difficulty of drug discovery and increased FDA regulatory stringency. The industry may not again equal the rate of innovation achieved in the 1950s even if it should greatly increase its expenditures in order to increase the rate of innovation above the present level. The increases of recent years appear to have done little more than offset the effect of increases in the prices of research inputs; they probably have not offset the effects of increased regulatory demands, to say nothing of the increase in the intrinsic difficulty of discovery. The firms are unlikely to raise their expenditures substantially unless the expected rate of return from such investment is at least equal to that from other investments. We will return to this question in chapter 7. The next chapter discusses size of firm in relation to research.

CHAPTER 5

RESEARCH ACTIVITY
AND SIZE OF FIRM

INTRODUCTION

Schumpeter asserted that since modern industrial research requires large re-sources,[1] large firms would do proportionally more research than small ones and so produce proportionally more innovations. Other writers suggest three additional reasons for expecting large firms to be more innovative relative to their size: (1) by undertaking several research projects simultaneously they can reduce their risks; (2) their diversification permits them to exploit the unexpected benefits of research; (3) they can achieve economies of scale in research.[2]

This chapter tests the following three hypotheses: (1) The quantity of resources devoted to research in the pharmaceutical industry increases more than proportionally with size of firm; (2) economies of scale are present in research; (3) research output increases more than proportionally with size of firm.

Studies of pharmaceutical research so far have disagreed with Schumpeter. According to Edwin Mansfield and Henry Grabowski, large drug companies do not spend proportionally more money on research than smaller ones. W. S. Comanor observes diseconomies of scale in research. Jerome Schnee concludes that leading companies do not produce proportionally more innovations than other firms. Our own results, however, lead to directly opposite conclusions and confirm Schumpeter's thesis.[3]

Since we are concerned with the implications of the study for U.S. government policy, and the competitive behavior of the industry may vary among countries, we examine only the behavior of firms whose principal markets, head office, manufacturing facilities, and research laboratories are located in the U.S. Further, limiting the study to U.S.-based firms permits the use of data on employment in U.S. pharmaceutical laboratories as a measure of research inputs. Drug companies usually locate their principal laboratories in their home countries, and data on laboratory employment by company are unavailable for other countries. The tests, therefore, refer to the U.S. drug industry.

Like other writers on drug research, we use U.S. ethical drug sales to measure firm size, largely because world ethical sales by company are difficult to estimate.

RESEARCH EFFORT AND SIZE OF FIRM

The examination of the effect of size of firm on research effort will use two measures of research effort. The first is based on laboratory employment, and the second is the number of publications in scientific journals.

EMPLOYMENT MEASURE OF RESEARCH EFFORT. We will first test the hypothesis that research effort increases more than proportionally with size of firm with the following linear logarithmic equation:

$$\ln E = a + b \ln S,$$

where E = laboratory employment less auxiliaries in each U.S. company in 1969, as reported by National Academy of Sciences–National Research Council, *Industrial Laboratories in the United States,* 1970.

S = U.S. ethical sales in 1968 for each company as reported by *US Pharmaceutical Market, Drug Stores and Hospitals,* IMS America, Ltd.

This form is chosen because the relationship is expected to be logarithmic. In addition, the hypothesis itself suggests the form: a regression coefficient significantly greater than 1 constitutes confirmation. The logarithmic form has the other important advantage of coping with the heteroscedasticity of the data.

The measure of effort, total employment exclusive of auxiliaries, is chosen over the more inclusive measure because it provides a more consistent measure of research effort among firms. Some companies charge maintenance to adjacent production facilities and therefore do not report all auxiliaries as part of laboratory employment.

Data on R & D expenditures, the major other type of measure of research effort, is available only for those few larger firms which publish figures on R & D expenditures in annual reports. The coverage is very incomplete even for the larger firms. Another serious defect is that the data include nonpharmaceutical research expenditures. The NAS/NRC data on laboratory employment are for individual laboratories which can be identified as pharmaceutical or other. Even predominantly pharmaceutical laboratories conduct other research, but this is as close as we can get to measuring R & D inputs. Unfortunately, a number of companies did not supply employment data for one or more laboratories and had to be omitted from the sample. PMA estimates of expenditures per scientist increase with size of firm. This suggests that employment data understates the increase in research effort with size of firm.

The measure of firm size, by U.S. ethical drug sales, is for 1968; the employment data are for 1969. We are interested in the effect of firm size on research effort; the one-year lag is designed to allow some time for decisions to take effect.

Consider the results. The first test, which is based on a linear-logarithmic equation (equation 5.1 of table 5-1), does not favor the hypothesis that research effort increases more than proportionally with firm size. The value of the regression coefficient, .57, is well below unity. This result may be due to a high minimum laboratory employment required for the design of production processes and the disproportionate use of laboratory employees by small firms for the design of new dosage forms and combinations. We have evidence that small firms do devote their R & D resources disproportionally to the design of new dosage forms and combinations.

The leading twenty firms by sales in 1965 accounted for 82 percent of new single entities between 1966 and 1972 and for only 36 percent of the new combination drugs.[4] In addition, these twenty firms produced only half of all new dosage forms. Most of the new dosage forms produced by large companies follow shortly after the introduction of the new single entity. The small firms, on the other hand, produce new formulations of old drugs whose patents have expired. The R & D work done by small firms thus is limited to developmental projects where the degree of uncertainty of technical failure is small. They choose old, standard drugs for new combination and new dosage forms, so the toxicology and clinical tests either are unnecessary or perfunctory.

If these are the reasons, then a second-degree logarithmic equation should fit the data better. This indeed turns out to be the case. Two such equations have

TABLE 5-1
Regression Analysis of Variation in Laboratory
Employment among Forty Firms in 1969, with Size of
Sales in 1968 as Independent Variable

$\ln E = 2.99 + .57 \ln S$		5.1
$(t = 8.56)$		
$(SE = .07)$	$r^2 = .67$	
$\ln E = 2.66 + .15 (\ln S)^2$		5.2
$(t = 9.25)$		
$(SE = .016)$	$r^2 = .71$	
$\ln E = 2.40 + .35 \ln S + .10 (\ln S)^2$		5.3
$(t = 6.64)$ $(t = 7.28)$		
$(SE = .052)$ $(SE = .013)$	$r^2 = .87$	

Sources: Sales from *U.S. Pharmaceutical Market, Drug Stores and Hospitals*, IMS America, Ltd. Employment from National Academy of Sciences–National Research Council, *Industrial Laboratories in the United States*, 1970.

Note: E = Total employment in laboratories exclusive of auxiliaries 1969.

S = U.S. ethical sales 1968.

been fitted, and equation 5.3, which contains a linear as well as a quadratic term, does much better than either equation 5.2, which includes only a quadratic term, or equation 5.1, the linear equation.

The results support the hypothesis that research efforts increase more than proportionally with size of firm. The fit of equation 5.3 is extraordinary: it explains as much as 87 percent of the interfirm variance of the relation between research employment and size of firm. We shall therefore assume that equation 5.3 is correct.

The regression coefficients are positive and highly significant and indicate a large and increasing elasticity of research effort with respect for firm size. The elasticity refers to the percentage increase in research effort associated with an increase of 1 percent in size: if the elasticity equals 1, it signifies a proportional increase in effort with size of firm. The formula for the elasticity is $E_e = d \ln E/d \ln S$. Applied to equation 5.3, this formula yields $E_e = .35 + .20 \ln S$. The elasticity of research effort thus increases with the logarithm of size. Research effort begins to increase more than proportionally with sales (at which $E_e = 1$) at a sales-size of $26 million, which is hardly large. The largest firms thus devote relatively the largest effort, and, what is more, as firm-size increases, the relative research effort continues to increase.

RESEARCH EFFORT MEASURED BY NUMBER OF PUBLICATIONS. Scientists in pharmaceutical laboratories want to publish their work, and their employers, who share some of the benefits, encourage publication. Acceptance by a journal signifies that the work meets the usual scientific standards, so it provides an outside check on the quality of the work in the laboratory. There is also the benefit of inviting further validation or contrary evidence from other scientists, which is important in so empirical a field as pharmaceutical research. Additional leads may be obtained; reports or results with a compound for other samples and other species may be very illuminating. Research-oriented firms willingly risk revelations that may aid competitors in the rivalry to develop a new drug, since their success depends more on a well-developed program of research, an accumulation of knowledge, and a highly motivated group of scientists than on secret bits of information. Rarely is a single publication of crucial importance, and encouraging publication stimulates greater effort.

The number of publications is an index of output and therefore of input. Scientists themselves regard articles as the end-product of research whether or not they report drug discoveries, and reports of findings relating to physiological processes may be more valuable ultimately than those directly concerned with individual drugs. The research-oriented firm, in fact, may turn out many valuable scientific reports and few drugs; other firms may profit from the drugs which eventually result from the reports. To the extent that scientists seeking advancement publish articles reporting trivial experiments, the measure is deficient. But the error need not bias the estimate of the effect of firm size on research effort.

TABLE 5-2
Regression Analysis of Variation in the Number of
Publications among Forty-four Firms in 1965–70,
with Size of Sales in 1968 as
Independent Variable

$\ln P = -4.08 + 1.62 \ln S$		5.4
$(t = 5.24)$		
$(SE = .309)$	$r^2 = .40$	
$\ln P = -5.62 + .48\,(\ln S)^2$		5.5
$(t = 7.88)$		
$(SE = .060)$	$r^2 = .58$	
$\ln P = -6.16 + .63 \ln S + .38\,(\ln S)^2$		5.5
$(t = 2.03)$ $(t = 5.16)$		
$(SE = .310)$ $(SE = .074)$		
	$r^2 = .62$	

Sources: Number of publications obtained from
count of publications dealing with pharmaceutical and
related subjects classified by companies by the Ringdoc System, Derwent Publications Ltd., London. Sales
and employment sources same as table 5-1.
Note: P = Number of publications by employees of
companies 1965–70.
S = U.S. ethical sale of companies 1968.

We now test the hypothesis that the number of publications rises more than
proportionally with the size of firm. The count of the number of publications is
based on the list of publications on pharmaceutical research appearing in 350
professional journals between 1965 and 1970 compiled by Derwent Publications
of London in their Ringdoc System. Size of firm is measured as before by U.S.
ethical sales.

The linear logarithmic regression equation (5.4, table 5-2) shows that the
number of publications increases more than proportionally with sales size. The
regression coefficient significantly exceeds unity; the estimate of the elasticity of
the number of publications with respect to size of firm is 1.62. An increase of 1
percent in sales size is estimated to yield an increase in research effort of 1.62
percent.

The quadratic logarithmic equations 5.5 and 5.6 provide better fits, and both
show that the elasticity of research effort increases with size of firm.

ECONOMIES OF SCALE IN RESEARCH

An unweighted count of discoveries by companies between 1965 and 1970 is the
initial measure of research output. Other measures, which we discuss later, will
weight the number by various indexes of importance. Still another measure is
the number of U.S. patents issued. Objections can be made to any of the
weighting systems and to the number of patents as a measure of output, so we

begin with the unweighted count. This count is based on de Haen's list of NCE's, but it eliminates new salts, esters, new uses, and new compounds later withdrawn.[5] A new salt or ester of an existing drug may represent a useful therapeutic advance, most often through improved pharmokinetics, which can permit greater convenience in dosage schedules and improvement in safety. The primary reason for excluding such derivatives of existing drugs is the much smaller research investment which they entail compared to basic new agents for the same or similar therapeutic indications. A new derivative which represents a new use of a drug which is already available is identical to the first; the only research required is that represented by the abbreviated NDA for its approval for this use. Drugs withdrawn from the market are excluded because they are withdrawn for the same reasons that keep others from being marketed in the first place; the only difference is the later perception of a deficiency.

The measure of input again is laboratory employment in 1969, exclusive of auxiliaries. The use of employment rather than expenditure data to measure inputs tends to understate the increase in inputs associated with increases in size of firm.[6] A resulting bias is to overstate the economies of scale. The observed economies of scale, therefore, have to be large to provide convincing evidence of their presence.

We have a problem here with the dates of our data for employment and number of new chemical entities. A research input will precede the introduction of the resulting new products. But the employment data are for 1969 and the number of NCE's is for 1965–70. The economies of scale will tend to be understated for the following reason: Suppose a firm is successful and discovers several new drugs. It will increase the size of its laboratory. The laboratory, at the time it is observed, will be larger than when the research was done to produce the new entities. Hence the observed elasticity of the number of new entities with respect to employment size will be less than the actual elasticity.

We also have the problem of zero values for many of the observations of new entities: many firms discovered no NCE's in 1965–70; and logarithmic equations cannot handle zero values. To exclude the zero observations, as sometimes is done, biases the results and reduces sample size. Therefore, we adopt the inelegant but expedient solution of substituting an arbitrarily small value (.0001) for zero (see Appendix A).

Some drugs are more beneficial than others or are more difficult to discover and develop. Economists like sales weights because they are a market measure of importance. In addition, we want an estimate of the economies of scale, and the measure of output should in some way be related to sales. One objection to sales weights is that sales value may be increased simply by increasing prices. It is often suggested that the demand for individual drugs is inelastic at the current price. Moreover, that part of sales which is the result of marketing activities may be falsely ascribed to laboratory size, since both are correlated with firm size. The equation attempts to estimate the increase in sales resulting from increases in employment of laboratories. But part of the increase in sales may be due to the associated increase in promotional expenditures. Another objection to the use of sales to measure output is that sales may not be a good measure of the importance of a drug, if doctors are gullible and therefore susceptible to promotional efforts. In addition, doctors may over-prescribe drugs because patients have been oversold on their virtues; they cannot feel they have been helped unless they take a prescription along when they leave the doctor. In short, weighting by sales volume seems fraught with many difficulties.

Skeptics of sales weights might prefer using the number of prescriptions as a measure of the usefulness of a drug. The number of prescriptions does not increase with price; but the number of prescriptions may respond to marketing activities. Other skeptics may prefer a weighting system based on the medical importance of drugs as judged by a panel of eminent and knowledgeable physicians. Or, they may prefer novelty as a criterion: drugs that are path-breakers are the most valuable. The number of patents is another measure of research output, although this measure will err with differences among firms in the propensity to patent discoveries and in the importance of patents.

Since summing up the pros and cons of the methods is inconclusive, we will resolve the problem by using different sets of weights. We will analyze variation in the number of new single entities (1) unweighted, (2) sales-weighted, (3) weighted by an index of novelty developed by Dr. J. G. Carpenter, (4) weighted by an index of medical importance, and (5) weighted by the number of prescriptions written in 1971. We will also (6) substitute for the number of new single entities another measure of research output: the number of patents. We will have trouble if the results of the different analyses substantially disagree; as it turns out, however, they do not.

UNWEIGHTED NEW ENTITIES. That economies of scale are large in research is confirmed by the regression coefficient of the linear logarithmic equation relating the number of new entities, N, to laboratory employment, E. The value of the regression coefficient is no less than 2.25 (equation 5.7 in table 5-3). The large coefficient of determination (.61) supports the conclusion.

The positive and highly significant regression coefficients of the squared terms in both quadratic equations indicate that the elasticity of the number of new entities with respect to size of laboratory increases with the size of laboratory.

SALES-WEIGHTED NEW ENTITIES. Sales in 1972 are the weights of the new entities. They include sales of the new entities themselves and sales of derivatives including duplicates produced under license by other firms, new dosage forms, salts, and esters. The importance of a new single entity increases with sales of its derivatives as well as its own sales.

The results of this analysis (table 5-4) strikingly resemble those of the

TABLE 5-3
Results of Regression Analysis of Variation in the
Unweighted Number of New Single Entities among
Forty U.S. Firms between 1965 and 1970, with
Laboratory Employment Exclusive of Auxiliaries in
1969 as Independent Variable

$\ln N = -15.64 + 2.25 \ln E$		5.7
(t = 7.68)		
(SE = .293)	$r^2 = .61$	
$\ln N = -11.41 + .26 (\ln E)^2$		5.8
(t = 8.308)		
(SE = .031)	$r^2 = .64$	
$\ln N = -8.41 -1.50 \ln E + .42 (\ln E)^2$		5.9
(t = -.860) (t = 2.175)		
(SE = 1.744) (SE = .192)	$r^2 = .64$	

Sources: New entities discovered by company from
Paul de Haen, *New Product Survey* and *Nonproprietary
Name Index,* and *Merck Index.* Laboratory employment
from NAS/NRC, *Industrial Laboratories,* 1970.
Note: N = Number of new entites introduced 1965–
70.
    E = Laboratory employment exclusive of aux-
    iliaries 1969.
Many firms did not introduce any new entities. In
order to retain them in the sample, I assumed that each of
them introduced .0001 new entities.

preceding one, in which innovative output was measured by the unweighted
number of new single entities.

The use of sales weights does not alter the conclusion that the economies of
scale are large. Moreover, the results of the quadratic equations again indicate
increasing scale economies with size of firm.

NOVELTY-WEIGHTED NEW ENTITIES. J. G. Carpenter has assigned indexes of novelty to new entities appearing in the United Kingdom in 1958–67.[7]
The index is based on differences in chemical structure between each drug and
its chemically most similar predecessor, whether introduced by the same firm or
another. We transferred the index to the same drugs appearing in the United
States. When a drug was not rated by Carpenter, it was assumed to belong to the
median class of novelty. The period 1965–67 was used because 1967 was the last
year for which Carpenter made the estimates.

The results are reported in table 5-5. Again, we have confirmation of large
and increasing economies of scale in research.

NEW ENTITIES WEIGHTED BY MEDICAL IMPORTANCE. The Centre for
the Study of Industrial Innovation, London, has developed a set of weights on
drugs based on medical importance as judged by a panel of physicians.[8] These

TABLE 5-4
Results of the Regression Analysis of Variation
in Sales-Weighted Number of New Single Entities among
Forty Firms between 1965 and 1970,
with Laboratory Employment Exclusive of Auxiliaries in
1969 as Independent Variable

$$\ln N_S = -16.04 + 2.46 \ln E \qquad\qquad 5.10$$
$$(t = 7.696)$$
$$(SE = .320) \qquad r^2 = .61$$
$$\ln N_S = -11.37 + .28 (\ln E)^2 \qquad\qquad 5.11$$
$$(t = 8.16)$$
$$(SE = .034) \qquad r^2 = .64$$
$$\ln N_S = -9.45 - .96 \ln E + .38 (\ln E)^2 \qquad 5.12$$
$$(t = -.49) \quad (t = 1.76)$$
$$(SE = 1.978) \quad (SE = .218) \quad r^2 = .63$$

Sources: New entities, duplicates, salts, dosage forms, from Paul de Haen, *New Product Survey* and *Nonproprietary Name Index.* Sales and employment sources same as table 5-1.

Note: N_s = Sales of new single entities introduced 1965–70 including duplicates, salts, and new dosage forms.

E = Laboratory employment exclusive of auxiliaries 1969.

TABLE 5-5
Results of Regression Analysis of Variation in the
Number of New Single Entities, 1965–67, Weighted by
an Index of Novelty among Forty Companies, with
Laboratory Employment Exclusive of Auxiliaries in
1969 as Independent Variable

$$\ln N_n = -15.10 + 2.22 \ln E \qquad\qquad 5.13$$
$$(t = 6.29)$$
$$(SE = .35) \qquad r^2 = .51$$
$$\ln N_n = -10.79 + .25 (\ln E)^2 \qquad\qquad 5.14$$
$$(t = 6.36)$$
$$(SE = .04) \qquad r^2 = .52$$
$$\ln N_n = -12.11 + .67 \ln E + .17 (\ln E)^2 \qquad 5.15$$
$$(t = .30) \quad (t = .70)$$
$$(SE = 2.25) \quad (SE = .25) \quad r^2 = .52$$

Sources: See table 5-1.

Note: Weighted for novelty based on chemical structure assigned by Dr. J. G. Carpenter, Pfizer, Inc., Sandwich, England. New entities assigned weights 1 to 5. Products not included by Carpenter assigned weight of 3.

TABLE 5-6
Results of Regression Analysis of Number of New
Single Entities Weighted by Medical Importance
among Forty Companies in 1965–70, with Laboratory
Employment Exclusive of Auxiliaries in 1969
as Independent Variable

$$\ln N_m = -15.84 + 2.43 \ln E \qquad\qquad 5.16$$
$$(t = 7.63)$$
$$(SE = .319) \qquad r^2 = .60$$
$$\ln N_m = -11.17 + .27 (\ln E)^2 \qquad\qquad 5.17$$
$$(t = 7.92)$$
$$(SE = .034) \qquad r^2 = .62$$
$$\ln N_m = -10.76 - .21 \ln E + .30 (\ln E)^2 \qquad 5.18$$
$$(t = -.10) \quad (t = 1.34)$$
$$(SE = 2.00) \quad (SE = .22) \quad r^2 = .61$$

Sources: See table 5-1.

Note: N_m = Number of new single entities weighted by medical importance assigned by a panel of physicians for the Centre for the Study of Industrial Innovation, London.

E = Laboratory employment exclusive of auxiliaries.

weights were applied to the new single entities introduced between 1965 and 1970 in the U.S. When a drug introduced in the United States did not appear in the list, it was assigned to the lowest class of importance.

The results, reported in table 5-6, indicate large and increasing economies of scale.

TABLE 5-7
Regression Analysis of Variation in Number of New
Single Entities, 1965–70, Weighted by Number of
Prescriptions in 1971 among Forty Companies, with
Laboratory Employment Exclusive of Auxiliaries in
1969 as Independent Variable

$$\ln N_r = -18.91 + 3.40 \ln E \qquad\qquad 5.19$$
$$(t = 7.73)$$
$$(SE = .439) \qquad r^2 = .61$$
$$\ln N_r = -12.53 + .39 (\ln E)^2 \qquad\qquad 5.20$$
$$(t = 8.37)$$
$$(SE = .046) \qquad r^2 = .65$$
$$\ln N_r = -7.90 - 2.33 \ln E + .64 (\ln E)^2 \qquad 5.21$$
$$(t = -.88) \quad (t = 2.18)$$
$$(SE = 2.659) \quad (SE = .294) \quad r^2 = .65$$

Sources: See table 5-1. Number of prescriptions from *National Prescription Audits, Therapeutic Category Report,* IMS America, Ltd.

Note: N_r = Number of new single entities weighted by number of prescriptions.

TABLE 5-8
Regression Analysis of Variation in the Number of U.S.
Patents, 1968–70, among Forty Companies, with Total
Laboratory Employment Exclusive of Auxiliaries in
1969 as Independent Variable

$\ln PA = -10.84 + 2.40 \ln E$	5.22
$(t = 5.61)$	
$(SE = .429) \qquad r^2 = .45$	
$\ln PA = -6.04 + .26 \, (\ln E)$	5.23
$(t = 5.46)$	
$(SE = .048) \qquad r^2 = .44$	
$\ln PA = -11.30 + 2.65 \ln E - .027 \, (\ln E)^2$	5.24
$(t = .96) \quad (t = .09)$	
$(SE = 2.754) \quad (SE = .304)$	
$\qquad\qquad\qquad r^2 = .44$	

Sources: See table 5-1.
Note: PA = Number of patents as reported by US
Patent Office, *Index of Patents* (annual).

NEW ENTITIES WEIGHTED BY THE NUMBER OF PRESCRIPTIONS.   Each
new single entity appearing between 1965 and 1970 is weighted by the number
of prescriptions sold in 1971. As in the case of sales weights, the number of
prescriptions includes those of derivatives as well as those of the original new
single entities.

The results (table 5-7) indicate large and increasing scale economies in
research.

OUTPUT MEASURED BY NUMBER OF PATENTS.   The number of patents is
the final measure of research output. The number of patents issued to pharmaceutical manufacturers between 1968 and 1970 is the dependent variable.

The results (table 5-8) again indicate large and increasing economies of scale.
The linear logarithmic equation shows large economies of scale, and the quadratic containing only the squared term shows increasing economies of scale.
When the linear term is introduced, the coefficient of the quadratic term
becomes negative, but it is not statistically significant.

INNOVATION AND SIZE OF FIRM

To examine the relation between innovative output and size of firm may appear
to be redundant, but some economists may disagree with the judgments in
dealing with measurement problems, notwithstanding the precaution of using
different measures of the same variable. Tests which deal directly with the
relationship between the number of innovations and size of firm may be
necessary additional evidence.

We will keep the same measures of innovative output. The first one is the

TABLE 5-9
The Results of the Regression Analysis of Variation in
Unweighted Number of New Single Entities among
Sixty U.S. Firms between 1965 and 1970, with
Sales-Size in 1965 as Independent Variable

$\ln N = -12.54 + 2.40 \ln S$	5.25
$(t = 8.47)$	
$(SE = .284)$ $r^2 = .56$	
$\ln N = -10.11 + .44 \, (\ln S)^2$	5.26
$(t = 9.28)$	
$(SE = .047)$ $r^2 = .61$	
$\ln N = 9.75 - .32 \ln S + .49 \, (\ln S)^2$	5.27
$(t = -.29)$ $(t = 2.51)$	
$(SE = 1.118)$ $(SE = .195)$ $r^2 = .59$	

Sources: See table 5-1.
Note: N = Number of new single entities in 1965–70.
       S = U.S. ethical sales in 1965.

unweighted number of new single entities over the period 1965 to 1970. The measure of firm size is U.S. ethical sales in 1965. The year for this measure precedes that for innovations so as to ensure that it is not influenced by the dependent variable.

UNWEIGHTED NEW ENTITIES. The linear logarithmic equation (table 5-9) shows that large companies will produce proportionally more innovations than smaller ones.

The coefficients of the squared terms in both quadratic equations are positive and highly significant, indicating an increasing elasticity of the number of discoveries with increases in firm size.

SALES-WEIGHTED NEW ENTITIES. The linear logarithmic equation (table 5-10), in which the dependent variable is the number of new single entities weighted by sales, does not support the hypothesis that innovative output increases more than proportionally with sales-size. The indicated elasticity, .62, is well below unity. This result, however, does not tell the story, for the equation gives a poor fit: the coefficient of determination is only .09.

The relationship is quadratic in the logarithms rather than linear. The equation which contains both linear and quadratic terms fits the data best. The coefficient of determination, which is .62, shows an excellent fit. The equation indicates that the elasticity of research output with respect to size of firm increases with size of firm. The output increases more than proportionally with size of firm and increasingly so as the firm grows.

NOVELTY-WEIGHTED NEW ENTITIES. The results of the analysis of variation in novelty-weighted new entities (table 5-11) are similar to those of the

TABLE 5-10

Results of Regression Analysis of Sales-Weighted
Number of New Entities in 1965–70 among Sixty
Companies, with Sales-Size in 1965 as Independent
Variable

$\ln N_S = -6.85 + .62 \ln S$	5.28
$(t = 2.459)$	
$(SE = .250)$ $r^2 = .09$	
$\ln N_S = -7.40 + .17 (\ln S)^2$	5.29
$(t = 4.54)$	
$(SE = .037)$ $r^2 = .26$	
$\ln N_S = -11.49 + 1.31 \ln S + .26 (\ln S)^2$	5.30
$(t = 7.10)$ $(t = 8.65)$	
$(SE = .184)$ $(SE = .030)$ $r^2 = .60$	

Source: List of new entities, from Paul de Haen, *New Product Survey* and *Nonproprietary Name Index.* Sales from *U.S. Pharmaceutical Market, Drug Stores and Hospitals,* IMS America, Ltd.

Note: N_S = number of new single entities 1965–72 weighted by 1972 sales of duplicates, salts, esters, new dosage forms as well as of the new single entities themselves.

S = sales in 1965.

analysis of sales-weighted new entities (table 5-10). The linear logarithmic equation and the quadratic equation with only the quadratic term fail to explain the variation. On the other hand, the fit of equation 5.33, which includes both the linear and quadratic terms, is quite good. Thus, when we use the novelty-weighted number of new entities as a measure of output we also find that the elasticity of output with respect to size of firm increases with size of firm.

TABLE 5-11

Results of Regression Analysis of Number of New
Entities, 1965–67, Weighted by Novelty among Sixty
Companies, with Sales-Size in 1965 as Independent
Variable

$\ln N_n = -8.20 + .95 \ln S$	5.31
$(t = 4.38)$	
$(SE = .22)$ $r^2 = .25$	
$\ln N_n = -7.03 + .09 (\ln S)^2$	5.32
$(t = 2.22)$	
$(SE = .04)$ $r^2 = .08$	
$\ln N_n = -11.59 + 1.46 \ln S + .19 (\ln S)^2$	5.33
$(t = 7.77)$ $(t = 6.21)$	
$(SE = .19)$ $(SE = .03)$ $r^2 = .54$	

Source: See table 5-10.

Note: N_n = number of new single entities weighted by novelty index constructed by J. G. Carpenter, Pfizer Inc., Sandwich, England.

TABLE 5-12
Regression Analysis of Number of New
Single Entities Weighted by Medical Importance
among Sixty Companies in 1965–70, with Sales-Size
in 1965 as Independent Variable

$\ln N_m = -6.52 + .49 \ln S$		5.34
$(t = 1.97)$		
$(SE = .251)$	$r^2 = .06$	
$\ln N_m = -7.53 + .18 (\ln S)^2$		5.35
$(t = 5.24)$		
$(SE = .035)$	$r^2 = .32$	
$\ln N_m = -11.30 + 1.21 \ln S + .27 (\ln S)^2$		5.36
$(t = 6.81)$ $(t = 9.26)$		
$(SE = .178)$ $SE = .029)$ $r^2 = .62$		

Source: See table 5-10.
Note: N_m = number of medically weighted new single
entities 1965–70 (see table 5-6 for details).
S = sales in 1965.

NEW ENTITIES WEIGHTED BY MEDICAL IMPORTANCE. The quadratic equation that includes a linear term again fits the data best (table 5-12), indicating an increasing elasticity of medically weighted discoveries with respect to sales-size of firm.

NEW ENTITIES WEIGHTED BY NUMBER OF PRESCRIPTIONS. Table 5-13 shows that the quadratic equation including the linear term fits the data best. We again obtain a positive and highly significant coefficient of the quadratic term.

OUTPUT MEASURED BY NUMBER OF PATENTS. Sales-size is less closely correlated with the number of patents than with the other measures of research

TABLE 5-13
Regression Analysis of Number of New
Single Entities, 1965–70, Weighted by Number of
Prescriptions in 1971 among Sixty Companies, with
Sales-Size in 1965 as Independent Variable

$\ln N_r = -6.47 + .94 \ln S$		5.37
$(t = 2.77)$		
$(SE = .34)$	$r^2 = .12$	
$\ln N_r = 6.68 + .20 (\ln S)^2$		5.38
$(t = 3.81)$		
$(SE = .052)$	$r^2 = .20$	
$\ln N_r = -12.34 + 1.81 \ln S + .33 (\ln S)^2$		5.39
$(t = 6.72)$ $(t = 7.45)$		
$(SE = .270)$ $(SE = .044) r^2 = .55$		

Source: See table 5-10.
Notes: N_r = number of new entities weighted by
number of prescriptions (see table 5-7 for details).

TABLE 5-14
Regression Analysis of Variation in Number of U.S.
Patents, 1968–70, among Sixty Companies, with
Ethical Sales in 1966 as Independent Variable

$\ln PA = 1.50 + .92 \ln S$ 5.40
$(t = 2.78)$
$(SE = .330)$ $r^2 = .12$
$\ln PA = -.90 + .16 (\ln S)^2$ 5.41
$(t = 3.06)$
$(SE = .053)$ $r^2 = .14$
$\ln PA = -3.82 + 1.06 \ln S + .18 (\ln S)^2$ 5.42
$(t = 3.52)$ $(t = 3.76)$
$(SE = .300)$ $(SE = .049)$ $r^2 = .28$

Source: See table 5-10.
Note: PA = number of patents (see table 5-8 for details).

output. The coefficient of determination for equation 5.42 of table 5-14 is the highest of the three, but it is only .28. This equation is consistent with the previous results in indicating that the elasticity of research output increases with size of firm.

CONCLUSIONS. The tests demonstrate that the largest firms discover relatively more new drugs than do smaller firms, regardless of the measure of the number of discoveries. This conclusion disagrees sharply with the writings of other students of research and innovation in the drug industry. In the rest of this chapter we shall discuss some of the sources of the disagreements.

PREVIOUS STUDIES

RESEARCH EFFORT. Edwin Mansfield[9] rejects the hypothesis that R & D expenditures increase among drug firms more than proportionally with sales size on the basis of a linear-logarithmic regression analysis of variation in total R & D expenditures (including nonpharmaceutical) among eight major drug firms with variation in total sales (including nonpharmaceutical). Our own results indicate that a linear logarithmic equation may well show a less than proportional increase in R & D effort with sales size. Only when we use a quadratic equation is the hypothesis confirmed.

Another source of the disagreement may be Mansfield's inclusion of nonpharmaceuticals in total R & D expenditures and nonpharmaceuticals in total sales. The larger firms tend to be more diversified, and this diversification results in a lower ratio of total R & D expenditures to total sales. Pharmaceutical research represents a larger share of pharmaceutical sales than research relating to other activities represents of other sales.

Henry Grabowski[10] analyzes R & D expenditures of ten major drug firms and obtains

$$R_t/S_t = 1/S_t \, (-6.21 + .17 \, S_t - .4 \times 10^{-3} \, S_t{}^2)$$
$$(1.29) \quad (.02) \quad (.1 \times 10^{-3})$$

(standard errors in parentheses).

Where S_t = total sales, including nonpharmaceutical sales, in year t;
   R_t = total R & D expenditures, including nonpharmaceutical R & D expenditures, in year t.

The coefficient of the squared term is significantly negative. Grabowski concludes that research intensity initially increases with firm size but declines over most of the relevant range.

Similar comments concerning the inclusion of nonpharmaceutical in total R & D expenditures and nonpharmaceutical in total sales apply to Grabowski's results as to Mansfield's. Grabowski recognizes that his results for the drug industry may reflect diversification of large firms into nonpharmaceutical products where "the opportunities for R & D applications are low."[11]

ECONOMIES OF SCALE. W. S. Comanor[12] measures research output by sales (Y) of new single entities introduced in 1955–60; he uses the sales during the first two years after introduction. His measure of research input is the number of professional research personnel (R), and he also introduces a measure of firm size, (S), sales of ethical drugs; (D) is a measure of product diversification. He obtains the following regression equation:

$$Y/S = .422 - 4.671R/S + .547R^2/S + .0000344S - .0000001281 - .130D \quad R^2 = .40$$
$$(.136) \quad (1.285) \quad (.107) \quad (.0000083) \quad (.000000031) \quad (.040)$$

(standard errors in parentheses).

The letter I stands for an interaction variable, the product of R and S.

The coefficient of firm size (S) is significantly positive, indicating a more than proportional increase in innovative output with increases in firm size. Comanor attributes this finding to the influence of the firm's marketing and distribution activities on sales; it will be recalled that the measure of R & D output, Y, is the sales of rather than the number of new single entities.

Comanor emphasizes the negative coefficient of the interaction variable I. He interprets this coefficient to signify that the marginal productivity of research personnel is inversely related to size of firm.[13] Comanor computes the elasticity of Y with respect to R for given values of S and finds that at small sales (less than \$10 million) the elasticity falls below unity, signifying diseconomies of scale in research for relatively small firms.

The negative coefficient of I probably reflects collinearity with R^2/S and S rather than the diseconomies of scale in research at large sizes. John Vernon and

Peter Gusen inform me that in a sample of fifty pharmaceutical companies, the Pearsonian correlation coefficient between R^2/S and I for 1965–70 is .86, and between S and I it is .82. It is unreasonable to introduce an interaction variable as well as R^2/S and S when collinearity is as high as it is. Comanor does not consider the problem of collinearity in his justification of the interaction variable.

This justification is limited to a reference to the possible organizational effects of large size of firm on research productivity. Earlier we argued that the organization of research in the pharmaceutical laboratories was not subject to bureaucratic interference. Comanor's argument is not persuasive. In fact, the discussion is so brief and casual as to give the impression that the variable was thrown in as an afterthought, despite its ultimate importance in the results. Comanor is not the first economist to introduce variables casually in regression equations, trusting to the econometric analysis to provide the test. But, in this case at any rate, the econometrics cannot be decisive owing to the collinearity.

INNOVATIVE OUTPUT AND SIZE OF FIRM. Jerome Schnee rejects Schumpeter's hypothesis that large firms will produce proportionally more innovations than small firms on the basis of two different analyses. One approach depends on an arithmetic regression which yields the following equation:

$$n = .31 + .07\ S - .0003\ S^2 \qquad r^2 = .66$$
$$(.22)\ (.02)\quad (.0002)$$

(standard errors in parentheses).

where n = number of new chemical entities introduced in the period 1950–62 of
       each of fifty-eight companies, and
where S = U.S. pharmaceutical sales of each of fifty-eight companies in 1950.

Schnee ignores the statistical nonsignificance of the coefficient of the squared term, and estimates the optimal size of the firms with respect to the number of innovations as $20 million, which, he states, corresponds to the twelfth largest firm. The results for economically weighted and medically weighted innovations are similar. Schnee concludes that "the firms that have contributed the most innovations relative to their size are not the largest firms, but somewhat smaller ones." And, he adds, "it is also important to note that this is true in the other industries included in Mansfield's previous studies."[14]

This conclusion is vulnerable, for it depends on the negative sign of the squared term, which, as we have seen, is statistically nonsignificant. Another objection is that the results may reflect heteroscedasticity in the data: the dispersion in both firm sizes and the number of new single entities per firm is large. Still another objection is that some of the so-called medium-sized firms performed well because they are parts of large foreign-based firms. Inspection of

TABLE 5-15
The Percent of Innovations and Industry Sales
Accounted for by Four Largest Ethical Pharma-
ceutical Firms, according to Schnee

	Unweighted	Medically weighted	Economically weighted
1935–49			
Innovations	37	45	50
Total Sales	50	–	–
1950–62			
Innovations	27	48	33
Total Sales	33	–	–

Source: Jerome Schnee, "Innovation and Discovery in the
Ethical Pharmaceutical Industry," chapter 8, in *Research and
Innovation in the Modern Corporation,* ed. Edwin Mansfield
et al. (N.Y.: W. W. Norton, 1971), p. 169.

Schnee's list of innovations shows many to have originated in British and Swiss firms, which at the time of the study were not at the top of the list of firms ranked according to U.S. sales, which is Schnee's measure of size of firm.

Schnee also rejects Schumpeter's hypothesis on the basis of a comparison between the four leading firms' share of the innovations between 1950 and 1962 and between 1935 and 1949 and their share of sales. Table 5-15 reproduces his findings.

The results are not as consistent as Schnee's conclusion leads us to believe, for the leading firms' share of medically weighted innovations in 1950–62 is much greater than their share of sales. His other results, however, apparently are unfavorable to Schumpeter's hypothesis. Our comments are methodological and pertain to the validity of the overall analysis. If one wants to determine the effect of firm size on the number of innovations, the obvious method is to start with a list of firms of different sizes and count the number of innovations from each firm. Schnee, however, relies on an invalid though popular method of analysis. His method begins with a list of innovations, which are classified by various characteristics of innovators, and expresses the number of innovations in each class as a percent of the total. Jewkes, Sawers, and Stillerman used this technique to support their argument that largeness of size in a firm is not conducive to innovation. Daniel Hamberg did the same thing and came to the same conclusion.[15] Mansfield applied the method to analyze innovations by size of firm and found that the largest steel companies produced a smaller share of steel innovations than their share of sales.[16]

Now the analysis of the effect of firm size says: if the x leading firms account for y percent of innovations, and y is less than z, the share of total sales, then increases in size of firm will reduce the total number of innovations. This is an invalid inference. Nor is it valid to infer that splitting up the firms will increase the number of innovations. First, Schnee's method credits small firms with all of the discoveries not accounted for by large firms. This includes the part due to random factors rather than characteristics of small firms. Thus, if an innovation results in a new firm being founded, then the innovation will be credited to small firms. The analysis wrongly presupposes in this case that the line of causation is from small size to innovation. To answer the question concerning the effect of size of firm, we should limit the sample of firms to those in existence at the beginning of the period. In other words, we should start with a list of firms rather than a list of innovations. Firms should be included in the sample regardless of whether or not they innovate, for it is the effect of firm size on the number of innovations that we want to estimate.

Second, each firm should have an equal weight in the analysis, since it is the behavior of firms that is in question. But the method used by Schnee weights firms by the number of their innovations.

Third, there is no reason to expect the x leading firms' share of innovations to exceed their share of sales, even if they exert proportionally more effort than smaller firms and enjoy economies of scale. Firms may enter and devote considerable resources to research. In addition, foreign firms may supply some of the innovations, and their share of sales in the U.S. may be small, despite their large size abroad. Finally, affiliates of large nonpharmaceutical firms may devote a more than proportional share of sales to research.

The error arising from what may be called random factors is the most interesting and possibly the most important in view of their large role in research success. Random factors include, besides luck, all those elements in research success that are not systematically related to size of firm, the single explanatory variable. These unspecified elements include research skills, intellectual tradition, strong motivation, good research leadership. Small as well as large firms may benefit from such advantages. Merely because one or a few small firms have such advantages does not mean that other small firms will; nor can we expect large firms suddenly to acquire them after they are split up. Such special advantages receive a large weight in any analysis which begins with a list of innovations and distributes them among firms of different sizes. A logarithmic regression analysis of the variation in the number of innovations among a sample of firms is free of this type of error.[17]

CONCLUSIONS

The three hypotheses tested in this chapter have been confirmed. First, research effort increases more than proportionally with size of firm in the pharmaceutical industry. Second, large firms enjoy economies of scale in pharmaceutical research. Third, the number of drug discoveries increases more than proportionally with firm size.

An examination of the results of previous studies, the conclusions of which disagree with those of the present study, reveals that the disagreements are due to the use of poor data for the measurement of firm size or to faulty analysis of the data by these other studies.

Our conclusion thus is that large firm size encourages innovation in the pharmaceutical industry.

CHAPTER 6

COMPETITION BY INNOVATION AND SOME CONSEQUENCES

INTRODUCTION

A pharmaceutical manufacturer has a choice between two basic competitive strategies: cutting prices or seeking innovations. The firm which pursues the price strategy will imitate other companies' drugs, and it will undercut their prices. Indeed, unless a firm innovates, it must cut prices in order to gain a significant share of a market, for it can make no special claims for its own drugs. However skillful the promotion may be, it cannot be counted on to work miracles. A firm must cut its price or be able to claim some quality advantage over rival products to obtain large sales.

The innovative strategy calls for investment in a research program which will produce drugs for diseases previously unsuccessfully treated with drugs, or new drugs which are in some way better than those previously used. This strategy is more difficult to pursue than the price strategy. The firm must usually make a large investment in R & D in order to discover and develop a new product which may win large sales but which also runs a great risk of failure.

Nevertheless, the latter has been the prevailing strategy of large pharmaceutical manufacturers. One reason for the choice is that patents have protected most drugs against imitation. The opportunity for the price strategy has been very limited, for few important drugs have been unprotected by patents during most of the period since World War II. Moreover, as drugs become older they are often outmoded; consequently, the sales of old drugs which have no patent protection have usually been too small to be attractive.

The opportunity for price competition has increased with the expiration of patents for large-selling drugs and the decline in the rate of innovation. As we will see in chapter 12, the large manufacturers competed vigorously in price during the 1960s and early 1970s in antibiotics. As other large-selling drugs

103

TABLE 6-1

R & D Funds as a Percentage of Net Sales by Industry in 1971

Food and kindred products	0.5
Textiles and apparel	0.4
Lumber, wood products, and furniture	0.6
Paper and allied products	0.9
Chemicals and allied products	3.8
Industrial chemicals	4.0
Drugs and medicines	7.6
Other chemicals	1.9
Petroleum refining and extraction	0.9
Rubber products	1.8
Stone, clay, and glass products	1.6
Primary metals	0.8
Ferrous metals and products	0.7
Nonferrous metals and products	1.1
Fabricated metal products	1.3
Machinery	3.9
Electrical equipment and communication	7.3
Radio and TV receiving equipment	2.4
Communication equipment and electronic components	8.4
Other electrical equipment	6.4
Motor vehicles and other transportation	3.1
Aircraft and missiles	16.6
Professional and scientific instruments	5.3
Scientific and mechanical measuring instruments	3.0
Optical, surgical, photographic, and other instruments	6.1
Other manufacturing industries	0.8

Source: National Science Foundation, *Research and Development in Industry*, 1971 (Washington, D.C.: National Science Foundation, 1972), NSF 73-305.

Note: The estimates of R & D funds on which the percentages reported here are based include government as well as company funds. In the case of drugs and medicines, companies provide nearly all of the funds, in contrast to other industries showing large percentages, including aircraft and missiles, and electrical equipment and communications.

come off patent we can expect the companies to manufacture duplicates and undercut the prices of original brands. However, for most drugs the opportunity for price competition up to the present has been limited, and the chief competitive strategy for large drug manufacturers therefore has called for a search for new drugs.

The innovative strategy has been attractive for other reasons. During the 1950s investment in R & D was highly productive. Many new drugs were produced, and they included a large number of major advances. A sufficient number of the new drugs resulted in large enough sales to generate a high rate of return on the investment in R & D. Not only were the sales large, but the costs of research at the time did not require the huge investment which they presently do, as we pointed out in chapter 3. The 1950s were truly a golden age of discovery. That decade saw the introduction of the tetracyclines, the tranquilizers, erythromycin, the oral antidiabetic drugs, and the thiazide diuretics. The investment in the R & D which led to the discovery of these drugs was highly profitable. These successes led to the expectations of further successes. Both society and the industry came to expect that drugs eventually would be found to deal with virtually all diseases.

Further pressure to increase investment in R & D was created by the high rate of obsolescence among drugs. As new discoveries were made, old drugs were displaced. In order for a firm to be able to maintain its position in the pharmaceutical market, it was forced to continue to invest in R & D and even to increase the investment. The industry's R & D expenditure therefore increased and became very substantial. Total expenditures in 1973 by the U.S. industry amounted to $870.7 million, constituting 14.7 percent of sales of ethical drugs.[1] The share of total sales spent on R & D by the industry exceeds that of most other industries (table 6-1).

The innovative strategy has not been without difficulties, especially in recent years. Pharmaceutical research is replete with both technical and commercial uncertainty, as we have already seen in describing this process. Some of the largest firms have introduced very few new drugs over an extended period (1962–68), as table 6-2 shows. We have also described some examples of large pharmaceutical research projects which continued for long periods before they yielded new products.

It is commercial success which is important, and the probability of such success is low. Very few of the drugs which were introduced obtained sufficient sales to yield an adequate rate of return on the research investment. If we consider an investment return of 10 percent after taxes to be the minimum acceptable level, then, as we will see in chapter 7, the gross margin and the commercial life of drugs combined with the estimate of the average cost of research per drug imply that the annual U.S. sales of an NCE must be at least $16.0 million. Very few of the drugs introduced between 1962 and 1968 achieved this level in 1972. Table 6-3 reveals that only eight of the seventy-nine introduced did so. Table 6-3 also shows that the sales of thirty-three of these drugs were less than $1 million. A majority had sales of less than $2 million. The sales of the very top drugs have been large, and the average is raised considerably above $2 million as a result. The average sales in 1972 of all NCE's introduced between 1962 and 1968 was $7.5 million, and this average was raised by $2.2 million by the sales of the single drug, Valium. Only a few drugs, then, are commercially successful, and it is these which carry the R & D and other costs for all products. They attract the unfavorable comments concerning prices in relation to costs, but their success must be viewed in a total setting in which many products fail. They represent the pot of gold that makes investment in R & D at all attractive.

TABLE 6-2

1972 U.S. Sales of New Single Chemical Entities Introduced 1962–68
That Were Discovered by the Ten Leading Firms (1972)

	Sales ($000)		Sales ($000)
Bristol Myers		**Pfizer**	
Oracon + Oracon 28	6,493	Navane	4,289
Mucomyst + Mucomyst 10%	3,869	Vibramycin Hyclate	23,557
Abbott		+ Vibramycin Monohydrate	
Eutonyl and Eutron	1,725	Rondomycin* Monohydrate	3,318
Tham + Tham E	122	**Roche**	
Vercyte	32	Valium	182,269
Squibb		Taractan	1,103
Hydrea	254	Fluorouracil	1,756
Upjohn		**Merck**	
Maolate	1,418	Edecrin + Edecrin Lyovac	1,714
Tolinase	10,282	Vivactil HCL	1,766
Lincocin	10,388	Mintezol	299
Uracil Mustard	3	Cuemid	112
Lilly		Cosmegen Lyovac	124
Loridine	15,495	Indocin	42,242
Aventyl	3,081	Aldomet Tabs + Aldomet Ester HCL	30,892
Dymelor	5,023	Cuprimine	202
Anhydron + Anhydron K	320	Alpha-redisol	199
Oncovin	2,625	**Ciba-Geigy**	
Keflin	63,189	Desferal Mesylate	35
Novrad + Novrad w/ASA	91	Hypertensin	22
American Home Products		Tegretol	1,148
Serax	10,426		
Unipen	2,949		
Protopam Cl	9		

Source: Based on Paul de Haen, *New Product Surveys* and *Nonproprietary Name Index*; and *U.S. Pharmaceutical Market, Drug Stores and Hospitals*, IMS America, Ltd.

Note: Sales of combinations containing new single entities introduced during this period and of new esters and salts of single entities introduced during this period are added to the sales of the new single chemical. Drugs withdrawn from the market are not included. Ciba and Geigy merged in 1972. The products which they introduced separately from 1962 to 1970 are listed under Ciba-Geigy. Drugs are listed by discovering firm, whether that firm or another firm introduced the drug.

TABLE 6-3
Number of New Single Chemical Entities Introduced
1962–68, by 1972 U.S. Sales of Entities

Sales $000	Number of drugs	Sales $000	Number of drugs
0– 999	33	20,000–29,999	2
1,000– 1,999	14	30,000–39,999	2
2,000– 3,999	9	40,000–49,999	2
4,000– 5,999	5	50,000–59,999	0
6,000– 7,999	3	60,000–99,999	1
8,000– 9,999	1	100,000+	1
10,000–14,999	4	Total	79
15,000–19,999	2		

Source: Paul de Haen, *New Product Survey* and *Nonproprietary Name Index;* and *U.S. Pharmaceutical Market, Drug Stores and Hospitals,* IMS America, Ltd.

Note: Sales of combinations containing new single entities introduced during this period and of new esters and salts of single entities introduced during this period are added to the sales of the new single chemical entity. Drugs withdrawn from the market are not included.

We can see in table 6-2 that individual companies, even among the ten leading firms, have few commercial successes. During the period 1962–68 Merck had only two NCE's whose sales in 1972 were sufficient to yield a return of 10 percent on the R & D investment; Pfizer, Roche, and Lilly each had only one.

In addition, the cost of R & D has increased, and the number of new drugs introduced per year has declined. In the latter part of the 1960s, R & D expenditures continued to be large, but the flow of new drugs fell off sharply. Part of the decline has been due to a more restrictive FDA policy after the 1962 drug amendments toward the introduction of new drugs. The reduced flow of new drugs may also have been due to a relatively larger share of the total R & D effort being devoted to areas of research which are intrinsically more difficult than the antibiotics, tranquilizers, and other fields which saw the earlier successes. Some of the investment in the 1960s was devoted to such areas as cardiovascular disease and arthritis, which continue to be difficult. These diseases are not well understood, and it is difficult to model the diseases in test animals. As we shall see later (in chapter 7), the expected return on investment in R & D has declined to a level which is below the expected return from alternative investments. Nevertheless, the industry continues to pursue the innovative strategy rather than the alternative.

This situation may change if the flow of new drugs remains small and if the opportunity for price competition expands as patents expire and as drugs which are not protected by patents begin to account for a larger proportion of total sales. After 1972 this segment of the market accounted for 35 percent of total sales (table 6-4). If we look at total prescriptions, the figure is even more striking: 44 percent after 1972 (table 6-5). A substantial part of the total

TABLE 6-4
Sales in 1972 of Leading Drugs Not Protected by
Patents after 1972, 1975, 1980

	Percentage
1972	35
1975	41
1980	69

Source: Sales data for individual products obtained from *U.S. Pharmaceutical Markets, Drug Stores and Hospitals,* IMS America, Ltd., 1972.

Note: Estimates based on dates of expirations of patents of 165 of 200 leading drugs by sales in 1972 for which dates could be obtained from Legal Division of Pfizer Inc. Drugs which have not been covered by patents are also included.

pharmaceutical market thus is now open to price competition, and this portion is growing. In fact, unless the number of new drugs introduced each year increases substantially, by 1980 a major part of the total market will be open to competition through imitation and reductions in prices. The figures reported in the tables do not permit a more precise estimate, since they assume no new drugs after 1972.

THERAPEUTIC FIELDS

The innovative strategy has resulted in the concentration of sales among firms within therapeutic classes. Much of the literature on the economics of the industry accepts the therapeutic classes as markets. The concentration thus has been taken as evidence of monopoly power. Before we can evaluate the sources of concentration by sales within therapeutic classes, it will be appropriate to discuss the concept of therapeutic classes.

Essentially we are interested in the problem of defining markets. Since this is a familiar problem in economics, we can be guided by economic theory. The market is defined as an area of competition. Within markets small price changes will result in the substitution of one product for another. By contrast, large price changes are required for substitution between products which are classified as belonging to different markets. Problems of classification arise when products are not homogeneous, and drugs are one such group. Even drugs which are prescribed for the same disease, and which therefore provide what is presumably similar therapy, are different in certain respects which may be important for particular patients and for some doctors. The problem may be particularly severe in the case of drugs because doctors are likely to be influenced more by differences in product characteristics than are consumers who purchase goods in other markets. Price to doctors is a secondary consideration. They are primarily

TABLE 6-5
Prescriptions in 1972 of Leading Drugs
Not Protected by Patents after 1972, 1975, 1980

	Percentage
1972	44
1975	51
1980	80

Source: Data on number of prescriptions by product obtained from *National Prescription Audit,* IMS America, Ltd., 1973.
Note: See table 6-4 concerning patent expirations.

concerned with therapeutic properties and with the possible risks of toxicity and other side effects. Thus even large price differences between drugs which provide essentially similar therapy may not influence demand if there are some differences in the therapeutic properties.

Nevertheless, drugs do compete. For the reasons just given, competition tends to focus on product characteristics rather than on price. When a new drug is introduced into a market, it will displace other drugs if it is therapeutically more effective or if it causes patients less discomfort. This becomes apparent when we examine the changes in prescribing patterns for various diseases. This examination also will illuminate the significance of the grouping of drugs into therapeutic classes. In general we would expect the drugs which provide similar therapy and which are grouped in the same therapeutic field to be closer substitutes than those which are classified in different therapeutic fields. The therapeutic fields therefore often are treated as though they are product markets.

But doctors can and do substitute a drug belonging to one therapeutic classification for another which is classified in another group. That this is so can best be seen from a discussion of the treatment of particular diseases. The following discussion concerns the treatment of angina pectoris, hypertension, and urinary tract infections.

However, before proceeding further with this discussion of competition between drugs classified in different therapeutic groups—competition which stresses product characteristics rather than price differences—we should note that chapter 12 shows that in some therapeutic classes, price competition has been severe among drugs offering similar therapy despite the apparent indifference of doctors to prices. As we shall see, pharmacists have substituted low-priced drugs for high-priced ones.

ANGINA PECTORIS. Angina pectoris, which is a pain associated with coronary artery disease, is caused by an inadequate supply of oxygen to the heart. The pain itself is a visceral sensation and is often described by patients as being heavy or dull. Attacks of angina are often precipitated by physical exertion or emotional stress. When physical exertion is the immediate cause, the pain becomes less severe if the patient rests. An attack often is dangerous and prompt treatment is mandatory.

Angina is treated by limiting the patient's exercise and by administering drugs, the most important of which are coronary vasodilators. Ataractics (tranquilizers) provide concomitant therapy to lower the risk of emotional upset. Basically, the organic nitrites and the organic nitrates are the two types of coronary vasodilators which are used.

The organic nitrates are the most frequently used drugs. This group can be broken down into the subgroups: short-acting and long-acting nitrates. Nitroglycerin is the only short-acting nitrate, and it is also the most popular. Reaction usually occurs within thirty seconds after the drug has been placed under the tongue. Other nitrates also are administered sublingually, but their action is not rapid. Isordil and Sorbitrate, for example, have sublingual dosage forms, but the onset of action is delayed for as long as ten minutes.

The long-acting nitrates have two disadvantages. First, difficulties in conducting clinical trials, including a high placebo response, raise questions concerning their effectiveness in preventing an attack. Secondly, repeated doses of long-acting nitrates build up a tolerance in the patient, and the therapeutic effect becomes weaker. By contrast, repeated usage of nitroglycerin does not reduce its efficacy. Recent studies have raised some doubts about the efficacy of another nitrate, PETN, and this has reduced the market share of the product Peritrate.

The problems in the use of the nitrates have led physicians to other drugs. Thus, the development of a sustained release dosage form has renewed the acceptance of papavarin by many physicians. This dosage form is much more convenient than the original dosage form, since it is taken only twice daily. The beta-adrenergic blocking agent, propranolol, which was recently approved for use in angina in the United States, has received recognition in other countries as an effective agent in reducing the number of attacks of angina. Diuretics and antihypertensives also are prescribed as concomitant therapy in hypertensive patients with angina. The control of the hypertension may relieve the angina.

In short, the treatment of angina pectoris usually requires the use of a coronary vasodilator from the subtherapeutic category of nitrates. Drugs from other therapeutic classes, including ataractics, diuretics, and antihypertensives, are also used in particular types of angina.

HYPERTENSION. The form of hypertension for which no recognizable cause can be ascertained is called "essential hypertension" and is the most common form of high blood pressure. Hypertension can also be due to renal or endocrine problems, some of which are surgically correctable. We will confine our remarks to essential hypertension.

Treatment such as weight reduction and limitation of salt intake is available.

But non-drug treatment usually is inadequate, and the physicians' options thus consist of using drugs from one or more of the following therapeutic classes: (1) rauwolfia-diuretics; (2) antihypertensives; (3) antihypertensive-diuretics; (4) rauwolfias; (5) diuretics; (6) sedatives-barbiturates; (7) ataractics.

The selection of a specific drug and course of therapy depends on both the severity of the hypertension and the patient's reaction. To demonstrate how the products in these therapeutic classes compete in the treatment of hypertension, we will follow a hypothetical case in which the mild form becomes progressively more severe and will note how specific drugs are added or substituted to achieve a satisfactory treatment.

The physician usually begins the pharmacologic treatment of mild essential hypertension with a thiazide diuretic. The initial lowering of blood pressure is probably the result of sodium depletion and the reduction in the volume of blood plasma. But since the plasma volume and the sodium level rise later in therapy, the continued antihypertensive effect of thiazide diuretics is thought to be largely due to lower peripheral blood vessel resistance.

One of the problems in the use of the thiazide diuretics is the resulting depletion of potassium. The physician has three alternative methods of dealing with this depletion depending on the severity of the potassium loss: (1) supplemental potassium, (2) potassium-rich foods, or (3) a combination of a thiazide and a potassium-sparing diuretic such as spironolactone or triamterene. The thiazide diuretic however, is necessary, since spironolactone and triamterene are not very effective as sole agents in the treatment of hypertension.

Another diuretic, furosemide, has increased its share of prescriptions for the treatment of hypertension. Furosemide is more potent than the thiazides and therefore requires less frequent administration. It also has the advantage of rapid onset of action and so necessitates less frequent urination.

If a diuretic alone is unsuccessful in reducing blood pressure, the physician may add reserpine to the regimen. He may simply add reserpine, or he may eliminate the diuretic and instead use a combination rauwolfia-diuretic, which usually is assigned to another therapeutic classification. The effect of reserpine on hypertension may be due partly to its weak tranquilizing effect. But since reserpine may bring about depression and peptic ulceration in some individuals, physicians do not usually prescribe reserpine as a tranquilizer. If they seek such an effect, they prescribe either sedatives or tranquilizers as adjunct agents.

Suppose now that our hypothetical patient's hypertension is moderate to severe, and that the previous efforts have not been particularly successful. The physician then will choose a course of therapy which employs more potent antihypertensives such as methyldopa, propanolol hydralazine, or guanethidine. These agents may be used alone or in combination with diuretics. These agents have more serious side effects than the less potent drugs used to treat mild hypertension. The physician tries to balance their therapeutic efficacy against their side effects and usually does so by adding a diuretic and lowering the dose of the hypertensive agent to achieve the desired response, while maintaining patient convenience.

Since the treatment of hypertension is likely to be necessary throughout the rest of a patient's life, successful therapy depends on a patient's cooperation and therefore on his convenience. Adjustments in therapy may also have to be made as tolerance develops or as side effects become unacceptable. The physician, therefore, must use a variety of drugs from several therapeutic classes to obtain maximum therapeutic efficacy. Moreover, some patients respond well to one drug, while others respond well to another. Thus there is no particular "best" drug for the treatment of high blood pressure. According to Dr. W. S. Peart, physicians treating hypertension should become accustomed to the actions and side effects of several drugs and use them selectively, exploiting each one to the limit of side effects before adding the adjunct or shifting to a new major drug. In the higher range of drug dosage, in which side effects increase, Dr. Peart encourages the use of several drugs. According to Dr. Peart, some patients do better on a alpha-methyldopa plus guanethidine plus chlorothiazide than on either of the main drugs alone.[2]

URINARY TRACT INFECTIONS. Urinary tract infections are caused by a variety of organisms. A large number of drugs in four therapeutic classes are appropriate to treat such infections. The specific choice of drug is frequently based on culturing the urine to determine the sensitivity of the infecting organisms. The most widely used category of drugs are the antibacterial agents, of which the most popular are the nitrofurantoins, methenamine mandelate, and nalidixic acid. The nitrofurantoins exert a bacteriostatic effect: they prevent the organism from growing. Methenamine mandelate has a similar effect: the formaldehyde which is released from the methenamine by low pH of the urine (due to the mandelic acid) inhibits bacterial multiplication. Nalidixic acid, which is well absorbed, stops the growth of bacteria by impeding the replication of bacterial genetic information.

The sulfonamides are the second most frequently prescribed drugs for urinary tract infections and have been successfully used for many years. The sulfonamides tend to have a similar therapeutic spectrum but vary in their solubility, absorption, and rate of excretion. Their mechanism of action is also bacteriostatic, and they have the advantage of a comparatively low cost. To achieve additional bacteriostasis, they are sometimes prescribed together with an azodye for acidification of the urine. These qualities have led the sulfonamide sulfisoxazole to be the most frequently used single drug for urinary tract infections.

The third most frequently employed agents are the broad and medium-spectrum antibiotics, among which the most widely used is tetracycline. Tetracycline and similar drugs are effective against a wide range of urinary tract pathogens with the exception of Proteus and Pseudomonas. These organisms are infrequent in new urinary tract infections, and since the tetracyclines are well absorbed orally and produce good urinary tract levels, they are desirable agents for this indication.

The fourth principal therapeutic group is the penicillins, the most popular of which is ampicillin. This drug is effective against a wide spectrum of bacteria, particularly gram-negative pathogens of the urinary tract. Ampicillin is excreted unchanged in the urine in high concentrations.

As these illustrations demonstrate, alternative drugs are available for the therapy of particular indications even when they are grouped into different therapeutic classes. They also indicate that the development of new drugs can lead to the displacement of previously used drugs.

We can also see the importance of product competition in the changes in prescribing patterns for individual diseases.

CHANGES IN PRESCRIPTION PATTERNS. We will rely on the data supplied by the National Disease & Therapeutic Index (NDTI), which is supplied by IMS. The data are collected from a sample of 1,500 physicians each quarter. The physicians record their diagnoses and the drugs prescribed. The number of visits to physicians and the number of prescriptions written for each drug are shown under each disease or indication. Consequently, we can determine the percentage of all visits resulting in a particular diagnosis for which doctors prescribed a particular drug.

The drugs which are prescribed for the treatment of anxiety reaction are classified frequently in three different therapeutic classes: minor tranquilizers, major tranquilizers, and sedatives. Sometimes the three classes are grouped together; at other times only the major and minor tranquilizers are grouped together. That there may be considerable overlapping among all three classes can be seen from the changes in the usage of drugs for the treatment of anxiety reaction. In 1963 the minor tranquilizers Librium and Equanil were widely used, but minor tranquilizers were not the only form of drug therapy. Stelazine, which is a major tranquilizer, was also prescribed, as was phenobarbital, which is a sedative. This pattern of prescribing may or may not indicate a high degree of substitution among the three classes of drugs; the distribution may reflect the imprecision of the diagnostic category "anxiety reaction," which may cover large differences in the severity of the disturbance. The uncertainty of diagnosis in such cases, however, may lead to some doctors preferring to use a minor rather than a major tranquilizer. In other words, the boundary line between appropriate uses of these drugs itself becomes imprecise.

That this is likely to have been the case is suggested by the change in the pattern of prescribing for anxiety reactions over the period of 1963–73. In 1973 the minor tranquilizers Valium, Librium, and Tranxene accounted for a majority of prescriptions. Mellaril was the only major tranquilizer among the four leading drugs prescribed in 1973 for this indication, and phenobarbital was no longer among the leading drugs.

The extent of the substitution within classes of drugs, of course, is much greater than between classes. Thus, in 1963 Librium and Equanil were the two minor tranquilizers among the four leading drugs used in the treatment of anxiety reaction. The data for 1973 reveal that by that year Valium had become very popular and had reduced the importance of Librium considerably. Equanil no longer was among the four leading drugs, and Tranxene had gained some importance.

Patients suffering from the indication "hypertensive heart disease" account for a large number of visits to doctors. In 1963 the leading antihypertensives prescribed included the generic drug reserpine, Rautrax N (a brand-name reserpine), and the rauwolfia-diuretic combination drugs Diupres and Hydropres. In 1973 the leading antihypertensives included Aldomet, a new type of antihypertensive; Aldoril, which combines Aldomet with a diuretic; Ser-Ap-Es, a triple combination drug including reserpine, another antihypertensive drug (hydralazine), and a diuretic; and Hydropres. Since 1963 many antihypertensive-diuretic combinations have been introduced, with the result that of the leading drugs of 1963, only one was still among the leaders in 1973.

Marked changes have also taken place in the treatment of various forms of arthritis, another group of prevalent diseases. We will look specifically at the drugs prescribed for the treatment of rheumatoid arthritis and osteoarthritis. In 1963 the four leading drugs for the treatment of rheumatoid arthritis accounted for only 25 percent of the total number of prescriptions. These drugs were prednisone, Butazolidin, Decadron, and Medrol. Three out of these four drugs were corticoids. By 1973 sales had become much more concentrated, with the leading four drugs accounting for 59 percent of total sales. Of the leading four drugs in 1963, only prednisone remained among the leaders in 1973. Myochrydine, Indocin, and Solganal had displaced the other leading drugs of 1963. In 1963 the leading drugs for treatment of osteoarthritis were Butazolidin, Tandearil, generic prednisolone, Hydeltra-TBA, and Aristocort. These drugs accounted for 31 percent of prescriptions. In 1973 the new drug Indocin alone accounted for 40 percent of all such prescriptions. Butazolidin still was among the leading four drugs, but the other three drugs which had been popular in 1963 no longer were among the leading drugs in 1973.

Sharp shifts also took place in the treatment of gastritis and duodenitis. In 1973 the four leading drugs accounted for 47 percent of total prescriptions, compared to 35 percent in 1963. The four leaders were the same drugs but the fact that their share increased so markedly indicates a shift away from other drugs. In addition, the increase in the share obtained by Librax was much larger than that obtained by the other leading drugs: Librax more than doubled its share.

Similarly, large changes are observed in prescribing for bronchopneumonia and influenza pneumonia. Ampicillin displaced penicillin as the leading drug in the treatment of the former. The only drug which remained among the four leaders over this period was penicillin G. None of the four leading drugs for the treatment of influenza pneumonia in 1963 were among the leaders in 1973. The four leaders in 1973 included Keflex, Vibramycin, and Cleocin, none of which had been introduced in 1963.

TABLE 6-6
Percentage of Office Visits, by Indication, Resulting in
Mentions of Specified Leading Drugs, 1963 and 1973

Indication	Drug	Therapeutic Field	Percentage
Anxiety Reaction			
1963	Librium	Minor tranquilizer	28
	Stelazine	Major tranquilizer	9
	Phenobarbital	Sedative	7
	Equanil	Minor tranquilizer	7
Total			51
1973	Valium	Minor tranquilizer	37
	Librium	"	14
	Mellaril	Major tranquilizer	4
	Tranxene	Minor tranquilizer	4
Total			59
Rheumatoid arthritis			
1963	Prednisone	Corticoid	9
	Butazolidin	Antiarthritic	6
	Decadron	Corticoid	5
	Medrol	"	5
Total			25
1973	Myochrysine	Corticoid	19
	Indocin	Antiarthritic	17
	Prednisone	Corticoid	16
	Solganal	Antiarthritic	7
Total			59
Osteoarthritis			
1963	Butazolidin	Antiarthritics	13
	Tandearil	Antiarthritics	8
	Prednisolone (generic)	Corticoid	5
	Hydeltra TBA or Aristocort	Corticoid	5
Total			31
1973	Indocin	Antiarthritic	40
	Butazolidin Alka	"	12
	Butazolidin	"	6
	Depo-Medrol	Corticoid	4
Total			62

TABLE 6-6 (continued)

Indication	Drug	Therapeutic Field	Percentage
Gastritis & duodenitis			
1963	Donnatal	Antispasm + Anticholinergics	20
	Pro-Banthine	"	6
	Librax	"	5
	Combid	"	4
Total			35
1973	Donnatal	Antispasmodics + Anticholinergics	23
	Librax	"	13
	Pro-Banthine	"	6
	Combid	"	5
Total			47
Bronchopneumonia			
1963	Penicillin G	Penicillin	21
	Declomycin	Broad & Medium	9
	Chloromycetin	Broad & Medium	8
	Terramycin	"	8
Total			46
1973	Ampicillin	Penicillin	18
	Penicillin G	"	10
	Tetracycline	Broad & Medium	7
	V-Cillin K	Penicillin	4
Total			39
Influenza pneumonia			
1963	Penicillin G	Penicillin	27
	Terramycin	Broad & Medium	23
	Penicillin-Streptomycin	Penicillin comb.	10
	Ilosone	Broad & Medium	10
Total			70
1973	Tetracycline	Broad & Medium	30
	Keflex	"	14
	Vibramycin	"	10
	Cleocin	"	8
Total			62
Hypertensive heart disease (Hypotensives)			
1963	Reserpine	Rauwolfia	10
	Diupres	Rauwolfia comb.	10
	Hydropres	"	9
	Rautrax N	Rauwolfia	8
Total			37
1973	Aldomet	Other hypotensive	19
	Aldoril	Hypotensive comb.	11
	Ser-Ap-Es	Rauwolfia comb.	10
	Hydropres	"	8
Total			48

TABLE 6-6 (continued)

Indication	Drug	Therapeutic Field	Percentage
(Diuretics)			
1963	Diuril	Diuretic	24
	Hydrodiuril	"	22
	Renese	"	9
	Mercuhydrin	"	6
Total			61
1973	Lasix	Diuretic	22
	Hydrodiuril	"	15
	Aldactazide	"	12
	Diazide	"	11
Total			60
Streptococcal sore throat			
1963	Penicillin G	Penicillin	29
	Pentids	"	8
	V-Cillin K	"	7
	Penicillin-G Procaine	"	7
Total			51
1973	Penicillin G	Penicillin	17
	V-Cillin K	"	9
	Pentids	"	8
	Penicillin VK	"	7
Total			41

Source: National Disease and Therapeutic Index, Reference File, Diagnosis, IMS America Ltd., 1963, 1973.

Note: The drugs listed in this table for a given indication are those with the same therapeutic goal (e.g., relief of inflammation). Other drugs prescribed for the same disease which have other therapeutic goals (e.g., analgesia), are not shown. And, of course, they are therefore not included in the total number of prescriptions which is used for computing the percentage. The title refers to "mentions," which include, in addition to written prescriptions, telephone orders for drugs and drugs dispensed by physicians.

This discussion of changes in prescribing practices suggests that the evidence of a high degree of concentration in therapeutic markets has little significance for the analysis of the competitive behavior of pharmaceutical firms. The development of new drugs, as we have seen, has resulted in the displacement of established drugs.

A commonly used measure of the degree of monopoly power is the concentration ratio, which is the percentage of total sales in a market supplied by some small number of sellers. Thus if the four leading firms control a large portion of the total sales in the market, economists will suspect that the four firms can and do maintain prices at a level which is above that which would prevail under conditions of competition. This line of reasoning is reflected in the frequent discussion of the degree of concentration of sales among pharmaceutical firms within the therapeutic classes. These therapeutic classes, which are constructed by market research firms for the analysis of changes in the distribution of sales among competing products, are taken to be economic markets.

The usual problems in defining markets are encountered in classifying drugs. Different observers use different definitions which are more or less inclusive. Thus, as we mentioned, minor tranquilizers are sometimes grouped together with major tranquilizers. On the other hand, they are sometimes classified separately. Some analysts would use a group which included sedatives as well as both major and minor tranquilizers.

Similar problems are encountered in the classification of antibiotics. The broadest group—the anti-infectives—includes sulfonamides, penicillins, and broad- and medium-spectrum antibiotics. For most purposes however, market research analysts find it convenient to work with narrower groupings. Thus, tetracyclines are frequently distinguished from penicillins. In fact, the different generic classes of penicillin are analyzed separately. Market analysts will look closely at trends in sales of different brands of penicillin VK, and similarly for ampicillin, penicillin G, and the cephalosporins. The narrower the definition of the group, the greater is the possibility of substitution among the products. We can expect that a reduction in the price of a particular drug will have a greater effect on the sales of drugs in the same generic class than on other drugs within any broader classification. This also holds for increases in promotional expenses. On the other hand, price reductions which are initially limited to a particular generic class may spread to other generic classes which provide similar therapy. Indeed they may spread beyond therapeutic classes as frequently defined. The price reductions in both tetracyclines and in ampicillins in the 1960s indicate that there were substitutions between these groups and that price was a factor.[3]

The boundaries between therapeutic classes of drugs break down after the introduction of important new drugs. Apparent boundaries marking off groups of substitute drugs become less significant in the face of such developments. Thus when new drugs are introduced, they frequently displace drugs which are assigned to other therapeutic classes. We have seen that Valium displaced phenobarbital and Stelazine in the treatment of anxiety reactions. Synthetic penicillins have displaced nonsynthetic penicillins and tetracyclines. New antihypertensives have displaced rauwolfias. In addition, we have seen that rauwolfia-diuretics have tended to displace rauwolfias which are not components of combination drugs. Indocin has displaced corticoids and ACTH-corticoids in the treatment of rheumatoid arthritis.

Thus, the concentration ratio of sales of therapeutic classes is likely to be an unreliable measure of monopoly power owing to substitution between therapeutic classes and the displacement of established drugs by new drugs whether they are inside or outside the same therapeutic class.

CONCENTRATION OF RESEARCH EFFORT
AMONG FIRMS WITHIN THERAPEUTIC FIELDS

The uncertainty of success in pharmaceutical research has led the large manufacturers to seek some protection against the possibility of total failure by distributing their efforts among many projects in different therapeutic fields. The description of pharmaceutical research in chapter 3 indicated another reason for the dispersion of research effort among some, if not all, fields. Each laboratory must maintain some competence in several fields in order to be able to conduct the animal screening tests for possible side effects in fields other than the primary one for a proposed drug. The number of patents issued to each of the ten leading firms within each therapeutic field provides one measure of the distribution of these firms' efforts. Questions have been raised as to the validity of using the number of patents as a measure of research effort, but these objections concern differences between various firms' propensities to patent inventions rather than the validity of this measure for assessing the distribution of a given firm's efforts. Table 6-7 reports the number and percent of patents issued to each of the ten leading firms in each therapeutic field in the years 1965–70. The data show that the individual firms distributed their efforts widely.

The consequence is that a substantial number of firms are engaged in research in the major therapeutic fields. Table 6-8 reports the number of companies which obtained ten or more patents in each of the therapeutic fields during the period 1965–70. For this purpose the number of patents can be used to identify the firms which have substantial programs; we are concerned not with the relative research effort of different firms, but with the number of firms which conduct programs. These numbers, however, understate the total number of firms doing research in each field, since they are limited to those with ten or more patents. This limitation is intended to indicate the number of firms which had substantial research programs. We can see that in the therapeutic classes which have large sales, the number of active firms is large: antibiotics, antiparistics, antibacterials, hypotensives, tranquilizers and sedatives, stimulants and antidepressants, analgesics, anti-inflammatories and antipyretics, and estrogens, androgens, and progesterones.

In addition, the industry includes many firms which make large R & D expenditures.[4] Twenty firms spent more than $10 million on R & D in 1971. PMA data also reveal that twenty leading firms account for only 55 percent of total R & D expenditures.[5] These observations suggest that research effort in therapeutic markets is not concentrated among a few firms.

On the other hand, there are numerous therapeutic markets. The number varies depending on the classification used. But most classifications list a large number (table 6-7 shows thirty-two therapeutic fields). The therapeutic fields

TABLE 6-7

Number and Percentage of U.S. Patents by Therapeutic Fields Issued in 1965–70 to Each of the Ten Leading Pharmaceutical Firms

Therapeutic Field	American Home Products		Lilly		Hoffman LaRoche		Merck		Bristol Myers		Pfizer		Johnson & Johnson		Abbott		SmithKline & French		Upjohn	
	No.	%	No.	%	No.	%	No.	%	No.	%	No.	%	No.	%	No.	%	No.	%	No.	%
Anti-infective																				
Antibiotic	15	2.4	65	21.2	9	1.7	31	3.5	24	13.9	26	9.4			9	6.1	2	0.8	53	12.2
Antifungal[a]	30	4.9	30	9.8	30	5.5	86	9.6			27	9.7			6	4.1	13	5.4	21	4.8
Antibacterial	49	8.0	4	1.3	32	5.9	63	7.0	49	28.3	36	12.9			21	14.3	5	2.1	38	8.8
Antiviral	9	1.5	8	2.6	2	0.4	12	1.3			3	1.1			2	1.4	23	9.5	11	2.5
Cardiovascular																				
Vasoactive	3	0.5			1	0.2	1	0.1	1	0.6	7	2.5			2	1.4				
Hypotensive	20	3.3	9	2.9	30	5.5	19	2.1	3	1.7	14	5.0			3	2.0	21	8.7	5	1.2
Antianginal	1	0.2									2	0.7			2	1.4				
Cardiotonic	4	0.7																		
Antiarrhythmic	1	0.2	2	0.7			13	1.5												
Blood																				
Coagulation agents							5	0.6			5	1.8			14	9.5				
Hypolipemic	11	1.8	1	0.3	3	0.6	12	1.3	5	2.9	4	1.4					3	1.2	14	3.2
Hypoglycemic	4	0.7	8	2.6	13	2.4	4	0.4			4	1.4							5	1.2
Neurological																				
Tranquilizers and sedatives	97	15.8	10	3.3	44	8.1	11	1.2	10	5.8	1	0.4	1	2.0	9	6.1	38	15.7	27	6.2
CNS stimulants	45	7.3	2	0.7	22	4.1	13	1.5	5	2.9	7	2.5	2	3.9	10	6.8	22	9.1	19	4.4
Anticonvulsant	30	4.9			37	6.8													6	1.4

Category	No.	%	No.	%	No.	%	No.	%	No.	%	No.	%	No.	%	No.	%	No.	%	No.	%
Anesthetic	2	0.3															10	4.1		
Analgesic	19	3.1			9	1.7	10	1.1	16	9.2									34	7.8
Hormones																				
Prostaglandin			1	0.3													1	0.4	1	0.2
Corticosteroid	87	14.2	11	3.6	61	11.2	35	3.9	6	3.5							14	5.8	29	6.7
Estrogen, progestogen, androgen													19	37.3						
Other hormones			1	0.3	1	0.2	2	0.2							1	0.7				
Other																				
Antihistamine	9	1.5			5	0.9					3	1.1			1	0.7	3	1.2		
Bronchodilator	44	7.2							1	0.6	6	2.2					7	2.9		
Anti-inflammatory, antipyretic			11	3.6	4	0.7	128	14.3	9	5.2	15	5.4			12	8.2	15	6.2	22	5.1
Immunosuppressant	10	1.6	3	1.0											2	1.4				
Vaccines	4	0.7					9	1.0	1	0.6	1	0.4								
Anticancer	2	0.3	9	2.9	5	0.9	4	0.4	1	0.6	8	2.9							14	3.2
Anorexic	7	1.1			3	0.5	2	0.2	1	0.6	1	0.4					5	2.1	5	1.2
Gastrointestinal	5	0.8			4	0.7	7	0.8	4	2.3					4	2.7	13	5.4	4	0.9
Diuretic	3	0.5					72	8.0	1	0.6	2	0.7					8	3.3	2	0.5
Muscle Agents	1	0.2			1	0.2	3	0.3												
Miscellaneous[b]	99	16.1	131	42.8	227	41.8	352	39.2	37	21.4	106	38.1	29	56.9	37	25.2	39	16.1	124	28.6
Total	615	100.5	306	99.4	543	100.0	896	99.8	173	100.1	278	100.0	51	100.1	147	100.1	242	99.9	434	100.1

Source: *Derwent Central Patent Index*, prepared by Derwent Information Service, England. Patents are listed the first time they are granted in one of the following countries: U.S., Great Britain, Netherlands, Belgium, France, South Africa, Canada, West Germany, East Germany, Japan, Switzerland, and the Soviet Union. Patents are for pharmaceutical compounds and processes primarily. Each patent is counted only once and listed with the first use given.

Note: Ten leading firms determined by 1973 U.S. sales.

aIncludes antiprotozoal, antimalarial, and antiparasitic agents.

bMiscellaneous includes minor therapeutic categories not listed above and processes and diagnostic tests.

TABLE 6-8
Number of Companies Obtaining Ten or More Patents
in Each Therapeutic Class between 1965 and 1970

Therapeutic field	Number of companies	Therapeutic field	Number of companies
Anti-infectives		Hormones	
Antibiotics	9	Prostaglandins	1
Antiparisitic	11	Corticosteroids	1
Antibacterial	15	Estrogens, androgens,	15
Antiviral	6	progesterones	
Cardiovascular		Other hormones	0
Vasoactive	1	Other	
Hypotensives	7	Antihistamines	1
Antianginal	1	Bronchodilators	0
Cardiotonic	0	Anti-inflammatory	15
Antiarrythmic	2	and antipyretic	
Blood		Immunosuppressants	1
Coagulants and anticoagulants	1	Anticancer	2
Hypolipemic	6	Vaccines	0
Hypoglycemic	3	Gastrointestinal	3
Neurological		Anorexic	1
Tranquilizers and sedatives	13	Diuretic	2
Stimulants and antidepressants	10	Muscle Relaxants	0
Anticonvulsants	3		
Anesthetics	0		
Analgesics	9		

Source: Derwent Central Patent Index, prepared by Derwent Information Service, England. Patents are listed the first time they are granted in one of the following countries: U.S., Great Britain, Netherlands, Belgium, France, South Africa, Canada, West Germany, East Germany, Japan, Switzerland, and the Soviet Union. Patents are for pharmaceutical compounds and processes primarily. Each patent is counted only once and listed with the first use given.

having small sales will have a high degree of concentration of research effort. We can also see, in table 6-9, that patents issued in the period 1965–70 are concentrated among a few firms; this is true even in fields where a substantial number of companies are engaged in research, as indicated by the number of companies receiving ten or more patents (table 6-8). The concentration of patents was large even in such fields as antiparisitics, antibiotics, tranquilizers and sedatives, stimulants and antidepressants, and in anti-inflammatory drugs. The data on concentration suggest that the distribution of research effort among companies within fields was highly unequal.

CONCENTRATION OF SALES OF INDIVIDUAL COMPANIES AMONG PRODUCTS

Another factor contributing to the concentration of sales in each therapeutic field among a few firms is that few drugs win large sales. We will look first at the

TABLE 6-9
The Percentage of Patents Issued to Four Leading
Firms by Number of Patents within Therapeutic
Classes, 1965–70

Therapeutic field	Percent	Therapeutic field	Percent
Anti-infectives		Hormones	
Antibiotics	53	Prostaglandins	94
Antiparisitic and antifungal	52	Corticosteroids	50
Antibacterial	49	Estrogens, Angrogens	48
Antiviral	46	and Progesterons	
Cardiovascular		Other hormones	0
Vasoactive	57	Other	
Hypotensives	62	Antihistamines	26
Antianginal	78	Bronchodilators	0
Cardiotonic	0	Anti-inflammatory	56
Antiarrythmic	55	Immunosuppressants	48
Blood		Vaccines	0
Coagulants and anticoagulants	38	Anticancer	44
Hypolipemic	58	Anorexic	30
Hypoglycemic	59	Gastrointestinal	42
Neurological		Diuretic	63
Tranquilizers and sedatives	70	Muscle Relaxants	0
Stimulants and antidepressants	56		
Anticonvulsants	69		
Anesthetics	0		
Analgesics	54		

Source: See table 6-8.

concentration of sales by a company among products. Each company, even among the large ones, will have few large-selling drugs. We have already seen that only a few large sellers were introduced in the years 1963–70, and no company introduced more than two drugs which obtained sales greater than $10 million in 1972 (table 6-2).

Each of the large pharmaceutical manufacturers therefore depends on a small number of its products for the major part of its sales. This can be seen in table 6-10, where we show the products which accounted for 50 percent of the sales of leading manufacturers. In 1960 Lilly sales were concentrated in Ilosone, V-Cillin-K, Darvon, NPH Iletin, Trinsicon, and Micebrin. Four products made up over 50 percent of SKF's sales, and three products accounted for more than half of Parke Davis's and Lederle's sales. No company required more than eight products to account for 50 percent of its total sales.

This concentration of sales in a few products has exposed each company to the danger of losing a large part of its sales to rivals' new products. The existence of substantial product rivalry is revealed by the shifts in the distribution of each company's sales among different products. Thus, as table 6-10 shows, the leading products of each company in 1960 generally accounted for a much smaller proportion in 1973. In some cases the decline in the percentage was due to the development of other drugs, which in 1973 accounted for a large part of total sales, rather than the decline in sales of the leading drugs of 1960. In absolute terms, the sales of the leading products of 1960 in Lilly's case increased greatly over the intervening years. The decline in the percentage of total sales represented by these drugs obviously was due to the introduction and development of new drugs since 1960 (table 6-11). By contrast, the absolute sales of the leading drugs of Parke Davis declined sharply, as did those of SKF and Lederle. Even though the important drugs of 1960 may not have become obsolete due to the development of new drugs or because of information about side effects (as in the case of Chloromycetin, Parke Davis' product), the possibility of these developments was sufficiently strong to provide inducement to the pharmaceutical manufacturers to continue their research efforts.

TABLE 6-10
Sales in 1960 and 1973 of Products Comprising 50 Percent of Firm Sales in 1960

	Sales			
	$(000) 1960	Percent 1960	$(000) 1973	Percent 1973
Lilly				
Ilosone/Ilotycin	21,505	15.6	26,035	·6.8
All Darvons	15,543	11.3	82,289	21.4
All Iletins	14,930	10.9	27,969	7.3
V-Cillin/V-Cillin-K	10,406	7.6	22,765	5.9
Trinsicon/Trinsicon M	5,923	4.3	3,933	1.0
Total	68,307	49.7	162,991	42.4
Upjohn				
Orinase	25,711	20.4	31,493	16.8
Medrol/Sol Medrol/Depo Medrol	14,262	11.3	24,687	13.2
Panalba	14,179	11.3	a	a
All Unicaps	12,745	10.1	10,586	5.6
Total	66,897	53.1	66,766	35.6
Parke Davis				
Chloromycetin	52,501	44.7	7,172	7.4
Myadec	5,412	4.6	8,483	6.3
Dilantin	4,011	3.4	15,797	11.8
Total	61,924	52.7	31,452	25.5
SmithKline & French				
Thorazine	20,595	17.5	22,816	14.1
Dexamyl/Dexadrine	26,932	22.9	6,945	4.3
Compazine	17,862	15.2	12,279	7.6
Total	65,389	55.6	42,040	26.0
American Home Products				
Equanil/Equagesic/Equanitrate	32,413	27.8	25,097	7.5
Premarin	9,581	8.2	48,155	14.5
Sparine	8,255	7.1	3,686	1.1
Bicillin	7,298	6.3	6,511	2.0
All Phenergans	7,160	6.1	22,571	6.8
Total	64,707	55.5	106,067	31.9
Lederle				
Achromycin/Achromycin V/ Achrocidin	43,827	38.0	9,600	9.4

TABLE 6-10 (continued)

	$(000) 1960	Percent 1960	$(000) 1973	Percent 1973
		Sales		
Declomycin/Declostatin	27,528	23.9	8,619	8.5
Total	71,355	61.9	18,219	17.9
Merck				
Diuril/Diupres	23,768	24.0	23,307	7.7
Hydrodiuril/Hydrodiuril NA/ Hydropres	14,532	14.7	35,648	11.8
All Decadrons and Neodecadrons	13,838	14.0	19,531	6.5
Tetrazets	2,175	2.2	1	b
Total	54,313	54.9	78,217	26.0
Squibb				
Rauzide/Raudixin/Rautrax N/ Rautrax	11,370	13.3	12,740	7.2
Mysteclin V/Mysteclin F	10,210	11.9	7,397	4.2
All Theragrans	9,223	10.8	21,733	12.2
Pentids	6,970	8.2	8,268	4.6
Kenalog/Kenacort	4,003	4.7	12,401	7.0
Naturetin K	3,113	3.6	2,080	1.2
Sumycin	2,636	3.1	10,568	5.9
Total	47,525	55.6	75,447	42.3
Abbott (& Ross)				
All Similacs	9,894	12.5	25,585	12.9
All Vidaylins	6,439	8.1	3,842	1.9
Dextrose 5 percent in water	6,201	7.8	8,371	4.2
Sucaryl	5,733	7.2	1,031	0.5
Erythrocin	4,699	5.9	25,287	12.7
Compocillin	3,880	4.9	3,309	1.7
Nembutal	3,698	4.7	3,520	1.8
Pentothal Sodium	2,928	3.7	3,483	1.8
Total	43,472	54.8	74,428	37.5
Pfizer (& Roerig)				
Terramycin/Terrastatin	14,888	22.7	12,054	6.4
Cosa Tetracyn	6,686[c]	10.2	2,143[c]	1.1
Diabinese	4,094	6.2	28,381	15.1
Atarax	3,414	5.1	6,065	3.2
Vistaril	2,919	4.4	18,733	10.0
TAO	2,792	4.2	1,548	0.8
Signemycin	2,637	4.0	d	d
Total	37,430	56.8	68,924	36.6

Source: U.S. Pharmaceutical Market, Drug Stores and Hospitals, 1960, 1973, IMS America, Ltd.

Note: Sales drawn from the ten leading firms (by sales) in 1960. Sales of salts, esters, various dosage forms, and combinations of the primary chemical entity in these products have been combined with the sales of the leading form of the drug.

[a]Withdrawn from the market.

[b]Sales loss of 0.1 percent.

[c]Cosa Tetracyn and Tetracyn in 1960; in 1973 Tetracyn only because Cosa Tetracyn was discontinued.

[d]Discontinued.

TABLE 6-11
Sales in 1973 and 1960 of Products Comprising 50 Percent of Firm Sales in 1973

	Sales			
	$(000) 1973	Percent 1973	$(000) 1960	Percent 1960
Lilly				
All Darvons	82,289	21.4	15,543	11.3
Keflin	68,587	17.8	*	*
Keflex	49,052	12.7	*	*
Total	199,928	51.9	15,543	11.3
Upjohn				
Cleocin	31,530	16.8	*	*
Orinase	31,493	16.8	25,711	20.4
Sol Medrol/Medrol/Depo Medrol	24,687	13.2	13,741	10.9
Tolinase	11,269	6.0	*	*
Total	98,979	52.8	39,452	31.3
Parke Davis				
Dilantin	15,797	11.8	4,011	3.4
Norlestrin	14,052	10.4	*	*
Myadec	8,483	6.3	5,412	4.6
Chloromycetin	7,172	5.4	52,501	4.5
Amcill	6,513	4.9	*	*
Benadryl	9,481	7.1	4,493	3.8
Benalin expectorant	5,238	3.9	1,437	1.2
Fluogen	4,653	3.5	*	*
Total	71,389	53.3	67,854	17.5
SmithKline & French				
Stelazine	21,275	13.1	8,943	7.6
Thorazine	22,816	14.1	20,595	17.5
Dyazide	19,886	12.3	*	*
Ornade	14,148	8.7	2,700	2.3
Combid	12,365	7.6	6,256	5.3
Total	90,490	55.8	38,494	32.7
American Home Products				
Premarin	48,155	14.6	9,581	8.2
Ovral	35,687	10.7	*	*
Atromid S	20,108	6.0	*	*
Isordil	18,349	5.5	221	0.2
Fluothane	17,220	5.2	2,595	2.2
Equanil/Equagesic/Equanitrate	25,097	7.5	32,413	27.8
Inderal	14,511	4.4	*	*
Total	179,523	53.9	44,810	38.4
Lederle				
Aristocort/Aristocort Forte/ Aristoderm	12,283	12.1	10,520	9.1
Achromycin/Achromycin V/ Achrocidin	9,600	9.4	43,827	38.0
Minocin	9,164	9.0	*	*
Mycin/Declostatin	8,619	8.5	27,528	23.9
Diamox	6,995	6.9	3,744	3.2
Pathibamate	5,947	5.9	3,965	3.4
Total	52,608	51.8	89,584	77.6
Merck				
Indocin	45,132	14.9	*	*

TABLE 6-11 (continued)

	Sales			
	$(000) 1973	Percent 1973	$(000) 1960	Percent 1960
Aldomet	43,912	14.5	*	*
Triavil	31,954	10.6	*	*
Aldoril/Aldochlor	27,828	9.2	*	*
Elavil	26,581	8.8	*	*
Total	175,407	58.0	0	0
Squibb				
Mycolog, Kenalog, Kenacant, and Mycostatin[a]	41,797	23.4	6,711	7.9
All Theragrans	21,733	12.2	9,223	10.8
Principen	11,809	6.6	*	*
Sumycin	10,568	5.9	2,636	3.1
Pentids	8,268	4.6	6,970	8.2
Total	93,093	52.7	25,540	30.0
Abbott (& Ross)				
All Similacs	25,585	12.9	9,894	12.5
Erythrocin	25,287	12.8	4,699	5.9
Dextrose in water	8,371	4.2	6,201	7.8
Surbex T/Surbex/Surbex WC	8,224	4.1	1,922	2.4
Selsun Blue/Selsun	7,581	3.8	1,811	2.3
Tranxene	7,000	3.5	*	*
Enduronyl/Enduronyl Fate	5,884	3.0	*	*
Placidyl	4,383	2.2	1,167	1.5
Total	99,537	46.5	25,694	32.4
Pfizer (& Roerig)				
Vibramycin	28,653	15.2	*	*
Diabinese	28,381	15.1	4,094	6.2
Sinequan	18,896	10.0	*	*
Vistaril	18,733	10.0	2,919	4.4
Total	94,663	50.3	7,013	10.6

Source: See table 6-10 for source and note on selection of drugs.
Note: The ten firms which led in sales in 1960 are those shown in this table.
*Product not available in 1960.
[a]The active ingredient of Kenalog is triamcinolone acetonide, and that of Mycostatin is mystatin. Mycolog contains both active ingredients.

CONCENTRATION OF SALES IN THERAPEUTIC FIELDS

Important new drugs displace the earlier drugs in the same therapeutic fields or they open up new therapeutic fields. At any time, therefore, a therapeutic field is usually dominated by a few products. Another factor which contributes to the high degree of concentration in sales among brands within therapeutic fields is the large number of therapeutic fields. Manufacturers' ethical sales as a whole amounted to only $5 billion in 1973, and the total number of therapeutic fields was as many as thirty-two, according to our classification. The sales of antibiotics and tranquilizers amounted to 12.3 percent and 11.2 percent of the total, respectively, because of the wide range of illnesses that can be treated by such drugs. But the demand for drugs in most therapeutic classes is small.

As can be seen in table 6-12, the five leading analgesics in 1973 accounted for 59.6 percent of total sales in that therapeutic category. Among penicillins the percentage was 41.9 percent; among diuretics, 76.3 percent; oral ataractics, 72.6 percent; broad and medium spectrum antiobiotics, 50.7 percent. We can also see that concentration has been the result of innovative competition in the data showing shifts in the distribution of sales among drugs. If we look at the data for oral diuretics (table 6-12), we can see that two of the five leading drugs in 1973 had not been introduced in 1960. Among broad and medium antibiotics, four of the five leading drugs in 1973 had not yet been introduced in 1960. Looking at the five leading oral diuretics in 1960 (table 6-13), we can see that their share dropped from 85.8 percent of diuretic sales to 30.8 percent in 1973. The five leading broad- and medium-spectrum antibiotics of 1960 accounted for 73.5 percent of sales in that year and only 12.9 percent in 1973. Similar patterns can be seen in other therapeutic fields.

Because innovative competition has led to a situation in many therapeutic classes in which a few products have a large share of sales, individual companies also have large market shares of sales in these fields. The pharmaceutical manufacturers which were successful in their efforts to develop important new products obtained large sales. Thus, Merck's development of Indocin resulted in the company winning a large share of the sales of antiarthritics (table 6-14). Hoechst achieved a large share of the diuretic market after it introduced Lasix. Lilly rapidly obtained a large share of the broad- and medium-spectrum market after it introduced its new line of cephalosporin products. Roche had similar success in the ataractic field with its new product Valium.

Table 6-15 shows the converse effect of product competition on market sales of individual companies. The shares of leading companies in 1960 were smaller in 1973. Lederle declined from 32.2 percent of sale of broad- and medium-spectrum antibiotics to 7.0 percent; SmithKline and French from 31.6 percent of sales of oral ataractics to 9.2 percent; Merck from 61.5 percent of sale of oral diuretics to 22.4 percent. Occasionally this pattern was reversed: Lilly's share of penicillin sales grew from 13.1 percent to 21.0 percent, and its share of analgesics grew from 12.9 percent to 32.3 percent. But in general the shares of leading firms declined.

The concentration of sales of many therapeutic classes in the hands of a few firms reflects successes of individual products and companies in innovative competition. These are the winners in a competitive struggle to gain the favor of doctors. The discussion of the significance of this concentration has been so limited to its apparent consequence for monopoly power that scholars have overlooked the fact that innovative success is the source of the concentration. Nor should it be overlooked that the concentration of sales reflects the public policy of encouraging innovation through the grant of patents. Public policy thus has had the intended effect of inducing innovation by offering to protect

TABLE 6-12
Leading Products in 1973 and Their Percentage of Sales in 1973 and 1960,
by Therapeutic Class

	% of Sales in 1973	% of Sales in 1960		% of Sales in 1973	% of Sales in 1960
Total antibiotics			Butazolidin/	19.5	47.0
Keflin	10.9	*	Butazoldin alka		
Keflex	7.8	*	Zyloprim	15.2	*
Garamycin	6.4	*	Benemid/	9.8	11.2
Vibramycin	4.6	*	Col Benemid		
Erythrocin	4.0	1.5	Tandearil	6.5	*
Total	33.7	1.5	Total	93.0	58.2
Broad- and medium-			Antihistamines		
spectrum antibiotics			Benadryl	23.9	17.9
Keflin	16.4	*	Chlortrimetron	21.3	21.7
Keflex	11.7	*	Teldrin	14.3	14.7
Garamycin	9.6	*	Dimetane[b]	9.0	7.6
Vibramycin	6.9	*	Polaramine	7.3	6.2
Erythrocin	6.1	2.1	Total	75.8	68.1
Total	50.7	2.1	Analgesics, ethical systemic		
Penicillins			All Darvons	30.8	11.3
V-Cillin K/	12.7	16.1	Tylenol	8.2	0.4
V-Cillin			All Empirins	7.9	9.2
Polycillin/	12.6	*	Talwin	7.8	*
Polycillin N			Percodan/	4.9	3.1
Principen/	6.4	*	Percobarb		
Principen N			Total	59.6	24.0
Omnipen/	5.7	*	Psychostimulants		
Omnipen N			Elavil	34.0	*
Pentids	4.6	11.8	Tofranil	25.6	28.0
Total	41.9	27.9	Ritalin	14.9	10.1
Oral Ataractics			Norpramin	6.4	*
Valium	40.8	*	Deprol	4.9	*
Librium/	14.2	12.1	Total	85.8	38.1
Libritabs			Oral hypoglycemics		
Mellaril	7.6	2.4	Orinase	31.1	82.7
Triavil	6.0	*	Diabinese	28.0	13.2
Stelazine	4.0	6.7	DBI-TD[c]	22.6	4.1
Total	72.6	21.2	Tolinase	11.1	*
Oral diuretics			Dymelor	4.8	*
Lasix	22.2	*	Total	97.6	100.0
Aldactone[a]	20.3	12.1	Sedatives		
Hydrodiuril	13.0	22.2	Dalmane	16.7	*
Dyazide/Dyrenium	12.0	*	Butisol	11.7	15.4
Diuril	8.8	39.3	Doriden[d]	10.8	12.1
Total	76.3	73.6	Placidyl	7.2	3.2
Antiarthritics			Quaalude	6.2	—
Indocin	42.0	*	Total	52.6	30.7

Source: See table 6-10 for source and note on selection of drugs.

*Product not available in 1960.

[a]Plus Aldactazide.

[b]Does not include Dimetapp, which is in the cough/cold therapeutic category.

[c]DBI and DBI-TD were sold to Geigy by USV during this period. USV still markets the product under the name Meltrol.

[d]Doriden was sold to USV by Ciba during this period.

TABLE 6-13
Five Leading Products in 1960 and Their Percentage of Sales in 1960 and
1973, by Therapeutic Class

	% of Sales in 1960	% of Sales in 1973		% of Sales in 1960	% of Sales in 1973
Total antibiotics			Pabalate	12.7	1.8
Chloromycetin	17.2	1.1	Benemid/	11.2	9.8
Achromycin/	14.4	1.5	Col Benemid		
Achromycin V			Aralen	6.7	0.1
Declomycin	9.0	1.4	Plaquenil	5.6	0.7
Ilosone/Ilotycin	6.5	4.1	Total	83.2	31.9
Panalba[a]	4.7	0.4	Antihistamines		
Total	51.8	8.5	Chlortrimeton	21.7	21.3
Broad- and medium-			Benadryl	17.9	23.9
spectrum antibiotics			Teldrin	14.7	14.3
Chloromycetin	23.9	1.7	Pyribenzamine	12.1	4.8
Achromycin/	20.0	2.3	Dimetane[b]	7.6	9.0
Achromycin V			Total	74.0	73.3
Declomycin	12.5	2.1	Analgesics, Ethical		
Ilosone/Ilotycin	9.0	6.2	Systemic		
Panalba[a]	8.1	0.6	All Darvons	11.3	30.8
Total	73.5	12.9	compound		
Penicillins			All Empirins	9.2	7.9
V-Cillin-K/V-Cillin	16.1	12.7	Demerol	5.7	3.0
Bicillin	12.7	3.6	Percodan/Percobarb	3.1	4.9
Pentids	11.8	4.6	Fiorinal/Fiorinal	1.8	4.5
Syncillin	7.4	0	with codeine		
Compocillin VK	6.4	1.8	Total	31.1	51.1
Total	54.4	22.7	Psychostimulants		
Oral ataractics			Tofranil	28.0	25.6
Equanil	22.9	2.8	Niamid	14.4	0
Thorazine	13.9	3.9	Nardil	11.9	0.3
Librium/Libritabs	12.1	14.2	Ritalin	10.1	14.9
Compazine	10.9	1.2	Marplan	9.7	0.4
Miltown	9.6	1.1	Total	74.1	41.2
Total	69.4	23.2	Oral hypoglycemics		
Oral diuretics			Orinase	82.7	31.1
Diuril	39.3	8.8	Diabinese	13.2	28.0
Hydrodiuril	22.2	13.0	DBI[c]	4.1	22.6
Esidrix	8.6	4.0	Total	100.0	81.7
Diamox	8.1	3.9	Sedatives		
Naturetin/	7.6	1.1	Butisol	15.4	11.7
Naturetin K			Doriden[d]	12.1	10.8
Total	85.8	30.8	Nembutal	10.2	5.8
Antiarthritics			Seconal	9.1	4.5
Butazolidin/	47.0	19.5	Tuinal	7.2	4.8
Butazolidin Alka			Total	54.0	37.6

Source: See table 6-10 for source and note on selection of drugs.
[a]This combination drug was withdrawn from the market before 1973, but one of the main components continued to be sold as Panmycin.
[b]Does not include Dimetapp, which is in the cough/cold therapeutic category.
[c]DBI and DBT-TD were sold to Geigy by USV during this period.
[d]Doriden was sold to USV by Ciba during this period.

TABLE 6-14

Firms Leading in Selected Therapeutic Categories in 1973 and Their
Percentage of Sales in These Categories in 1973 and 1960

	% of Sales in 1973	% of Sales in 1960		% of Sales in 1973	% of Sales in 1960
Total antibiotics			Antihistamines		
Lilly	37.8	17.8	Schering	28.6	28.2
Upjohn	10.1	15.6	Parke Davis	24.3	18.8
Pfizer/Roerig	9.6	10.1	Smith Kline &	14.4	16.3
Schering	11.8	0.3	French		
Lederle	7.0	23.3	Robins	9.0	7.7
Total	76.3	67.1	American Home	7.0	6.3
Broad- and medium-			Products		
spectrum antibiotics			Total	83.3	77.3
Lilly	37.8	9.2	Analgesics, ethical		
Upjohn	11.8	8.6	systemic		
Pfizer/Roerig	11.0	13.6	Lilly	32.3	12.9
Schering	9.6	0	Johnson and	13.1	0.5
Lederle	7.0	32.2	Johnson		
Total	77.2	63.6	Winthrop	11.1	5.9
Penicillins[a]			American Home	9.0	3.5
Bristol	22.6	8.0	Products		
American Home	20.6	17.0	Burroughs	8.1	9.4
Products			Wellcome		
Pfizer/Roerig	13.4	2.4	Total	73.6	32.2
Lilly	13.1	21.0	Psychostimulants		
Squibb	13.0	13.8	Merck	36.1	
Total	82.7	62.2	Geigy	25.6	28.0
Oral ataractics			Ciba	14.9	12.2
Roche	55.2	12.1	Lakeside	6.4	1.3
SmithKline &	9.2	31.6	Carter Wallace	4.9	
French			Total	87.9	41.5
Sandoz	7.9	2.4	Oral hypoglycemics		
Pfizer/Roerig	7.6	4.5	Upjohn	42.1	82.7
Merck	6.0	0.5	Pfizer/Roerig	28.0	13.2
Total	91.9	51.1	Geigy[b]	22.6	
Oral diuretics			Lilly	4.8	
Merck	22.4	61.5	USV[b]	2.3	4.1
Hoechst	22.2		Total	99.8	100.0
Searle	20.4	4.0	Sedatives		
SmithKline &	12.0		Roche	22.1	6.2
French			Lilly	13.7	24.0
USV	6.9		Abbott	13.1	13.8
Total	83.9	65.5	Johnson &	11.7	15.4
Antiarthritics			Johnson		
Merck	52.2	12.1	USV	10.8	
Geigy	26.6	47.4	Total	71.4	59.4
Burroughs Wellcome	15.2				
Robins	2.0	12.7			
USV	1.2				
Total	97.2	72.2			

Source: See table 6-10 for source and note on selection of drugs.
Note: Sales of subsidiaries are added to those of each parent firm.
[a]Does not include Penicillin-DHS and/or Streptomycin combinations.
[b]DBI and DBI-TD were sold by USV to Geigy during this period. USV still markets the product under the name Meltrol.

TABLE 6-15

Firms Leading in Selected Therapeutic Categories in 1960 and Their
Percentage of Sales in These Categories in 1960 and 1973

	% of Sales in 1960	% of Sales in 1973		% of Sales in 1960	% of Sales in 1973
Total antibiotics			Antiarthritics		
Lederle	23.3	7.0	Geigy	47.4	26.6
Lilly	17.8	37.8	Robins	12.7	2.0
Parke Davis	11.8	2.7	Winthrop	12.7	0.7
Pfizer/Roerig	10.1	9.6	Merck	12.1	52.2
Squibb	8.5	4.6	Dorsey	4.7	0.2
Total	71.5	62.4	Total	89.6	81.7
Broad- and medium-			Antihistamines		
spectrum antibiotics			Schering	28.2	28.6
Lederle	32.2	7.0	Parke-Davis	18.8	24.3
Parke Davis	24.0	2.3	Smith Kline &	16.3	14.4
Pfizer/Roerig	13.6	11.0	French		
Lilly	9.2	37.8	Ciba	12.7	5.3
Upjohn	8.6	11.8	Robins	7.7	9.0
Total	87.6	69.9	Total	83.7	81.6
Penicillins[a]			Analgesics, ethical		
Lilly	21.0	13.1	systemic		
American Home	17.0	20.6	Lilly	12.9	32.3
Products			Burroughs	9.4	8.1
Squibb	13.8	13.0	Wellcome		
Bristol	8.0	22.6	Winthrop	5.9	11.1
Abbott	6.7	1.8	Sandoz	3.6	7.4
Total	66.5	71.1	American Home	3.5	9.0
Oral ataractics			Products		
SmithKline &	31.6	9.2	Total	35.3	67.9
French			Psychostimulants		
American Home	28.2	5.3	Geigy	28.0	25.6
Products			Pfizer/Roerig	14.4	0
Wallace	14.0	1.4	Roche	12.8	0.4
Roche	12.1	55.2	Ciba	12.2	14.9
Pfizer/Roerig	4.5	7.6	Warner Lambert	11.9	0.3
Total	90.4	78.7	Total	79.3	41.2
Oral diuretics			Oral hypoglycemics		
Merck	61.5	22.4	Upjohn	82.7	42.1
Ciba	8.6	4.0	Pfizer/Roerig	13.2	28.0
Lederle	8.2	4.7	USV[b]	4.1	2.3
Squibb	7.6	1.1	Total	100.0	72.4
Searle	4.0	20.4	Sedatives		
Total	89.9	52.6	Lilly	24.0	13.7
			Johnson &	15.4	11.7
			Johnson		
			Abbott	13.8	13.1
			Ciba[c]	12.1	0
			Roche	6.2	22.1
			Total	71.5	60.6

Source: See table 6-10 for source and note on selection of drugs.
Note: Sales of subsidiaries are added to those of each parent firm.
[a]Does not include Penicillin-DHS and/or Streptomycin combinations.
[b]DBI and DBI-TD sold by USV to Geigy during this period but still marketed by USV
under the name Meltrol.
[c]Doriden sold to USV by Ciba during this period.

the market positions of the resulting new drugs and in fact has protected these positions.

Further, the high concentration ratios give a false impression of the extent of monopoly power. The concentration ratios have been unstable owing to the innovative competition which continues; apparent monopoly power may be destroyed by a new product.

CONCLUSIONS

Patent protection against imitation of new products, plus the history of successful R & D efforts in the 1940s and early 1950s, have led pharmaceutical companies to compete through innovation. Since the technical as well as the commercial results of drug research are uncertain, the firms' efforts are dispersed among many therapeutic fields. Nevertheless, patent data reveal a high degree of concentration of research effort within each field and thus great inequality in research effort among companies. The concentration of research effort is also owing to the large number of therapeutic fields.

Concentration of research effort is one of the factors in the concentration of sales in therapeutic fields. Another factor is the large number of fields with small sales; size of field is a factor in the concentration of sales as it is in the concentration of research effort.

The most important factor in the concentration of sales is the inequality of sales of individual drugs. The dispersion of sales of drugs within fields is large. A big winner will take a large part of the sales in its field. Thus the concentration of sales among companies in therapeutic fields is the result of the successes in innovative competition. Those which succeed in a field do so in a big way.

The innovative rivalry, which the concentration ratios reflect, results in a high degree of uncertainty for firms, including those having a large share of total sales in any field. The large share does not mean that the company has a secure position. Other companies are constantly searching for drugs to displace the leading drugs. And the drugs which have large sales attract efforts by other companies to produce drugs which offer better therapy. We have seen that drugs having large market shares have been displaced by new drugs. We have also seen that the companies which have increased their sales sharply have been those which introduced new and highly successful drugs.

Under these conditions the concentration ratio is not an index of monopoly power: a high concentration ratio does not signify that the leading firms in a therapeutic field are secure from product competition. They cannot be said to possess monopoly power. The leaders within a therapeutic field therefore continue to strive to introduce new drugs which are superior to those which they already have. And many firms are actively engaged in R & D efforts. The high degree of concentration in therapeutic fields thus does not signify that R & D efforts are limited to a few firms.

Since high concentration ratios signify monopoly power only if they refer to properly demarcated market areas, we have examined the basis for the use of therapeutic fields as markets. We have observed that the boundaries between therapeutic fields are not clearly defined. A good deal of substitution occurs between drugs classified in different therapeutic fields. Such substitution is reflected by the frequent aggregation of several fields into broader fields. Finally, the introduction of new drugs creates patterns of prescribing which are not in accord with previously established boundaries. A new drug which is classified in a particular therapeutic field will be substituted for an older drug in another field.

The erroneous use of concentration ratios as an index of monopoly power rests on a theory of oligopoly which suggests that the tendency to collude increases as the number of firms declines. The theory suggests that a group of firms will seek to maximize their joint profits, and the ease with which such collusion can be practiced varies inversely with the number of sellers. The concentration ratio is the proxy for the number of sellers. The theory thus predicts that the average profit rate increases among industries with the concentration ratio. The empirical support for the theory that a high concentration ratio results in high profits is weak. The studies which have found a relationship between concentration and the profit rate fail to take into account other determinants of profits, such as the growth of demand. Stanely Ornstein thus includes in his equation independent variables representing economies of scale and the growth of demand as well as the concentration ratio, and he finds that concentration has no significant effect.[6] Shepherd obtains similar results. He also finds that the profit rate increases with the individual firm market share. The relationship can be ascribed to the advantages of firms which win large market shares. Were it due to monopoly power, then the concentration ratio would be seen to have an effect on the profit rate, but Shepherd does not observe this relationship.[7]

As we have mentioned, the stress on the concentration ratio as an index of monopoly power is based on the plausible hypothesis that a few firms will find it in their interest to collude and that a small number find it easier to reconcile their differences in interests and views on what the correct price should be. However, it fails to consider other conditions for successful collusion. Some writers have suggested that if entry is easy, then collusion will break down regardless of the level of concentration.[8] High profits will attract entry. In the case of the drug industry, we have seen that many firms engage in research in an effort to develop new drugs. These firms are already members of the drug industry, but in each of the therapeutic fields only a few have a significant share of total sales. Consequently there are many potential entrants to each field. The question has been raised about the validity of regarding therapeutic fields as markets; if the markets are broader, however, the concentration ratios are lower. Entry is not easy in the sense that new and better drugs are difficult to discover and develop. The difficulty of such research discourages potential competitors from attempting to introduce new drugs. Nevertheless, many firms do engage in R & D and thus make the attempt. These firms are already in the industry, but this makes no difference for the problem at hand, since the degree of concentra-tion within therapeutic fields is at issue.

The test of the proposition that the high concentration ratios have resulted in monopoly power is the expected profit rate on investment, which we use to measure the profitability of investment. This is not the same as the realized profit rate which is the more commonly used index of monopoly power. In the next chapter we will estimate the expected profit rate on investment in R & D in the drug industry, primarily for the purpose of determining whether it is sufficiently attractive to encourage the maintenance of such investment. The estimate turns out to be so low as to indicate that the profitability of R & D investment is below the level required for the present volume of investment to be maintained. Since R & D investment constitutes the major part of total investment in this industry, the expected rate of return on total investment also is low, which suggests that the pharmaceutical manufacturers do not exercise monopoly power. The chapter also includes an analysis of the realized profit rate which finds that the apparently high average profit rate earned by firms in this industry is the result of treating R & D costs as expenses instead of as investments, the high degree of risk involved in such investments, and the growth of demand.

The concentration ratios are inconclusive evidence of monopoly power in this as in other industries. The profitability of investment is a better index of monopoly power, so the discussion in the next chapter is critical for the monopoly issue.

CHAPTER 7

THE EXPECTED
RATE OF RETURN ON
PHARMACEUTICAL R & D

INTRODUCTION

The fact that most new drugs have come from industry laboratories is insufficient to warrant large industrial R & D expenditures in the future from the point of view either of society or of the industry. Research is an uncertain business. We must have evidence that large R & D expenditures will generate more new drugs before we advocate continuing or increasing industry spending. To my knowledge, only Martin Baily's study of pharmaceutical R & D directly asks whether increases in expenditures result in more discoveries, although the responsiveness of drug innovation to market prospects, reported by Sam Peltzman, implies a positive relationship between R & D activity and the production of innovations.[1]

As table 7-1 shows, Baily finds that the number of discoveries increases with R & D expenditures. Baily's estimates of the cost of R & D to develop a given number of drugs are based on a regression equation describing the relationship between R & D expenditures by the industry and the number of drugs introduced over a period of time by the industry as a whole. The number of new drugs increases less than proportionally with total industry expenditures, according to Baily, owing to the depletion of research opportunities.

Chapter 5 observed a positive relationship among pharmaceutical companies between the number of NCE's and a measure of laboratory employment. Our study of economies of scale in pharmaceutical research thus provides additional confirmation that more spending on R & D tends to produce more new drugs.

Although Sam Peltzman's study on consumer legislation did not directly explore the effect of increased R & D expenditures, its findings are directly relevant to this topic. For the pre-1962 period, Peltzman found that the number of NCE's introduced each year increased with increases in the expected size of

136

TABLE 7-1
Annual Expenditure Required to Develop a
Constant Number of New Drugs
(1957–59 $ Millions)

Number of NCE's	Before the 1962 Regulations Change		After the 1962 Regulations Change	
	Total	Cost per NCE	Total	Cost per NCE
5	12.35	2.47	29.09	5.82
10	29.94	2.99	70.55	7.06
15	54.45	3.63	128.3	8.55
20	88.03	4.40	207.4	10.37
25	133.4	5.34	314.4	12.58
30	194.1	6.47	457.4	15.25

Source: Martin Baily, "Research and Development Costs and Returns: The U.S. Pharmaceutical Industry," *Journal of Political Economy* 80 (January/February 1972):78.

the market for drugs (measured by the lagged number of prescriptions sold and lagged expenditures for physicians' services). These relationships imply that the firms increased their expenditures on R & D with forecast increases in the demand for drugs and that these extra expenditures added to the rate of pharmaceutical innovation.

The innovation rate is much lower today than it was in the 1960s, despite greatly increased expenditures. This fact may seem to contradict the thesis that an increase in R & D will result in the development of more new drugs. The apparent inconsistency is due to the increased costs of pharmaceutical R & D, to which we return later.

Investment in pharmaceutical R & D will be maintained at current levels only if the expected return on the investment at least equals that expected from alternative investments. In the following discussion, estimates are made of the expected rate of return from drug industry investment in R & D. This expected rate of return is then related to estimates of expected return for other industries. The estimates refer only to the return from investment in R & D. The income on which this return is computed is adjusted for production costs of the newly developed drugs, including the costs of financing plant and equipment and providing working capital. The estimates do not refer to the return from total investment in the drug industry.

The expected return must be distinguished from the familiar accounting rate of return on investment. The estimated expected return makes use of an expected stream of future investment and an expected stream of income. The investment is estimated according to the projected costs of the required services, goods, equipment, and so on. The income is estimated according to expected prices and the costs of producing the income. By contrast, the accounting rate of return for any year is calculated on the basis of the book value of investment (reflecting the historic cost of construction of plant and equipment or the cost of acquisition with no allowance for inflation and investment in R & D and market development) and the income in the year for which the estimate is made. The expected rate of return is forward looking, as the name suggests.

The expected rate of return is the relevant criterion for investment decisions, while the accounting rate is intended to measure the success of past investments. (As we will see later, it is a biased measure even of the success of past investment, since it is based on a measure of assets which excludes a part of investments. This part is a major portion of the total in the drug industry.) The criterion for evaluating the effect of public policy on investment decision, including its effect on investment in R & D, is the impact of policy on the expected rate of return. If a proposed public policy reduces the expected rate of return on investment in research and development below the level available from alternative investment, then it is likely to reduce investment in research and development. The accounting rate is frequently used as a measure of the expected rate, and the distinction between the two is not always made. In the drug industry the resulting error is likely to be large because of the long period for research and development for a new drug and the consequent long lag of income behind investment. One reason that the current accounting rate of return on investment is relatively high in the drug industry compared to what it is in other industries is the continued large sales of some major drugs introduced in the late 1950s and early 1960s. In recent years neither the number of innovations per dollar of total investment nor the sales of new drugs per dollar of total investment have been as large as they had been. As a result, the current expected rate of return on investment is not likely to be as high as the accounting rate of return on past investment.

The estimate of the expected rate of return will be made for the industry as a whole. The average, it should be noted, is weighted. Large firms are given greater weight than small ones. To obtain the average expected rate of return, we compute the average cost of R & D per NCE using industry aggregates. Since large firms contribute most of the total R & D expenditures and discover most of the NCEs, the average reflects their experience more heavily than does the experience of the small firms.

Since the investment in R & D for a new drug spans several years, the equation used here represents investment as a stream of discounted expenditures. These expenditures are offset by the stream of discounted income earned from the expenditures. The equation determines the rate of return yielded by the projected streams of investment and income. If this expected rate of return is higher than the expected rate available for other investments, then the investment is attractive. The formula is as follows:

$$\frac{c_1}{(1+i)} + \frac{c_2}{(1+i)^2} + \ldots + \frac{c_n}{(1+i)^n} + \frac{y_{n+1}}{(1+i)^{n+1}} + \frac{y_{n+2}}{(1+i)^{n+2}} + \ldots + \frac{y_{n+m}}{(1+i)^{n+m}} = 0,$$

where c = annual cost of research, y = annual net income after associated costs, i = discount rate, and the subscripts refer to years. The costs of research (c) have negative signs. The problem is to solve for i, given estimates of c and y for each year.

THE CURRENT EXPECTED RATE OF RETURN

ESTIMATING COST. If the goal of public policy is to encourage significant therapeutic discoveries, then we must estimate the current (1973) expected rate of return on investment directed to such discoveries. On the basis of this procedure, we estimated in chapter 3 that the current pre-tax average cost of R & D for an NCE is $24.4 million. The after-tax cost is approximately $12.2 million. In chapter 3 we also estimated the average R & D period to be ten years. Our estimate of each of the annual costs of R & D (c) in the equation for the expected rate of return is thus $1.22 million ($12.2 million divided by 10).

ESTIMATING INCOME. The anticipated net income per NCE must also be estimated. Average 1972 U.S. sales of the NCE's introduced in 1966–72 was $3 million.[2] The figure is low; first, because doctors take as long as two to three years to adjust their prescribing to new drugs, and, second, because very few large-selling drugs were introduced in this period. We should therefore estimate the average sales per NCE in 1972 for a group of NCE's introduced over a period beginning before 1966 and ending before 1972 so as to include in our calculation some drugs whose sales were relatively large. Experimentation with a few periods led to the selection of 1962–68 as one yielding a relatively high average. Following the rule of caution the decision was made in such a manner as to produce an overestimate of the expected rate of return. The average 1972 sales of NCE's introduced in 1962–68 were $7.5 million. By limiting the NCE's to those introduced between 1962 and 1968, one makes it possible for all the drugs included to have had ample time to achieve their full sales potential by 1972. Thus, 1972 represented the eleventh year of commercial life for the drugs introduced in 1962 and the fifth year for those introduced in 1968. In addition, the selection of this period results in a higher estimate of the expected rate of return than alternative selections, as table 7-2 shows.

We must also include foreign sales in our estimate. On the basis of PMA's estimate for 1972, we can add 47 percent to the estimate of that year's domestic sales, which brings the total to 147 percent of $7.5 million, or $11.0 million per NCE.

It is now time to calculate the net profit after taxes. Net profit must include the share of total sales revenues spent on R & D, since this expenditure represents new investment for future innovations. The estimated after-tax profit margin, including R & D expenditures is 15.4 percent of sales. To arrive at this estimate, we used a sample of six firms with over 60 percent of net sales from

TABLE 7-2
Average Sales in 1972 of NCE's Introduced
in Various Periods ($ Millions)

Period of introduction	Average sales per NCE in 1972	Period of introduction	Average sales per NCE in 1972
1956–66	$5.3	1962–68	7.5
1960–68	6.3	1962–70	6.8
1960–69	6.2	1965–69	5.6

Sources: Based on Paul de Haen, *New Product Survey* and *Nonproprietary Name Index;* and on *U.S. Pharmaceutical Market, Drug Stores and Hospitals,* IMS America, Ltd., various years.

pharmaceutical products, summed the profits before taxes and R & D expenditures for the six firms, and then expressed the sum as a ratio to the sum of net sales.

The gross margin as computed must be adjusted to exclude the cost of financing the required investment in plant and equipment, inventories, and receivables. When a new drug is developed and introduced to the market, there must be plant and equipment available to produce it, and funds are also required for working capital. It is estimated that 2.6 percentage points of the gross margin are required for these purposes, which leaves a profit margin of 12.8 percent of sales as the return on investment in R & D. The total investment required for plant and equipment for the six companies in the sample was estimated conservatively on the basis of the book value of plant and equipment after depreciation in 1972. The book value of new working capital was added to obtain the required capital investment. A total for all six companies taken together was obtained. An interest rate of 8 percent was applied to this total to obtain the cost of financing. Not all of this estimated cost of financing could be deducted from the profit margin computed earlier, since the net income figure was net of interest payments. Hence, we subtracted from this estimate of the cost of financing the interest payments that were actually made. The cost of financing so adjusted was subtracted from the profits previously calculated, and the result was expressed as a percentage of sales. This method is conservative inasmuch as the actual cost of financing exceeds 8 percent and the procedure makes no allowance for a return on investment in working capital in excess of the cost of financing.

The formula used to obtain y was as follows:

$$y = .5 \left[\text{Profits Before Taxes} + \text{R \& D} + \frac{.08 \text{ Debt}}{\text{Debt} + \text{Equity}} \text{(Working Capital} + \text{Net Plant)} - .08 \text{(Working Capital} + \text{Net Plant)}\right]$$

That is to say that y, which is the net income from investment in R & D, equals profits plus R & D expenditures less the cost of financing working capital and plant and equipment after the appropriate adjustment for taxes. The book value of Net Plant is taken as an estimate of the average investment in plant and equipment required to generate the indicated profits and R & D expenditures. The interest rate, as noted, is assumed to be 8 percent. Since profits are computed after interest payments, and such interest is already deducted in the term representing the cost of financing working capital and plant and equipment, a further adjustment is needed. We add back into profits the part of the cost of financing working capital and plant and equipment that is financed by debt. The entire expression is multiplied by .5 to adjust for taxes.

Certain objections can be made to this procedure. The estimate of necessary plant and equipment is based on the ratio of net plant to sales. The technically correct approach would be to estimate the current cost of the required plant and equipment and obtain an estimate of the cash flow each year after estimating the annual depreciation. Our procedure is likely to result in a higher estimate of the expected rate of return, since the book value of net plant and equipment does not allow for inflation in the cost of construction.

The assumed rate of return on plant and working capital (8 percent) is higher than the calculated expected rate of return (3.3 percent), because it is an estimate of the cost of financing such plant and working capital. One might argue that the appropriate rate for plant and working capital is return on total investment, which would fall between the two: the rate of return on plant and working capital should equal that on R & D. If this were assumed, it would increase the expected return on R & D. We have not adopted this procedure, because it is our intention to estimate the expected rate of return on R & D at the present level of investment in R & D. For this purpose it is necessary to assume that the cost of financing plant and equipment is determined by the market rather than by the firm's decision concerning the amount to be invested in R & D and the resulting expected rate of return from this investment. The result of the analysis, it should be noted, is that it suggests that firms should not continue to maintain their present rate of investment in R & D.

When we apply the 12.8 percent margin to annual sales of $11.0 million per NCE, we obtain $1.40 million in net profits per year per NCE. This is the estimated value, after sales level off, for each y in the equation. We assume that this leveling off occurs in the third year after introduction (year 13 of table 7-4). Some evidence suggests that the period of introduction is longer, especially for widely used drugs. In that case, the short introduction period tends to overstate the rate of return. We should also mention that we assume that sales in the year of introduction (year 11 of table 7-4) are one-third of the peak level (year 13 and the following years until the decline sets in) and two-thirds of this level in the year following the introduction. We assume that the decline which sets in in year 24 is symmetrical with the growth period after the drug is introduced. It is now necessary to estimate the period during which a company can expect to sell an NCE in reasonably large quantities. This commercial life is estimated at

TABLE 7-3

Financial Data for Six Pharmaceutical Companies, 1972 ($ Thousands)

	Net Sales	R & D	Profits Be-fore Taxes	Gross Plant	Net Plant	Current Assets			Curr. Liab.	Working Capital
						Inventory	Acc'ts Rec.	Other Current Assets		
Abbott	521818	31249	60116	340464	230372	113231	112372	67082	129295	163390
Eli Lilly	819718	74287	196361	489639	308215	168626	132604	211187	226928	285489
Merck	958266	79665	266456	556183	300041	195724	175880	92712	174409	289907
G.D. Searle	271878	35892	53388	108234	68781	53691	72130	92910	71074	147657
Upjohn	511337	50276	91456	335158	198575	116690	117435	66051	115091	185085
Syntex	160408	15342	42819	94588	68152	40527	34307	52139	50056	76917
TOTAL	3243425	286711	710596	1924266	1174136	688489	644728	582081	766853	1148445
Percentage of Net Sales	100.0	8.8	21.9	59.3	36.2	21.2	19.9	17.9	23.6	35.4

Source: Securities and Exchange Commission 10-K Reports and/or Annual Reports of companies.

Note: Companies in "Pink Sheet" pharmaceutical index with over 60 percent of net sales from pharmaceutical sales were chosen. All companies reported for calendar year ending December 31, 1972, except Syntex, whose figures are for year ending July 31, 1973.

TABLE 7-4
Estimated Stream of Cost of R & D and Net Income
for an Average NCE ($ Millions)

Year	R & D Cost = (c)	Year	R & D Cost = (c)	Year	Net Income = (y)	Year	Net Income = (y)	Year	Net Income = (y)
1	−1.22	6	−1.22	11	.47	16	1.40	21	1.40
2	−1.22	7	−1.22	12	.94	17	1.40	22	1.40
3	−1.22	8	−1.22	13	1.40	18	1.40	23	1.40
4	−1.22	9	−1.22	14	1.40	19	1.40	24	.94
5	−1.22	10	−1.22	15	1.40	20	1.40	25	.47

Source: See text for computations.

fifteen years. The estimated commercial life in 1960 was five years, according to a study by William E. Cox.[3] The general opinion is that the average life of new drugs has increased since then. Clymer assumes a life of fifteen years.[4] The explanation usually offered for the increase in average life is the decline in the number of new drugs introduced each year. This decline has been ascribed to increased difficulty in the obtaining of Food and Drug Administration approval of new drugs and to the increased difficulty of discovering and developing new drugs.

CALCULATING THE EXPECTED RATE OF RETURN. The final task is to solve the equation for i and so obtain the expected average rate of return. The estimated stream of c and y for an average NCE is shown in table 7-4. The expected rate of return on R & D investment obtained with this schedule is 3.3 percent. This calculated expected rate of return is in part based on the solution of the value of i in an equation setting the present value of a stream of expenditures and revenues equal to zero. This approach resembles ordinary cash-flow analysis. The method, however, departs from the cash-flow procedure in using estimates of the funds invested based on book values. It is thus a hybrid between cash-flow and an accounting rate of return. The hybridization results from the fact that we estimate the expected rate of return on investment in R & D only, but use a gross-margin estimate which includes the return on other investments. The objection may be made that the appropriate criterion for the decision to undertake research is the expected rate of return on total investment including plant and equipment rather than investment in R & D alone. A good case may be made for this position. The present procedure can be defended on the consideration that the focus of this paper is the return on investment in R & D rather than the return on the total investment required to introduce a new drug. Estimating this latter return raises a whole new range of problems. In any case, a complete cash-flow analysis would have required an estimate of the cost of a new plant and an estimated depreciation schedule for the production of the new drugs. These estimates would have required information on the cost of plants required for specific kinds of drugs and would have required assumptions on the distribution of the output of new drugs by type of drug. In addition, we would have had to make assumptions about the location of the plants and costs of construction. The present procedure is much simpler. A rough estimate using the book value of gross plant as the initial investment in plant and equipment suggests that this expected rate of return is close to our estimate for the expected rate of return on investment in R & D. No attempt has been made to estimate the expected rate on total investment using an estimate of the current cost of plant and equipment. An estimate using plant and equipment at current cost would be lower than an estimate using book values since construction prices have increased.

Before the significance of this estimate is discussed, we can examine alternative estimates made according to alternative assumptions on the gross margin. The objection may be made that the assumed gross margin is based on the total sales of the six companies and that their margins may be lower on nonpharmaceutical products than on pharmaceutical products. In addition, among pharmaceutical products the average gross margin for NCE's may exceed the average gross margin for all products. However, the use of the average for all pharmaceutical products is unlikely to be a source of large error, since most sales are sales of products that are still under patent and therefore are not yet in direct price competition with generically similar products. Nevertheless, since the estimate of 15.4 percent may appear to be too low, table 7-5 provides additional estimates made on the basis of assumed gross margins of 17.5 percent and 20.0 percent.

TABLE 7-5
Estimates of Expected Rates of Return
on Investment in R & D in 1973, Using
Alternative Gross Margins and Lengths
of Commercial Life

Length of Commercial Life	Alternative Gross Margins		
	15.4[a]	17.5	20.0
15 years	3.3	4.6	6.0
20 years	5.1	6.3	7.5

Source: See text for computations.
[a]This gross margin of 15.4 is based on six company reports, taking aggregate profits before taxes plus R & D expenditures and dividing by aggregate sales. The percentage arrived at is 30.8, which is then adjusted for taxes by dividing by two. See text for additional details.

We have reason to believe that 20 percent errs on the high side as an estimate of the true gross margin on pharmaceutical sales. The 10K reports indicate that the aggregate pharmaceutical sales of the companies in our sample account for 70 percent or more of their aggregate total sales (the higher this percentage is, presumably the higher is the over-all gross margin, since the assumed error is understatement of the gross margin on pharmaceutical products through the inclusion in total sales of other products). We can also assume that the after-tax gross margin on sales of nonpharmaceutical products is not less than 10 percent. These estimates yield a maximum estimate of the after-tax gross margin on total sales of 17 percent. But we have seen that the overall margin in fact was 15.4 percent.

Another reason the true gross margin is unlikely to be higher than those appearing in table 7-5 is that these gross margins are calculated after taxes, costs of administration, marketing, and other costs. Further, the assumption is made that the relationship between the total of these costs and sales is the same for new drugs as for old drugs. But the cost of marketing a drug is higher in the first few years of its commercial life than it is later. A company introducing a new drug must spend more on promoting its use by doctors when the drug is still unfamiliar; furthermore, sales take some time to build. The gross margin for a new drug in the first few years thus may be lower rather than higher than the gross margin for an old drug.

There is also the question of the commercial life of an NCE. Since our estimate of the commercial life has as its sole basis the fact that members of the industry have used the estimate in their own calculations, table 7-5 also includes estimates of the expected rate of return assuming a twenty-year commercial life.

To determine whether the estimated rates of return are sufficient to encourage the industry to continue investing in R & D, we must set up a benchmark against which to measure the rates. One decision criterion often used in other industries in the past was 10 percent after taxes. In the late 1960s this was the minimum rate required in farm machinery, textiles, and electrical equipment.[5] The minimum probably has increased with the steep rise in the rate of interest since then. The minimum required rate for pharmaceutical R & D probably should be above the minimum required rate for investment generally in other industries because investment in pharmaceutical R & D is more risky than other types of investment. The probability that a given research project conducted by a specific company will yield a successful product which will generate sufficient sales to recoup investment and some profit is small.

Even the probability of technical success—let alone commercial success—is small. We saw that, in 1970, only 1,013 substances reached the stage of clinical testing, compared to the 703,900 substances which were pharmacologically tested. The number that were technically successful (which means the number that passed all clinical tests, obtained approval from the FDA, and were introduced in the market) was only sixteen.[6]

It may be argued that a small number of successes out of many attempts does not signify a high degree of risk, if a given investment in R & D can be counted on to generate a specified number of successes with a high degree of certainty. Such certainty, as we saw in chapter 6, clearly is not characteristic of investment in pharmaceutical R & D.

In any case, it is commercial success that is important, and the probability of commercial success is low. Very few of the drugs introduced obtained sufficient sales to yield an adequate rate of return on the research investment. If a return of 10 percent on total investment is a minimum acceptable level, then our assumptions on the gross margin and commercial life of drugs, when combined with the estimate of the average cost of research per drug, imply that the annual world sales of an NCE must be at least $23.5 million to yield a minimum acceptable return. At this level of sales the net income (the y in the equation for the expected rate of return) would be $3.0 million. Given our estimate of the relationship of domestic to foreign sales, this $23.5 million total sales should include $16.0 million of domestic sales. Few of the drugs introduced between 1962 and 1968 achieved this level of domestic sales in 1972. Table 6-3 (in chapter 6) in fact shows that only eight of the seventy-nine introduced did so. A majority had sales of less than $2 million. The sales of the most successful drugs have been large and have raised the average sales of all NCE's to $7.5 million.

In sum, the few commercially successful drugs, which attract unfavorable attention, carry the R & D costs and other costs of all products. In addition, these successful drugs provide the incentive for R & D investment.

These data suggest a very high degree of risk in investment in pharmaceutical R & D. A benchmark for such investment above 10 percent could well be appropriate, particularly at the present time when the return on high-grade corporate bonds is not much less than 10 percent. Nevertheless, in accordance with the rule of caution that we have been observing, 10 percent is used as the criterion in the following estimate.

The estimates of the expected rates from investment in pharmaceutical R & D are well below the minimum rate required in other industries. The combination of the current cost of research, innovation rates, product prices, and sales yields an expected rate of return from current investment in research much lower than would be required to maintain such research at the current level. Indeed, the best estimate of the expected rate of return, based on a 15.4 percent gross margin and a fifteen-year commercial life, gives a 3.3 percent return, well below the required minimum.

One objection which can be raised to the estimates made here is that the sales of NCE's can be expected to grow with the market as a whole, which has been growing at an average rate of 7 percent per annum, whereas we assumed that the average sales of NCE's will remain at the 1972 level. The objection is not so serious as it may appear to be at first glance, inasmuch as it is the sales of all ethical drugs which have grown at the 7 percent rate, rather than the average sales of NCE's. Part of the growth in total pharmaceutical sales has come from new products that opened new markets. It is true that the average sales of NCE's have increased since the early 1960s, but their increase comes partly from the decline in the number of new drugs per year. It is hazardous, on this showing, for anyone to predict continued growth in average sales per NCE, and we have not made such a prediction.

The error resulting from a failure to provide for future growth in sales may be offset by other errors in the opposite direction: our disregard of the increase of 6 percent per annum in the prices of goods and services consumed in R & D; our omission of the rise in the costs of research as a result of the increased difficulty of R & D and the greater regulatory requirements for approval of new drugs; our disregard of all increases in the costs of the plant and equipment necessary for the manufacture of new drugs since the existing plant and equipment came on line; our use of book value of working capital rather than replacement costs; and our assumption of an 8 percent cost of financing plant and equipment and working capital. It is at least likely that these factors will counterbalance any possible error from our assuming no growth in sales.

The expected rate of return for the industry as a whole is only one point to be considered. Individual companies continue to increase their investments for a number of reasons: some firms expect to do better than the average because they have performed well in the past and because they can predict better-than-average prospects for specific ongoing research projects, particularly compounds that have reached the stage of clinical trials designed to determine efficacy (phase II). A firm's decision whether or not to continue a research project already under way will depend on information on the prospects of success that is specific to the firm rather than on the expected rate of return from investment in R & D for the industry as a whole. But the decision to inaugurate a new line of research may depend more on an evaluation of the prospects of success based on the industry's performance, especially inasmuch as any new project will take several years to complete. During this time there may be a turnover of personnel engaged in the project. In other words, over the long term, a firm cannot count on doing any better than other firms in the industry that have the same size, general location, and wealth.

Individual companies may hope for a breakthrough in their own or in other laboratories that will inaugurate another stream of innovations; and to be able to take advantage of such a breakthrough, each company must maintain research staff and research programs. Individual companies may be willing to gamble in the hope of beating the high odds against finding a drug that will have huge sales, just as bettors invest in a roulette wheel at a cumulative expected return of minus 3 percent in the hope of hitting their number and producing a 3600 percent return. These firms will maintain and possibly even increase their R & D expenditures on the basis of short-term expectations. They already have the staff and facilities for research and development, and they are not ready to abandon them, particularly if they are optimistic about current research projects.

Another, more general, objection to the estimates of the current expected return on industry investment in pharmaceutical R & D is that the estimates may appear to be merely the result of a fanciful chain of reasoning, inasmuch as the industry has continued to increase its investment in research and development. Thus, despite the apparent low expected rate of return from investment in R & D, expenditures on R & D have continued to increase even after correcting for increases in the wages and salaries of employees in laboratories and in the prices of purchased goods and services. Total employment in the laboratories also shows a continuing increase. Yet firms do in fact consider the ultimate profitability of R & D expenditures even if they do not use our estimating procedure. It may be noted that some financial analysts have recently made bearish forecasts of future industry earnings on the basis of similar appraisals of the effect of the increase in R & D costs and the decline in the number of new drug product introductions. The Futures Group, a consulting firm of Glastonbury, Connecticut, has predicted a sharp drop in the average after-tax margin of the industry before 1980 as a result of increased R & D costs and an increased share of sales to hospitals, clinics, and Health Maintenance Organizations. No account is taken of the drop in the number of NCE's.[7]

Our discussion of investment should not be taken to signify that the amount of research by the industry has grown. We can only say that more resources now are being employed in R & D than in the past. There is nothing wrong with recognizing that this increase represents an increase in investment, since measures of investment generally are based on estimates of the quantities of resources used. Nevertheless, we have a problem of interpretation. The increase in FDA regulatory requirements renders the measure inadequate for estimating changes in the amount of research. A given quantity of resources now cannot achieve as much as it did in 1960 owing to the greater restrictiveness of the FDA. A larger part of the effort must be spent in meeting these requirements rather than in advancing the investigations. A company may be favorably impressed with the results of some clinical tests and therefore may want to complete the research which it hopes will enable it to market a drug. But the FDA requires the company to spend more on the research than it originally planned and to prolong the R & D period. The company will spend the additional resources, but the increase does not represent more research. Martin N. Baily has estimated that the change in regulations after 1962 increased the cost of research by 136 percent (table 7-1). This estimate is so large that it suggests that the quantity of research has declined despite the increase in expenditures and in laboratory employment. In short, the number of new drugs which a given expenditure of resources can generate is much lower today than it was at the beginning of the 1960s.

A recent article by Dr. Sarett,[8] who is president of Merck, Sharp, and Dohme Research Laboratories, supports this view. Sarett predicts that the rise in the cost of research will have the effect of reducing the amount of research. He believes that most research directors will shift their expenditures from discovery research to the development of drugs. The regulatory requirements, which apply to development more than to discovery research, will accelerate the shift. Furthermore, companies will find it difficult to increase their total R & D expenditures at the same rate as costs. Sarett predicts a decrease in the number of research projects; indeed, he reports that the number of projects at Merck, Sharp, and Dohme decreased by 10 percent between 1969 and 1974. Sarett also predicts certain changes in the direction of research. Economic considerations will lead to greater emphasis on epidemiologically important diseases, and laboratories will reduce their search for drugs for rare diseases. In other words, research will be restricted to areas where the expected rate of return is relatively high.

THE EXPECTED RATE OF RETURN ON R & D PERFORMED IN 1960

It is reasonable to suppose that the pharmaceutical industry made large investment in R & D during the 1960s because the expected rate of return on research and development investment at the beginning of that decade was attractive.

To test this supposition, we have estimated the expected rate of return on R & D for the industry in 1960, using the number of new chemical entities appearing during the years 1955–58. Chapter 3 estimated the total R & D cost of an NCE in 1960 at $1.30 million before taxes. We can now distribute the after-tax cost, $.65 million, equally over the R & D period of five years. We have in fact been told by people who were members of industrial research laboratories at the time that the R & D period was much shorter. Moreover, Schnee estimates the development period then to have been two years. Sarett's estimate for 1958–62 is the same.[9] Our estimate, therefore, tends to understate the expected rate of return in that earlier period.

The income from each NCE is calculated in the following way. We have assumed that the gross margin was the same in 1960 as in 1973–that is, 15.4 percent. In addition, we have assumed that the cost of financing plant and equipment and working capital in 1960 represented the same percentage of sales as it represented in 1973–that is, 2.6 percent. Actually, the cost of financing plant and equipment and working capital probably accounted for a larger proportion of sales in 1973 than it accounted for in 1960 because of increases in the cost of construction of plant and equipment and in interest rates relative to the prices of drugs. The use of 2.6 percent as an estimate for 1960 therefore results in an understatement of the expected rate of return in that year. In 1960 the average sales per NCE among those introduced between 1955 and 1958 was

$2.2 million. Thus, the net income (the y) in the three-year plateau of the total five-year commercial life may be estimated at $.28 million.

The estimated stream of cost of R & D plus net income for an average NCE for those years is as follows ($ million):

Year		Year	
1	−.13	6	.14
2	−.13	7	.28
3	−.13	8	.28
4	−.13	9	.28
5	−.13	10	.14

Cox, from whose study the estimate of the expected commercial life of NCE's in 1960 is obtained, based his estimated on observations of those NCE's that were introduced in 1955 and 1956.[10] He defined the commercial life of a drug as terminating when sales declined to 20 percent of peak sales. Cox estimated the average on the basis of the number of years that elapsed following the year of introduction when 50 percent of the drugs introduced had reached this level. Informal oral sources within the industry agree that five years was the expected commercial life at that time. Cox's estimate is for all NCE's, and the commercial life of "important" drugs may have been longer. Since our list of drugs is more selective than Cox's, we may be understating the expected life of drugs in the category with which we are dealing.

The result of our calculations is an estimate of an expected rate of return of 11.4 percent. This is considerably larger than the current expected rate, but not very much above the minimum rate of 10 percent which we have postulated as required to attract continued investment. Using the same assumptions on gross margin, on the cost of financing plant and equipment and working capital, and on the length of commercial life for 1956 as for 1960, we find the estimate of the expected rate of return for 1956 is about the same as the estimate of the expected rate of return for 1960.

By performing calculations for 1960 similar to those for 1973 summarized in table 7-5, we can derive alternative estimates for the expected rate of return during 1960. As table 7-6 shows, these alternative estimates of the expected rate of return from investment in R & D in 1960, using assumed gross margins of 17.5 and 20.0 percent, are substantially higher than the 11.4 percent figure listed above. These alternative gross margin estimates yield expected rates of return of 14.9 percent and 18.4 percent. The expected rate of return may have been well above our best estimate of 11.4 percent owing to errors in the lengths assigned to the R & D period and to the commercial life of the NCE. We have suggested that the bias in both cases results in an underestimate of rate of return; therefore, the decline in the expected return on investment in R & D may have been larger than our estimates indicate.

We must inquire why the expected rate of return on investment in R & D

TABLE 7-6
Estimates of Expected Rates of Return from
Investment in Pharmaceutical R & D in 1960,
Based on Alternative Gross Margins

Gross Margin (percent of sales)	Expected Rate of Return (percent)
15.4	11.4
17.5	14.9
20.0	18.4

Source: See text for computation.

decreased between 1960 and 1973. The decrease comes from rising costs of R & D over this period and from the decline in the number of NCE's. It will be remembered that in 1960 the cost of R & D per NCE was $1.3 million compared to $24.4 million in 1973. The increase in sales per NCE was substantial, as was the increase in the commercial life of each drug, but the effects of these two changes taken together were insufficient to offset increases in the cost of R & D. It may be noted that the decline in the expected rate of return set in immediately after the 1962 Drug Amendments rather than gradually over an extended period.

The estimate of the expected rate of return for 1967 is negative. On the basis of Sarett's work[11] we assumed the length of the R & D period to be six years. We had no basis for the estimate of the commercial life, so we assumed that it was ten years, which is intermediate between the five-year estimate for 1960 and the fifteen-year estimate for 1973. The total pre-tax R & D cost per NCE was estimated at $7.9 million. The estimate was based on the number of new entities appearing in the years 1961–65. The costs of the required research were estimated on the basis of PMA figures on research expenditures during the years 1958–62. To take care of price increases, we estimated a 20 percent increase in prices of research goods and services between 1960 and 1966. As before, we assumed that 50 percent of total R & D expenditures could be allocated to discovery research. This part of the total was allocated entirely to the cost of R & D for NCE's. The development costs were distributed among NCE's and other new drugs. The after-tax cost of R & D ($7.9 million $\times$ .5) was distributed equally over the 6-year R & D period, so that each c in the formula was estimated at $.66 million. To arrive at the new income, we first estimated the average sales of NCE's in the U.S. at $2.7 million, which was the average sales in 1966 of NCE's introduced in the period 1957–64. Alternative average sales figures are given in table 7-7.

To arrive at total world sales, we multiplied the domestic sales by 1.33, since, according to PMA, foreign sales in the year 1966 were 33 percent of total domestic sales. The same margin (15.4 percent), which after correction for cost of financing plant and equipment and working capital become 12.8 percent, was

TABLE 7-7
Average U.S. Sales in 1966 of NCE's
Introduced in Various Periods

Period of Introduction	Average Sales in 1966 ($ million)
1958–64	$2.2
1957–64	2.7
1956–64	2.6
1955–64	2.5

Sources: Paul de Haen, New Product Surveys and Nonproprietary Name Index; and IMS America Ltd, Drug Stores and Hospitals.

applied to arrive at net income. The use of alternative gross margins of 17.5 and 20.0 percent resulted in very low positive rates of return: 1.1 and 3.1 percent respectively. The low expected rate of return on investment in R & D resulted from the sharp rise in the cost of R & D after 1962 and the decline in the number of NCE's introduced each year after 1962. The rise in the expected rate of return since 1967 is the result of the growth in the size of the market and the lengthened commercial life of drugs.

REALIZED PROFITS

Questions will be raised concerning the validity of the estimates of the expected rate of return on investment in R & D, because they do not seem to be in accord with estimates of the average rate of return on stockholders' equity. The estimate of the expected rate in 1973 is below the minimum rates generally required for investment in other industries and the estimate for 1960 is only slightly higher. This suggests that the overall realized rate of return on investment in the pharmaceutical industry is less than that in other industries, but the reported rate of return has been greater. In fact, much of the argument that the leading firms have exercised monopoly power rests on the evidence of relatively high realized accounting rates of return on stockholders' equity.

We have argued elsewhere that the appropriate criterion of monopoly power is the expected rate of return on investment and not the realized rates of return.[12] The essence of this argument is simple. If firms exercise monopoly power, then a firm which uses the optimum technology and scale of plant but which has no special advantages over other firms should expect to earn a high profit at current prices. If a firm cannot expect to earn excess profits from new investment at current prices, then we cannot infer the presence of monopoly power from high realized profits. High realized profits can be the result of many things. A high level of demand may be the source of high profits, and there may be other special conditions as well, such as relatively high level of risk, a continuing flow of innovations, and superior efficiency. In other words, monopoly power is not the only possible source of high profits. But unless there is some other explanation, persistent high expected profits are evidence of monopoly power. We have seen that the criterion of the expected rate of return would lead us to reject the hypothesis that the leading pharmaceutical manufacturers exercise monopoly power. Investment in R & D accounts for the major part of total investment in this industry, and the current low expected rate of return from such investment signifies that the overall expected rate of return is well below the expected rate from investment in other industries.

The discussion of monopoly power in this and other industries, however, usually is based on the record of realized profits which are measured by accounting methods. The data for the pharmaceutical industry which are usually cited indicate that the profits have been persistently higher than in other industries and therefore that the manufacturers have obtained monopolistic prices. Much of the case for proposals to control drug prices or for the compulsory licensing of drug patents depends on these data.

Data on accounting profits suffer from a number of serious deficiencies in relation to the monopoly issue. In the first place, individual firms may earn high profits persistently even when they do not possess monopoly power. Thus high profits may be due to superior efficiency and they may persist in a particular industry. In any industry the firms which are highly efficient can be expected to grow and obtain a large share of the market and to earn high profits. In industries where the differences in efficiency between firms are large, those of superior efficiency will earn relatively higher profits than firms in other industries and obtain a larger share of total output.[13]

The leading firms in the drug industry are likely to earn high profits and do so persistently because of the importance of innovation in this industry. The innovators are the largest firms and their relatively high profits will persist as long as they continue to innovate and their new products are protected against imitation by patents. The profits of other firms in the industry may be no higher than those of other firms in other industries, but the average for the drug industry may be high simply because the leading firms' innovations account for a large part of total industry sales. We have seen that a majority of drugs are still covered by patents, so that for this reason alone profits in the industry will be high.

In addition, the so-called average profit rate usually is an average which is computed for the larger and more successful firms rather than for the industry as a whole. As we have argued, the innovations which contributed to the growth of the larger firms to their current rank also contributed to their relatively high profits. The use of profit rates of leading firms to represent the average of the industry as a whole thus will lead to a larger overstatement of that average for the drug industry than for other industries. That the average accounting profit rate of the leading companies is above the average for a larger group of leading drug firms is seen in table 7-8. The table shows two series of profit-rate averages for the industry. One is for the twelve largest firms (column B). The other (column A) uses a larger sample of leading firms which still is a small part of the total number of firms in the industry. Despite the fact that the twelve leading firms are included in the larger sample of leading firms and the accounting rate of return shown (column A) is a weighted average which gives greater weight to the twelve leading firms, the accounting rate is noticeably higher for the twelve firms (except 1971). We would expect this in a competitive, risky industry, [14] and we find this to prevail in the pharmaceutical industry. When the average for the twelve leading companies (column B) is compared to that for all manufacturing, which is represented by the average for the FTC-SEC sample of manufacturing corporations (column C), it is found to be much higher; the average difference over the period 1968–72 is 8.8 percentage points. This is the chief evidence of monopoly power. The appropriate comparison, however, is between representative averages for the pharmaceutical industry and all manufacturing.

For the purpose of measuring the effect of monopoly power even the FTC-SEC sample average of the pharmaceutical industry (column A) is also biased, because of the weight of large companies in its computation. The large companies earn higher profits than other companies because they are more successful rather than because they are monopolistic, and the importance of such success is greater in an innovational industry like the drug industry than in other industries. But the average for this sample is more representative than that of the alternative sample.

TABLE 7-8
Comparison of Drug Industry Profit Rates with All Manufacturing Industry
Profit Rates on Stockholders' Equity in the United States

	Drug Industry (A)	Drug Industry (B)	All Manufacturing Industry (C)
1961	16.1	17.7	8.9
1962	16.0	17.1	9.8
1963	16.4	17.8	10.3
1964	17.7	18.9	11.6
1965	19.7	21.0	13.0
1966	19.6	21.1	13.4
1967	16.8	19.0	11.7
1968	17.5	18.8	12.1
1969	17.6	19.9	11.5
1970	17.2	19.6	9.3
1971	20.4	19.4	9.7
1972	17.6	18.5	10.6

Sources: (A) FTC-SEC *Quarterly Financial Report* (averages of four quarters for each year); Average profit on stockholders' equity of pharmaceutical companies included in FTC-SEC sample. (B) *Report of the Federal Trade Commission on Rates of Return in Selected Manufacturing Industries* (various years). (C) *Economic Report of the President, 1975*, table C-76, p. 337.

The FTC-SEC sample average for the pharmaceutical industry usually is below the average for the twelve leading firms. The difference in 1970 thus was 2.4 percentage points. The only year in which the difference was in the other direction was in 1971. The excess of the average profit rate for the drug industry is still much higher than the all-manufacturing profit rate. But, as we will see, the difference can be accounted for by factors other than monopoly power.

MONOPOLY AND PROFITS IN THE PHARMACEUTICAL INDUSTRY

This section will estimate how much each of three nonmonopoly factors (expensing of R & D, risk, and growth of sales) contributes to the difference between the average reported rate of profit in the drug industry and average rate for all manufacturing. It will be seen that these estimates throw doubt on the monopoly hypothesis even if they do not account for all of the difference in profit rates.

In order to remove the effect of year-to-year variation in the difference between the average profit rate of the industry and that by all manufacturing industries, we will compare the average for the drug industry for the years 1968–1972 (18.1) with the corresponding average (10.6) for all manufacturing industries. The difference to be explained thus is 7.5 percentage points.

EXPENSING OF R & D. Expensing the full costs of R & D in the year in which they occur is a conservative accounting convention which protects firms against the failure to realize any return from so uncertain an investment as R & D expenditures. It refuses to assume that R & D is an asset and also yields the tax benefit of what is in effect a form of accelerated depreciation. Such treatment is required by the rules of the accounting profession.

Since the profit rate is allegedly evidence of monopoly power, our primary concern here is to estimate the effect of expensing R & D on the accounting rate of profit rather than to debate the wisdom or tax consequences of this accounting procedure. Clearly from an economic standpoint the capitalization procedure is more appropriate than that of expensing, since R & D expenditures are intended to create a future flow of income.[15]

We can see the effect of expensing R & D expenditures in the following analysis. Let P_e equal the profit rate on stockholders' equity computed by expensing R & D costs. We will assume that R & D costs are the only costs. Then,

$$P_e = (S - R)/E_e$$

where S = sales,

R = R & D expenditures,

E_e = stockholders' equity computed under the expensing procedure.

Let P_c designate the profit rate computed by capitalizing R & D expenditures. Then,

$$P_c = (S - D)/(E_e + U)$$

where D = depreciation charges for R & D expenditures in past years and in the current year, and

U = the undepreciated part of R & D expenditures.

Thus absolute profits under expensing $(S - R)$ will exceed absolute profits under capitalization $(S - D)$ to the extent that D, the current year's depreciation, exceeds R, the current year's research expenditures. As research expenditures decline, they will reach a point where depreciation charges exceed the current level of research expenditures. When the absolute profits are equal under the two procedures, the rate of profit under the expensing procedure will be larger owing to the inclusion of U, the undepreciated part of research expenditures, in stockholders' equity under the capitalization procedure.

The problem is thus to estimate the effect that expensing drug R & D has on the drug industry's reported rate of profit. My estimate is based on Jesse Friedman's estimate for six of the largest manufacturers.[16]

Friedman estimates that capitalization of R & D expenditures would reduce the average rate for his six drug companies from 21.2 percent to 16.8 percent (a difference of 4.4 percentage points). We have started with a lower base, 18.1 percent, so we will use a proportionate decrease (3.8 percentage points). Since a comparable adjustment for all manufacturing industries would reduce their average profit rate only by .3 percentage points, according to Friedman, the net adjustment for the accounting procedure thus reduces the difference by 3.5 percentage points. The difference between the reported average profit rate for the drug industry and that for all manufacturing is 7.5 percentage points, so we are left with 4.0 percentage points still to be accounted for.

Since this large adjustment considerably reduces the estimate of the alleged monopoly effect on the average profit rate, Friedman's estimate needs evaluation. His crucial assumption is a twenty-year period for depreciation. This assumption corresponds to the estimates of the R & D period plus the commercial life of a new drug that we used in obtaining the expected rate of return on investment in R & D. In addition, a comparison of Friedman's estimate of the effect of expensing R & D on the reported rate of profit and that of Harry Bloch[17] indicates that Friedman's estimate is conservative.

RISK. Economists generally agree that profit rates increase directly with the riskiness of investments. The explanation runs as follows. Firms undertaking risky investment projects suffer from losses or low earnings more frequently than firms investing in relatively secure projects. Their inducement to undertake such risky investments is a relatively high average rate of return. This hypothesis is confirmed by Conrad and Plotkin, who found that the average profit rates of industries increase directly with the dispersion of profit rates among firms in those separate industries, which is the Conrad-Plotkin measure of risk. [18]

The Conrad-Plotkin equation for the average profit rate relates it to the index of risk and so provides a basis for estimating that part of the average profit rate of the drug industry that is due to a relatively high degree of risk. This equation indicates that 2.8 percentage points of the industry's average profit rate should be ascribed to risk, which reduces the residual difference from 4.0 to 1.2 percentage points.[19]

THE GROWTH OF SALES. Economists have overlooked the effect of steadily growing sales on the drug industry's profits, perhaps because of the belief that periods of market growth are short and therefore cannot produce high profits over a long period. General studies of industry profit rates, however, indicate that the growth in demand may be important even over a long period. Stanley Ornstein utilizes market concentration, firm size, economies of scale, capital requirements, and the capital-labor ratio, as well as the growth of sales as explanatory factors, and he finds that the growth in sales is by far the most important variable accounting for as much as 60 percent of the interfirm variation in profit rates. Another study, by W. G. Shepherd, also indicates the importance of this variable.[20]

Both domestic and foreign sales by the drug industry have grown continuously since the early 1950s. The increase in domestic sales is the result of the increase in the demand for medical services which in turn can be traced back to the growth of population, changes in the age composition of that population, the increase in the general level of income and to several familiar developments in the financing of medical care. Specifically, during the 1950s and 1960s nearly all families in the middle- and upper-income groups obtained some form of hospital insurance; by 1968 more than 90 percent of families with income over $10,000 had hospital insurance.[21] Thus, while in 1950 private health insurance paid for 8.5 percent of total medical bills, in 1971 it paid 25 percent. In the latter year it covered 41 percent of all medical costs not paid for by public programs. And private insurance was much more important in relation to hospital care than it was to medical care generally; it constituted 73 percent of consumer outlays for hospital care in 1971. And it is well known that the demand for medical care, and therefore drugs, increases with the number of families covered by medical insurance. This is one of the reasons total medical care expenses rose from 5.9 percent of personal consumption expenditures in 1960 to 7.7 percent in 1970.

The other elements in the growth of demand are also familiar. Since 1950 real personal incomes have risen significantly, and growth in personal income has traditionally been associated with an increase in expenditures for medical care. Also, during this period, Medicare and Medicaid were inaugurated, increasing demand among the aged and those with low incomes. Finally, the age structure of the population has continued to shift upwards creating an obvious increase in the demand for medical care. The contribution of this component may exceed that of all of the other components of the growth in demand.

The growth in consumer demand for medical care led to an increase in domestic drug sales measured in constant dollars between 1960 and 1972 of 148 percent, which is the equivalent of an average annual rate of growth of 7.9 percent. The increase in drug sales thus was much larger than the 62 percent growth of GNP (average annual rate of growth of 4.2 percent) over the same period.

The growth in sales abroad has been even more spectacular. The constant-dollar increase in the foreign sales of the industry between 1960 and 1972 was 331 percent,[22] or the equivalent of an average annual rate of growth of 12.4 percent.

We must estimate the effect of this growth of sales on the profit rate in the industry. Shepherd's equation provides a basis for such an estimate. This equation indicates that about 1.1 percentage points result from the growth of sales.[23] Subtracting this 1.1 percent from the 1.2 yields a final residual of .1 percentage points. This residual indicates that the excess of the average accounting rate of profit in the industry over the average for all manufacturing corporations is accounted for by other factors than monopoly power.

The results may be difficult to accept, for they suggest the anomalous conclusion that patents, which, as is well known, are more important for the pharmaceutical than other industries, have apparently not achieved their goal of permitting innovators a high rate of profit. But the mystery is only apparent: the availability of patents has encouraged individual companies to invest at such high rates that their average rate of profit is no higher than in other industries.

A patent prevents imitation of an innovation for a specified period and so permits the owner to retain the resulting profits. Withdrawal of some of the rights granted under patents will reduce the short-run rate of profit to be obtained from innovations, and the average rate of profit in the industry will also decline. But over any extended period there is no reason for the average profit rate from investment in R & D to be any higher than from other forms of investment, whether or not patents are available. A higher average rate of return will induce additional capital to enter, up the point where the rate of return is again equal to that available from other investments. Similarly, a lower rate of return will tend to divert investment elsewhere. Thus, a reduction in the protection offered by patents will reduce the profit rate from investment in R & D only temporarily; it will encourage the industry to reduce the quantity of its investment in R & D and thereby raise the profit rate on R & D.

The emphasis in this discussion has been on the average rate of return rather than on the rate of return of individual companies that succeed or fail in their searches for new products. Of course, the "winners" will earn high profits, and any reduction in the protection offered by patents will limit these profits. It is these winners and the high profits they generate that attract public attention.

But the important consideration from the standpoint of public policy is not the level of profits earned by successful innovators; rather, it is the magnitude of investment by the entire industry in R & D and the average rate of return it earns on such investment. Changes in the rules of the game, as defined by the patent system, enacted to limit high profits by the "winners," will most likely act to lower the overall quantity of industry resources invested in R & D.

The opportunities for investment in R & D, which is the principal form of investment in this industry, change over time as major discoveries occur and changes take place in the economic conditions of the industry and in its institutional framework, which includes the patent system and all of the associated rights. That changes in opportunities for profitable investment are reflected primarily by changes in the volume of investment rather than by changes in the profit rate is illustrated by the experience of the drug industry itself. Opportunities in this industry have been the result of important scientific breakthroughs in the 1940s and 1950s. Investment in R & D in the industry grew enormously starting in the early 1950s. By 1971 the industry R & D expenditures for human ethical drugs were twelve times as large as they were in 1950.[24] This can be compared to total gross private domestic investment in 1971, in the economy as a whole, of 2.8 times that in 1950. The growth in drug R & D expenditures, moreover, has outpaced the growth in drug sales.

The average realized rate of profit of pharmaceutical manufacturers has not exceeded the average realized rate of all manufacturing after adjustment for expensing R & D, riskiness of investment, and the growth of sales, despite the importance of patents for this industry. The patent protection has resulted in a large investment in R & D rather than a high expected rate of profit. The public policy of granting patents has had the intended effect of increasing investment in research which has reduced the profit rate to the same level as in other industries where patent protection is unimportant.

Not only have the patents failed to maintain a profit rate in excess of the average for all manufacturing but the expiration of patents threatens to reduce the average profit rate in this industry to a level which is below that of all manufacturing. The rate of innovation declined in the 1960s and the sales of new drugs have not been so large as to compensate for the decline in the rate. If the present rate of innovation continues, we can expect the realized rate of profit to decline as the patents on the drug introduced in the late 1950s and early 1960s expire. Maintenance of the rate of growth of demand in the industry will not prevent the realized rate from falling most of the way to the all-manufacturing average. The realized rate of profit may decline below that of all manufacturing as firms expand this output of generic products and engage in severe price cutting. As realized profits fall, firms will quickly come to understand that the expected rate has declined, if they have not already understood this, and investment in R & D then surely will decline. If the rate of profit falls below the all-manufacturing average, the decline in R & D investment will bring it back to that level. From the standpoint of public policy the important prediction is not that the profit rate ultimately will converge to that of all manufacturing but that *investment in pharmaceutical R & D will decline.*

CONCLUSIONS

If the drug industry is to maintain or increase its investment in R & D, the rate of return it expects from such investment must at least equal that obtainable from alternative investments. While the expected rate of return from investment in other industries probably exceeds 10 percent after taxes, the expected rate from investment in pharmaceutical R & D is estimated at 3.3 percent. This expected rate has declined from the level of 1960. It therefore seems likely that the low level and the decline in the rate from the previous high level will cause investment in pharmaceutical R & D to fall.

These are the primary considerations which must guide the development of public policy. Unfortunately, the debate over alleged monopoly power in the industry has dominated discussion and has largely obscured these considerations from public view. The attention given to the industry by the various federal agencies and congressional committees has been concerned primarily with the possibility that the prices of drugs are excessive and warrant changes in public policy to limit the resulting apparently high profits. The evidence, however, is very dubious. The discussion in the present chapter indicates that prices currently are not sufficiently high to yield a rate of return which will attract investment in pharmaceutical R & D.

Since R & D expenditures account for a major part of total investment by the pharmaceutical industry, the expected rate of return on investment in the industry, including plant and equipment as well as R & D, is unlikely to exceed the expected rate on investment in other industries. The average price of drugs thus is not sufficiently above costs to warrant the change of the exercise of monopoly power. Were prices monopolistic then the expected rate of return from investment in the industry would be above the expected rate in other industries.

The case for the proposition that prices in the industry have been excessive rests to a large extent on the evidence of the comparison of the average accounting profit rate on equity in the industry with that in other industries. A high average accounting rate of profit, however, by itself does not signify excessive prices, for it can be due to other things. The high current average in this industry is due to the noncapitalized investment in important innovations of the late 1950s and early 1960s, which are still protected by patents; the current high profits thus are the result of successful R & D investment many years ago which is not reported on the books of the companies. The lag between investment and profits in this industry is long. The cause of the high current accounting profit rate is not high prices but the practice of expensing R & D rather than capitalizing it. The effect of this practice on apparent profit rates is largely due to the great lag between investment and profits. Other factors include the continued growth in demand for drugs in the U.S. and in the world as a whole, and the high risk associated with investment in pharmaceutical R & D. The apparently high average profit rate thus can be explained without resorting to the hypothesis that firms exercise monopoly power.

Proponents of changes in public policy aimed at reducing the prices of drugs point to the profits earned in the manufacture and sale of certain prominent drugs. These drugs, however, have been exceptionally successful. The sales of most drugs are not large enough to result in high profits to their manufacturers. Nevertheless, it is the highly successful drugs which have been taken to be representative of the industry's products.

CHAPTER 8

THE LIFE OF
DRUG PATENTS

INTRODUCTION

The ever recurrent human impulse to kill the goose which lays our golden eggs has manifested itself once again, in recent years, in the form of proposals to shorten the term of patents for drugs or to require compulsory licensing for limited fees. The majority of our life-saving, illness-mitigating drugs have been produced by profit-motivated, industrial investment in research and development. Without patents to protect the industry's right to collect a return on this investment, the ability of physicians to aid their patients would be severely limited.

Nonprofit investment in drug research, which would occur even in the absence of a patent system, does occasionally produce a polio vaccine or a penicillin. Such investment supports most medical-related research. But nearly all of the nonprofit research is devoted to biological research which is only distantly related to drug discovery. The industry has the major responsibility for the discovery and development of new drugs: 91 percent of all new drugs introduced between 1960 and 1969 were the product of industrial R & D.

We are dependent upon the patent system to motivate that part of drug R & D which is responsible for the discovery of the vast majority of new drugs which have shortened stays in mental hospitals, nearly eliminated diseases such as tuberculosis which were once major causes of death, and are now making inroads on such current major killers as hypertension and heart disease.

Progress in drug therapy has slowed down, yet it continues. Such progress is our hope for a continuing reduction in human suffering and a further rise in healthful longevity. But that hope is being threatened by a continuing decline in the profitability of drug research—a decline which is partly the result of the falling effective life of drug patents.

162

EFFECTIVE VERSUS NOMINAL PATENT LIFE

A drug requires approval by the FDA to be marketed. Before such clearance, the patent is ineffective. We distinguish the *effective* life of a drug patent, which begins with the marketing of the protected drug, from its *nominal* life, which begins with the issuance of the patent. The effective life is shorter, because the date of marketing 'comes after the date of issuance and both the effective and the nominal life end with the expiration of the patent. This chapter estimates the average effective life and examines the trend in this average.

The effective life of a drug patent may be reduced by increasing the period needed to meet regulatory requirements for marketing as well as by legislating a shorter nominal life. We therefore investigate the change in the period from the date of submission of the application to the FDA for approval of an IND to the date of approval of the NDA. The approval of an IND authorizes clinical tests. The application for such approval marks the beginning of the regulatory period: it is when the FDA first becomes involved. The end of the regulatory period comes with the approval of the NDA, at which time the manufacturer is authorized to begin marketing the drug. In this chapter, data on the length of the regulatory period for drugs which came to market in the late 1960s and that for drugs which came to market in the 1970s are compiled and compared to determine whether this is the primary cause of the shortening which has occurred in effective patent life.

A patent is applied for shortly after the compound has been synthesized and has received the initial animal tests to determine whether it possesses the desired biological activity. The resulting drug usually is not marketed until several years later, if it is ever marketed. The time in between is taken up with additional and more intensive animal tests, clinical tests, and the FDA review of the evidence of efficacy and safety of the drug.

The sponsor of a potential drug must file with the FDA an IND application supporting the claim that the drug can be safely administered to humans under controlled conditions. If the FDA does not comment adversely within thirty days of the application, then clinical testing may begin. These phase I tests, which are usually conducted with a small number of normal volunteers, determine the maximum dosage of drug which is free from unacceptable side effects. A compound which successfully passes these early clinical trials becomes an active drug candidate; it is tested for long periods of time (often two or two-and-a-half years) for an indication of its long-term safety in animals with metabolic pathways similar to those in humans. At the same time it is also ready to be tested in human subjects with the target disease in order to determine its efficacy. These phase II tests are followed by phase III studies with large groups of outpatients in a search for low-incidence side effects. The sponsor can now submit an NDA to the FDA for its approval. The FDA seldom reviews the data submitted in the NDA within the legally required 180 days.

Some of the discussion of public policy assumes that the effective life of patents is the same as the nominal life. This assumption was one of the factors which induced Senator Estes Kefauver in 1961 to introduce a bill incorporating a provision requiring the compulsory licensing of drug patents. Senator Gaylord Nelson recently revived the Kefauver proposal in modified form.[1]

THE NATURE AND PURPOSE OF THE PATENT GRANT

Before estimating the effective life of drug patents, we will discuss briefly some related issues. Proposals which would reduce the life of a patent assume that it grants special rights which must be justified. Statements which describe the patent as a grant of monopoly power and defend it as being necessary to induce investors to accept the risk involved in R & D investment encourage the impression that the patent right is exceptional in some way. But investment in R & D receives no more special treatment than investment in construction. A patent is a deed reserving the collectible fruits of R & D investment for the investor just as a deed to an apartment building reserves the collectible fruits of the investment in construction for the investor. Others may also invest in apartment construction to compete in the rental market, but the deed prevents them from moving into someone else's apartment without payment to the investor. A patent simply prevents someone else from using the knowledge developed by R & D investment without payment to the investor on mutually acceptable terms. Others can invest in R & D programs which produce competing products.

There is special treatment of investment in R & D to the extent that the deed does not give the investor rights to his investment in perpetuity, as a deed to an apartment building does. The patent recognizes the rights of ownership of the fruits of R & D just as a deed recognizes the rights of ownership of a building. The parallel may not be obvious because of the intangibility of the knowledge which the patent covers and the difficulty in distinguishing new from old knowledge. The concept of ownership of a specified physical object is easier to grasp. One must bear in mind that it is the new knowledge represented by a patented product which creates the right; the designer of a new product which is an obvious application of old knowledge cannot under the law obtain a patent.

Acceptance of rights of ownership entailed by patents thus does not depend on a special evaluation of the resulting benefits: they are part of a wider class of ownership rights. But, since this inclusion is not widely recognized, patents have been defended as a distinctively different kind of property necessary for the encouragement of invention. It is obviously true that patents protect the manufacturer of a new product against imitation and thereby raise the expected rate of return from investment in R & D. This, of course, encourages such investment, but no more so than property rights encourage investment in buildings.

The social gains from innovations encouraged by patents will always exceed the private gains of patent holders; the private gains are only part of the total social gain. Consider, for example, the extreme case of a product covered by a patent which gives the patent holder an effective monopoly because the product has no good substitutes. Even then the patent holder will not capture the total benefit from the production and sale of a product. Whatever the price is, some purchasers would be willing to pay a higher price in order to gain the benefit from the product. These purchasers receive a net benefit equal to the difference between the price they are willing to pay and the actual price.[2] The patent holder could obtain the total social benefit only by charging each consumer the maximum price he would be willing to pay. Since the price is the same to all consumers, the patent holder does not obtain the total benefit. A high price may deprive some consumers of the product, but if the patent was required in order to induce the required R & D investment, it does not make such consumers worse off.[3]

A related issue concerns the importance of patent protection. The resistance of drug companies to proposals to limit the effective life of drug patents is obvious evidence of their importance. Nevertheless, some of the literature suggests that patents generally, including those for drugs, are an unnecessary incentive to innovation, because innovators generally are protected by other barriers to competition. One suggestion is that the lack of appropriate technology and of service organizations may prevent potential competitors from entering the market quickly, after the introduction of a new product, and undercutting the price.[4]

It is true that in some industries the necessary technical knowledge to manufacture a complex product is difficult to acquire. In addition, innovators are protected by the dependence of customers on technical services supplied along with the products and by the difficulty which competitors have in matching the quality of these services. Moreover, patent protection is of less value where new products are constantly being introduced.

In the case of the pharmaceutical industry, however, duplication of products by competitors is so easy as to make patent protection extremely valuable. A drug's label reports its formula, and many manufacturers can easily replicate the compound. Thus, when the patent on a large-selling product expires, many imitations enter. It is true that by the time a patent expires, the original producer has established a well-known brand name in which physicians have some confidence. But as other major manufacturers introduce duplicates, many physicians will shift to prescribing generically rather than specifying the brand name of the original product. Thus, over 30 percent of the total number of prescriptions of leading multiple-source drugs are written generically.[5] The generic manufacturers which base their appeal on price take a large share of the sales away from the original producer. The patent thus provides important protection against imitation in the drug industry.

Another quite different argument also suggests that patents are unimportant.

Edmund Kitch says that a good substitute for a patent is the requirement of NDA approval, which a company must obtain from the FDA before it markets a drug. Obtaining such approval is a very complex, time-consuming and expensive procedure. The application itself runs into thousands of pages because the FDA requires from the applicant all of the available information which is related to the effect of the compound. It is important to note that the FDA requires an NDA for all drugs which differ generically from previously marketed drugs. Two drugs are generically identical when the active ingredient is the same in both. The requirement applies to molecular modifications of an original drug having similar therapeutic effects and side effects as well as to drugs having no obvious predecessors. Further, sponsors of derivative drugs which are not duplicates cannot rely on evidence of efficacy and safety presented in the application submitted in behalf of the original drug but must supply fresh evidence. Thus, according to Kitch, the requirement that the manufacturer of a new drug submit an NDA provides the same type of protection as a patent.[6]

But Kitch exaggerates the effectiveness of the protection which the NDA can provide against imitation. The requirement does not apply to generic versions of drugs which have been on the market for some time. A manufacturer which proposes to duplicate a drug classified as old is required to submit only an Abbreviated New Drug Application, a brief document which describes the manufacturing process and refers to published literature on the efficacy and safety of the original drug. How old a drug must be before a generic version is exempt from the NDA requirements is not known. The FDA has not announced any general rules governing the acceptability of ANDA's. We do know that potential producers of generic versions can present ANDA's shortly before the expiration of a patent, and the FDA may be prepared to accept ANDA's within a much shorter time of the grant of the patent of the original drug than seventeen years. Compulsory licensing, in that case, would limit the effective life of patents, perhaps very considerably.

We will now return to the main question. What is the average effective life of drug patents? It is not certain that the average effective life is less than seventeen years. Deliberate delays in filing applications for patents so as to prolong their effective life, as well as delays in the Patent Office in granting applications, may extend the effective life. The delays may more than offset the period required for clinical testing and FDA approval.

Nevertheless, the effective life is likely to be less than the nominal life. The application for a patent is likely to come well before the marketing of a drug, because delay entails some risk to the validity of the claims of the innovator. Another firm working in the same field may file a patent application for the same drug first. In addition, public discussion of the new compound prior to one year before the filing of the application endangers the validity of the patent, since it places the compound in the public domain.[7] Therefore, a patent usually will be applied for early in the development of a drug, and thus it is likely to be issued before marketing.

ESTIMATES OF EFFECTIVE PATENT LIFE

The effective life of a drug patent is the difference between the date of expiration of the patent and the date at which the NDA is approved. An example of a short effective patent life as a result of the long regulatory period before a drug can be marketed is provided by Hyperstat, one of the new chemical entities introduced in the period 1966–73 (table 8-1). It was patented in 1961, and its patent expires in 1978. Since it was not cleared for marketing in the United States until 1973, ten years after its NDA was submitted to the FDA, and twelve years after the patent was granted, the effective life of its patent in the U.S. market is only five years (from 1973 NDA approval to patent expiration in 1978).

Our estimate of the average effective life of drug patents will be based on a list of NCE's introduced in the United States during the years 1966 through 1973. The list was constructed by Harold Clymer of the SmithKline Corporation. Mr. Clymer defined a new chemical entity as a compound of molecular structure not previously tested in man, excluding new salts, vaccines, and diagnostic agents.

For our estimate, we need the date of the approval of the NDA for each drug and the date of patent. No problem is presented by the date of the approval of the NDA; this information is published in the weekly list of drugs approved by the FDA, which is available in the *Food, Drug & Cosmetic Law Reports,* published by the Commerce Clearing House, Inc. To establish a patent date for each NCE, we first obtained a list of patents relating to each drug, together with their dates of issue. These lists were compiled by the patent consultant, Louis Leaman. The problem was to select the patent which provided the effective protection against imitation. It is generally true that process patents are not very effective, since it is usually easy for a pharmaceutical manufacturer to develop alternative processes without risking infringements. In addition, process patents are difficult to enforce, since it is not easy to obtain an exact description of the process used. The manufacturer is unlikely to supply such a description if he is infringing a process patent unless forced to do so by a court order. The patent covering the chemical composition of the active ingredient thus is the significant one. We have used the date of this patent for the estimation of what we designate as the Best Judgment Estimate. Since process patents may provide some protection, we will also provide an alternative estimate, which we designate as the High Estimate.

The Clymer list of NCE's introduced in the U.S. between 1966 and 1973 included ninety-five drugs. Of this list, fourteen were not protected by patents and one had been withdrawn from the market. Therefore the study was limited to the remaining eighty drugs (table 8-1).

After Leaman supplied the list of patents together with the patent numbers and dates of issue of patents for each of the drugs, the patent covering the chemical composition of the active ingredient was identified. Letters were then

TABLE 8-1
List of Eighty NCE's Introduced 1966–73

Company	Brand Names	Generic Name	Year Introduced
Abbott	Tranxene	Clorazepate	1972
American Home	Atromid-S	Clofibrate	1967
Products (Ayerst	Inderal	Propranolol	1967
and Wyeth)	Veracillin	Dicloxacillin	1968
	Ovral	Norgestrel	1968
Baxter Laboratories	Travase	Sutilains	1969
Boehringer Ingelheim	Alupent	Metaproterenol	1973
Bristol	Versapen	Hetacillin	1970
Burroughs Wellcome	Zyloprim	Allopurinol	1966
	Tabloid Brand Thioguanine	Thioguaine	1966
	Alcopara	Bephenium	1967
	Imuran	Azathiopine	1968
Dome	Tridesilon	Desonide	1972
Dupont (Endo)	Symmetrel	Amantadine	1966
	Narcan	Naloxone	1971
Fisons	Intal	Cromolyn	1973
Geigy	Tegretol	Carbamazepine	1968
Hoechst	Lasix	Furosemide	1966
Hoffmann-LaRoche	Matulane	Procarbazine	1969
	FUDR	Floxuridine	1970
	Dalmane	Flurazepam	1970
	Ancobon	Flucytosine	1971
	Bactrim	Trimethoprim + Sulfamethoxazole	1973
Johnson & Johnson	Retin-A	Tretinoin	1971
Lakeside	Triclos	Trichlorethyl phosphate	1972
Lederle	Levoprome	Methotrimeprazine	1966
	Myambutol	Ethambutol	1967
	Aristospan	Triamcinolone	1969
	Minocin	Minocycline	1971
Lilly	Loridine	Cephaloridine	1968
	Kafocin	Cephaloglycin	1970
	Keflex	Cephalexin	1971
	Capastat	Capreomycin	1971
	Darvon-N	Dextropropoxyphene napsylate	1971
McNeil	Haldol	Haloperidol	1967
	Innovar	Fentanyl + Droparidol	1968
	Sublimaze	Fentanyl	1968
Mead Johnson	Halotex	Haloprogin	1971
	Megace	Megestrol Acetate	1971
Merck	Vivactil	Protriptyline	1967
	Edecrin	Ethacrynic Acid	1967
	Mintezol	Thiabendazole	1967
Merrell National	Clomid	Clomiphene	1967
Ohio Medical	Ethrane	Enflurane	1972

TABLE 8-1 (continued)

Company	Brand Names	Generic Name	Year Introduced
Organon	Pavulon	Pancuronium Bromide	1972
Parke Davis	Steri-Vial Propoquin	Amopyroquin	1966
	Ponstel	Mefenamic Acid	1967
	Betapar	Meprednisone	1968
	Ketalar	Ketamine	1970
Pennwalt	Zaroxolyn	Metolazone	1973
Pfizer/Roerig	Rondomycin	Methacycline	1966
	Vibramycin	Doxycycline	1967
	Navane	Thiothixene	1967
	Sinequan	Doxepin	1969
	Geopen	Carbenicillin	1970
	Mithracin	Mithramycin	1970
	Antiminth	Pyrantel	1971
Robins	Sulla	Sulfameter	1966
	Pondimin	Fenfluramine	1973
Sandoz	Serentil	Mesoridazine	1970
	Sanorex	Mazindol	1973
Schering	Garamycin	Gentamycin	1966
	Tinactin Cream	Tolnaftate	1966
	Hyperstat	Diazoxide	1973
Searle	Ovulen	Ethynodiol diacetate + Mestranol	1966
SmithKline	Vontrol	Diphenidol	1967
	Ancef	Cefazolin	1973
Squibb	Hydrea	Hydroxyurea	1967
	Teslac	Testolactone	1969
Syntex	Lidex	Fluocinonide	1971
Unimed	Serc	Betahistine	1966
Upjohn	Cytosar	Cytosine Arabinoside	1969
	Cleocin	Clindamycin	1970
	Trobicin	Spectinomycin	1971
	Methosarb	Calusterone	1973
	Prostin Alpha	Dinoprost Tromethamine	1973
USV	Voranil	Clortermine	1973
Wampole	Urispas	Flavoxate	1970
Winthrop	Talwin	Pentazocine	1967
	Marcaine	Bupivacaine	1972

Note: Where the same chemical entity is marketed by more than one company under different brand names, only the company holding the patent is listed here.

sent to all of the patent holders requesting that the date of issue of each patent covering the active ingredient be confirmed. At the same time we requested confirmation of the date of approval of the NDA. Replies were not received for ten products. Since the dates of both the patents covering composition of matter and of the NDA approvals were confirmed for all of the products covered in the responses, we assumed that the dates were accurate for the products for which no responses were received.

THE AVERAGE EFFECTIVE PATENT LIFE OF NCE'S INTRODUCED 1966–73. The average effective life is considerably shorter than the nominal patent life. The Best Judgment Estimate of the arithmetic mean of the effective patent life of NCE's introduced in the period 1966–73 is 13.1 years, or 3.9 years less than the nominal life of seventeen years.

Table 8-2 shows a large dispersion of effective patent life. Eighteen percent of all products have effective lives of less than ten years, while, at the other extreme, 16 percent have a longer effective life than the nominal one. The patent in the latter group was granted after marketing. The remaining 66 percent are scattered over the range of ten to seventeen years, with a moderate degree of concentration in the intervals thirteen to fourteen and sixteen to seventeen years.

An analysis by therapeutic classes (table 8-3) reveals that although the FDA may be expected to be permissive towards NDA's for cancer drugs, the average effective life of drugs in this group is short. The short effective patent life of analgesics and anesthetics may be the result of difficulty in demonstrating efficacy. At the other end of the ranking are anti-inflammatories and psychotropics, which show the longest patent life.

Some of the classes may have too few drugs for the averages to be reliable. However, since such classes do give some indication of the interclass variation in effective patent life, any reduction in the number of classes would sacrifice information.

Two biases lead to underestimates of the average effective patent life. They also present serious problems for the later estimation of the average regulatory period and of the NDA approval period.

The first bias is the result of the exclusion from our list of those patented

TABLE 8-2
Distribution of NCE's Introduced 1966–73,
by Years of Effective Patent Life

Effective Life (years)	Number of Drugs	Percent of Total
More than 17	13	16
16–16.9	11	14
15–15.9	6	8
14–14.9	5	6
13–13.9	12	15
12–12.9	3	4
11–11.9	9	11
10–10.9	7	9
less than 10	14	18
Total	80	101

TABLE 8-3
Average Effective Patent Life for NCE's Introduced
1966–73, by Therapeutic Field

Therapeutic Field	Effective Patent Life (years)
Anti-infectives	13.7
Anti-inflammatories	15.3
Psychotropics	14.9
Analgesics and anesthetics	11.2
Cancer chemotherapy	11.5
Diuretics and cardiovascular	13.4
Antispasmodics and muscle relaxants	12.5
Other hormones	13.4
Miscellaneous	13.0
All fields	13.1

drugs which have not yet won NDA approval. According to Wardell and Lasagna, the delays of new cardiovascular drugs have been especially long.[8] Table 8-4, which is reproduced from Wardell and Lasagna's study, lists the dates of introduction of cardiovascular drugs in the U.K. and U.S. during the period 1962–71. The table shows that most drugs introduced in the U.K. still are not available in the U.S., and drugs which are available usually were first introduced in the U.K. One example is the antihypertensive drug, bethanidine, which Burroughs Wellcome marketed in the U.K. as long ago as 1963. According to Wardell and Lasagna, the β-blockers are a major development in the treatment of angina and hypertension. The delay in approving of the use of propanolol for the treatment of angina in particular has been out of line with expert medical opinion in the U.S. The other β-blockers, which are not available at all in the U.S., offer advantages over propanolol for some patients.

The second bias stems from the FDA's limitation of approval for use to a single indication. When the FDA approved of the marketing of propanolol in 1967, the agency restricted its use to the treatment of two specific types of cardiac arrythmias: pheochromocytoma and hypertrophic cubaortic stenosis. The FDA permitted the treatment of angina with propanolol six years later in 1973, much later than in many other countries. The restriction against the treatment of hypertension with this drug has not yet been lifted. According to Wardell and Lasagna, the drug is efficacious for both indications, and unwanted side effects are both predictable and manageable when proper precautions are taken. Moreover, expert opinion, as represented in 1971 by the *AMA Drug Evaluations*, advocated propanolol for the treatment of angina. Wardell and Lasagna also cite a textbook article of 1971 by Killip[9] hailing propanolol as the most significant advance in the treatment of angina since the advent of nitroglycerin. The same article also describes the use of propanolol in the treatment of hypertension. The fact that these publications are not periodicals indicates that expert opinion probably reached these views before 1971. Since American Home

TABLE 8-4
Introduction of Cardiovascular Drugs

	Date of Introduction		Lead in Years	
	U.K.	U.S.	U.K.	U.S.
Antihypertensive				
Pargyline (Eutonyl, Abbott)	1963	1963	0	0
Methyldopa (Aldomet, M.S.D.)	1962	1963	1	
Bethanidine (Esbatal, B.W.)	1963	–		
Guanoxan (Envacar, Pfizer)	1964	–		
Guanoclor (Vatensol, Pfizer)	1964	–		
The β-blockers[a]	1965	–		
Debrisoquin (Declinax, Roche)	1967	–		
Clonidine (Catapres, Boehringer)	1971	–		
β-adrenoreceptor antagonist				
Propranolol (Inderal, I.C.I.)	1965	1968	3	
Practolol (Eraldin, I.C.I.)	1970	–		
Oxprenolol (Trasicor, Ciba)	1970	–		
Antiarrhythmic				
Bretylium tosylate[b,c] (Darenthin, B.W.)	1959[d]	–		
β-blockers[a] other than propanolol	1970	–		
Antianginal, vasodilator, and miscellaneous				
Isoxuprine (Vasodilan, Mead Johnson)	1963	1959		4
Prenylamine[c] (Synadrin 60, Hoechst)	1961	–		
Benziodarone[b,e] (Cardivix, Genatosan)	1962	–		
Trimetazidine[b] (Vastarel, Servier)	1964	–		
The β-blockers[a]	1965	–		
Verapamil (Cordilox, Harvey)	1967	–		
Moxisylyte[b] (Opilon, Warner)	1968	–		
Hypolipedmic				
Dextrothyroxine (Choloxin, Flint)	1961	1967	6	
Cholestyramine (Cuemid, M.S.D.)	1970	1965[f]		5
Clofibrate (Atromid-S, I.C.I.)	1963	1967	4	

Source: William M. Wardell and Louis Lasagna, *Regulation and Drug Development* (Washington, D.C.: American Enterprise Institute for Public Policy Research, 1975), p. 60.

[a]Listed here but counted under a different heading in the numerical summary.

[b]International Nonproprietary Name.

[c]Listed but does not satisfy all criteria for inclusion in numerical summary.

[d]As antihypertensive.

[e]Subsequently withdrawn. Listed but not included in numerical summary.

[f]Not approved as hypolipidemic in U.S.

Products obtained a patent for propanolol in 1967, the effective patent life for its use in cardiac arrythmias is the full seventeen years which was the datum used in the estimates of average effective life. But for angina the life will be eleven years and for hypertension the life will be even shorter. The treatment of the two specified types of arrythmias are minor uses, so the resulting estimate of the effective life of the patent for propanolol is biased upwards. This bias affects the estimates for other drugs in the same manner.

The Best Judgment Estimate was based on the date of the patent covering the composition of matter of the active ingredient. As we suggested previously, patents covering manufacturing processes and medical use are considered to be generally ineffective. Nevertheless, we take the precaution of providing a High Estimate of the effective patent life based on the date of the last patent pertaining to a product. The High Estimate is 14.1 years, compared to 13.1 years for the Best Judgment Estimate. Even this High Estimate results in an estimated average effective life of 2.9 years less than the nominal life.

THE TREND. We also want to know whether the FDA restrictiveness has grown over time and has resulted in a downward trend in the average effective life of patents. We therefore compare the Best Judgment Estimate of the average effective life of drugs approved in 1966–69 with that for 1970–73. The average dropped by 1.5 years, from 13.9 years for the first period to 12.4 years for the second period. The comparison of High Estimates yields substantially similar results: a drop of 1.3 years, from 14.8 years to 13.5 years.

The pervasiveness of the decline in average effective life of patents among therapeutic classes (table 8-5) suggests that greater FDA restrictiveness is the source rather than greater intrinsic difficulty of research and development. Greater intrinsic difficulty is more likely to be restricted to one or two therapeutic classes.

THE REGULATORY PERIOD

The FDA is involved in the regulation of the discovery and development process between the submission of the IND and the approval of the NDA. We will estimate the average length of this regulatory period for drugs in the entire

TABLE 8-5
Changes in Average Effective Patent Life from 1966–69 to 1970–73,
by Therapeutic Field

| | Average effective life (years) | | Difference (years) | Change percent |
	1966–69	1970–73		
Anti-infectives	13.8	13.6	−.2	−1.2
Anti-inflammatories	17.3	7.4	−9.9	−57.0
Psychotropics	17.4	12.5	−4.9	−28.2
Analgesics and anesthetics	12.5	9.3	−3.2	−26.0
Cancer chemotherapy	11.4	11.6	−.2	−1.5
Diuretics and cardiovascular	15.4	5.3	−10.1	−65.4
Antispasmodics and muscle relaxants	13.9	11.2	−2.7	−19.3
Other hormones	13.4	13.3	−.1	−.6
Miscellaneous	11.6	13.9	−2.3	−19.4
All fields	13.9	12.4	−1.5	−10.8

TABLE 8-6
Distribution of Length of Regulatory Period
for NCE's Introduced 1966–73, by Years

	Number	Percentage
8 and over	6	8
7–7.9	4	5
6–6.9	10	12
5–5.9	9	11
4–4.9	16	20
3–3.9	26	32
2–2.9	9	11
Total	80	99

period 1966–73 as well as the difference between the average regulatory periods for NCE's approved in the same two subperiods which we used previously with a view to determining whether increased FDA restrictiveness has reduced the average effective patent life. The required data were obtained from the FDA and from companies which marketed the drugs.

THE AVERAGE REGULATORY PERIOD FOR NCE'S INTRODUCED 1966–73. The average regulatory period for NCE's introduced during the period 1966–73 was 4.8 years. Table 8-6 analyzes the number of NCE's by length of regulatory period. As many as 13 percent required more than seven years. Table 8-7 reports the average regulatory period for each therapeutic class. The longest regulatory period surprisingly was required by cancer drugs, despite the desperate need for such drugs and the high incidence of mortality within a short time of the onset of cancer. Any evidence of efficacy should be considered adequate, and the usual safety considerations should not apply. The regulatory delay may be offset for patients in major hospitals by the availability of experimental drugs which have not been approved for marketing. Such drugs, however, are not as readily available for other patients.

TABLE 8-7
Average Regulatory Period for NCE's Introduced 1966–73, by Therapeutic Field

	Regulatory Period (years		Regulatory Period (years)
Anti-infectives	4.3	Diuretics and	4.9
Anti-inflammatories	4.2	cardiovascular	
Psychotropics	5.0	Antispasmodics and	4.6
Analgesics and anesthetics	4.6	muscle relaxants	
Cancer chemotherapy	5.6	Other hormones	3.3
		Miscellaneous	5.9
		All fields	4.8

175

TABLE 8-8
Percentage Distribution of Approval Periods for NCE's
Introduced 1966–73, by Length of Approval Period

Approval Period (years)	Number of NCE's	Percent of Total
0–.9	14	18
1–1.9	27	34
2–2.9	21	26
3–3.9	9	11
4–4.9	3	4
5–5.9	1	1
6	5	6
Total	80	100

The manufacturer must obtain approval of an NDA before marketing a new drug. The period between the dates of submission and approval of the NDA is a measurable part of the whole regulatory period, and the time required by the FDA for such approval has attracted a great deal of attention. We call this the approval period. Our survey of companies obtained the dates of submission of NDA's for all NCE's introduced between 1966 and 1973 together with confirmation of the dates of approval of the NDA's. The average approval period is 2.4 years. Table 8-8 reports the percentage distribution of approval periods. As many as 48 percent required more than two years.

Table 8-9 shows that the approval period varies among therapeutic fields. The miscellaneous category required the longest average approval period (3.6 years). The bronchodilator drugs, which are included in this category, took an especially long time to win approval. The average approval period for the specified fields ranged from 2.0 years to 2.4 years. This range is not so large as to require special comment.

THE TREND. We have suggested that the lengthening rather than the acceleration of the regulatory period is more likely to be the principal source of the

TABLE 8-9
Arithmetic Mean Approval Time for Each Therapeutic Field of 1966–73 NCE's

	Mean Approval Period (years)		Mean Approval Period (years)
Anti-infectives	2.0	Diuretics and cardiovascular	2.2
Anti-inflammatories	2.3		
Psychotropics	2.0	Antispasmodics and muscle relaxants	2.4
Analgesics and anesthetics	2.2		
Cancer chemotherapy	2.0	Other hormones	2.4
		Miscellaneous	3.6
		All fields	2.4

reduction in effective patent life in the issue of patents. That the suggestion is correct is confirmed by our finding that the average regulatory period for drugs first marketed in 1970–73 was 5.6 years, or 1.6 years more than the average of 4.0 years for those first marketed in the subperiod 1966–69. Indeed, the increase in the regulatory period appears to be the only explanation for the reduction in effective patent life, since it is virtually the same: it will be recalled that the effective patent life declined by 1.5 years.

The estimate of the increase in the regulatory period between the two subperiods understates the full effect of the regulatory changes after 1962. All of the drugs introduced in the period 1966–69 were subject to the new regulations and the changed attitudes of agency officials. A better estimate of the delaying effect of the greater restrictiveness may be based on the average regulatory period of drugs introduced in 1970–73 and that of drugs introduced in 1966 for which the IND submission dates were early in 1963. Clinical tests for these drugs began before the IND's were required. Sponsors did not experience the full effect of the IND requirement, and the severity of regulatory demands increased later. The average regulatory period for the nine drugs approved in 1966 for which the IND submission dates came in the first six months of 1963 was 3.0 years, or 2.6 years less than the average of 5.6 years for the drugs introduced in 1970–73.

This difference tends to overstate the delaying effect of the new regulatory demands, since clinical testing began prior to IND submission in early 1963. But the overstatement is small, since such testing is unlikely to have gone on for more than six months. Mr. Harold Clymer, then vice-president of research and development of SmithKline, estimates that before the 1962 amendments, pre-clinical testing on the average took less than six months.[10] Indeed, by limiting the estimate of the regulatory period to the period between the date of IND submission and the approval of the NDA, we underestimate the increased delay. The IND requirement brought about an increase in the period required for preclinical animal testing. Thus, in 1969 Clymer estimated that the preparation for clinical testing, including the meeting of IND requirements, as well as the waiting period of thirty or more days following the IND submission before clinical testing was permitted, was 6 to 12 months.[11]

We can see that the increase in the average regulatory period was associated with a large increase in the proportion of NCE's having to wait more than seven years for NDA approval after the IND was submitted (table 8-10). The regulatory period having the largest percentage of NCE's approved in 1966–69 was 3 to 3.9 years. In the second subperiod the largest percentage showed up among those with a period of 7.0 years or more. The shift was large and involved a high proportion of NCE's.

The increase in the regulatory period was pervasive among therapeutic classes (table 8-11), confirming our earlier suggestion that the reduction in the average effective life between the two subperiods considered was the result of increased

TABLE 8-10
Distribution of Number and Percentage of NCE's Introduced in
1970–73 and 1966–69, by Length of Regulatory Period

Length of Regulatory Period (years)	Number of NCE's Introduced		Percentage of NCE's Introduced	
	1966–69	1970–73	1966–69	1970–73
7.0 and over	0	10	0	26
6–6.9	3	7	7	18
5–5.9	4	5	10	13
4–4.9	12	5	29	13
3–3.9	16	9	39	23
Less than 3	6	3	15	8
	41	39	100	101

FDA restrictiveness. The decline reported for anti-inflammatory drugs may be attributable to the small number of such drugs approved in both periods. Random influences on dates of the issue of patents in relation to IND submission and NDA approval dates may have overwhelmed the effect of greater FDA restrictiveness.

Part of the increase in the regulatory period may have come from an increase in the period required for NDA approval. But, in fact, the average NDA approval period declined by 0.8 years, from 2.8 years for drugs introduced in 1966–69 to 2.0 years in 1970–73.

TABLE 8-11
Changes in Average Length of Regulatory Period
from 1966–69 to 1970–73, by Therapeutic Class

	Average Regulatory Period (years)		Difference (years)	Change (percentage)
	1966–69	1970–73		
Anti-infective	3.3	4.7	1.4	42
Anti-inflammatory	4.8	3.3	−1.5	−31
Psychotropic	4.9	5.9	1.0	20
Analgesic and anesthetic	4.2	6.6	2.4	57
Cancer chemotherapy	4.9	6.6	1.7	35
Diuretic and cardiovascular	3.4	7.8	4.4	129
Antispasmodic and muscle relaxants	3.8	5.0	1.2	32
Other hormones	3.2	3.3	.1	3
Miscellaneous	4.6	6.7	2.1	46
Average	4.0	5.6	1.6	40

Table 8-12 shows that a substantial shift in the distribution of the lengths of approval periods towards the lower end. The percentage of drugs requiring less than one year for approval increased sharply from 7 percent to 28 percent. The proportion of those requiring 3 or more years dropped sharply from 28 percent to 15 percent.

As table 8-13 reports, the average approval period of all therapeutic fields except "Other hormones" declined between the two subperiods, and most of the declines were substantial. This analysis indicated that the reduction in the approval period was general rather than confined to one or two therapeutic classes.

One reason for the reduction in the approval period was the announcement in 1970 by the FDA of guidelines for adequate and well-controlled clinical investigations.[12] Both FDA officials and sponsors of drugs were able to speed up the process of approval with these more precise criteria for evaluating clinical investigations. In addition, the FDA published procedural requirements for requesting public hearings concerning issues of fact connected with an NDA. Dr. J. Richard Crout, Director of the Bureau of Drugs of the FDA, has stated that the FDA also improved managerial procedures designed to speed up decisions. According to Dr. Crout, moreover, the agency no longer suffers from the management instability which plagued it in the period 1962 to 1969.[13] This instability probably contributed to greater delays.

Since the regulatory period as a whole increased, the part preceding the submission of the NDA grew considerably. We can estimate the lengthening of the average pre-NDA submission part of the regulatory period. The average regulatory period as a whole increased by 1.6 years and the average NDA approval period fell by 0.8 years. The average pre-NDA part of the regulatory period thus increased by the sum, or by 2.4 years.

TABLE 8-12
Percentage Distribution of Approval Periods
for NCE's Approved in 1966–69 and 1970–73

Approval Period (years)	1966–69		1970–73	
	No. of NDA's	Percentage	No. of NDA's	Percentage
0–.9	3	7	11	28
1–1.9	14	34	13	33
2–2.9	12	29	9	23
3–3.9	5	12	4	10
4–4.9	3	7	0	0
5–5.9	1	2	0	0
6 and over	3	7	2	5
Total	41	98	39	99

TABLE 8-13
Arithmetic Mean Approval Period for Each Class
of NCE's Approved 1966–69 and 1970–73

	Years	
	1966–69	1970–73
Anti-infectives	2.5	1.6
Anti-inflammatories	2.6	1.1
Psychotropics	2.2	1.9
Analgesics and anesthetics	2.4	1.9
Cancer chemotherapy	2.3	1.4
Diuretics and cardiovasculars	2.2	2.0
Antispasmodic and muscle relaxants	4.3	1.3
Other hormones	1.4	3.1
Miscellaneous	4.6	2.9
Average	2.8	2.0

A NEW DELAY?

The FDA currently is considering a proposal which if enacted would further delay the marketing of new drugs and, more importantly, would render the discovery and development of new drugs much more difficult. The Health Research Group (HRG) has proposed that to protect human experimental subjects against risks of toxicity which animal tests may reveal, all of the usual animal tests should be completed and evaluated before an IND application is granted. The proposal would exempt compounds which promise a treatment for a fatal disease for which adequate alternative therapy is unavailable.

To evaluate this proposal it is necessary to review the discussion in chapters 2 and 3 of both clinical and animal tests in drug research. Drug research is organized by a series of provisional hypotheses which are refined after empirical tests. The assessment of the validity of hypotheses relating to the potency of synthesized chemical structures is very difficult in view of the inadequacies of animal models of human diseases; and the more innovative the potential therapeutic discovery, the more necessary is clinical validation. Governmental regulation which causes delays in clinical feedback to the discovery team thus can interfere seriously with research and bogs down the process of drug discovery, because the scientists are deprived of an indicator of the critical leads to new drugs.

Although the HRG seems to perceive great risks to the subjects of these early human trials, these tests have proven to be extremely safe. An article published by the Food and Drug Administration states: "the safety record of such research is excellent. FDA knows of no volunteer patient who has been permanently harmed as a result of phase I [early clinical] testing of hundreds of new compounds under the FDA procedures established in 1962."[14]

Drug research thus depends critically on early clinical tests for the evaluation of potential drugs. The evidence of animal studies concerning efficacy and safety, while valuable, is incomplete, and the development of a drug requires the possibility of clinical trials alternating with syntheses of new compounds and further animal tests. Furthermore, the limitation of research to animal studies alone until a late date may result in the rejection of potential drugs which would be accepted on the basis of clinical studies. In addition, tests of safety conducted with normal human volunteers have had adequate safeguards.

If the HRG's proposal is enacted, it would prevent the rapid evaluation of potential drugs by clinical tests and so render the whole process of drug research much more difficult than it already is. We have seen that drug research depends on the possibility of tests of numerous hypotheses through clinical trials. Rapid verification or rejection of hypotheses would become impossible, thus threatening to reduce the rate of drug innovation.

In addition, the cost of drug R & D would be increased enormously. We have seen in chapter 3 that, currently, the average time required to discover and develop a drug is at least ten years and the cost of R & D per NCE is $24 million. The current costs of R & D and the time required to produce a new drug are so high as to result in a low expected rate of return from investment in R & D. Chapter 7 estimated this rate to be 3.3 percent. Other factors in this low expected rate of return are the rate of innovation and the low average profit per drug. The acceptance of the HRG proposal would increase the time and costs required for R & D and reduce the expected rate of return further. Our description of drug research indicates that the completion of the presently required animal tests requires about two years. Of this time, we have seen that six to twelve months is required before the submission of an IND application. To require all of the usual animal tests to be completed and evaluated before an IND application is granted thus would extend the research period by at least twelve to eighteen months. The evaluation process by the FDA is likely to extend the period even more. According to a report by the Science and Technology Office of the National Science Foundation, carcinogenic testing in rodents would require two to three years.[15]

CONCLUSIONS

Owing to the delays required by clinical trials and other procedures for assuring efficacy and safety prior to marketing, when pharmaceutical manufacturers introduce new drugs, their patents do not protect them against imitation by competitors for the full seventeen years of nominal patent life. The average effective patent life of NCE's introduced in the years 1966–73 is estimated to be 13.1 years. Moreover, the effective patent life has declined over this period from 13.9 years for drugs introduced in 1966–69 to 12.4 years for those introduced in 1970–73.

Investment in R & D depends on the expected rate of return from such investment. We have suggested that this expected rate is inadequate to encourage the maintenance of the present level of expenditures by the industry. If more new drugs are to be introduced, then additional investment in R & D is necessary. Such an increase will require an increase in the expected rate of return. Appropriate public policy would include extending patent life, contrary to the proposals which have been made to reduce it.

One of the factors in the low expected rate is the reduction in effective patent life of drugs due to regulatory requirements for proof of efficacy and safety. Any benefits from the regulation of the marketing of new drugs may not be sufficient to compensate for the costs of meeting the requirements, including those arising from delays in the introduction of new drugs. The acceleration of regulatory procedures will reduce the cost of delays and any advance in the date of introduction of new drugs will increase the expected rate of return. The resulting addition to the effective life of a patent will increase the expected rate more than the same addition at the end of the patent life. One year more at the beginning of an effective patent life adds much more to the present value of a stream of income at the date of the investment decision than a year added at the end. The reduction in the effective patent life of 1.5 years over a relatively short period from the midpoint of 1966–69 to the midpoint of 1970–73 was associated with an increase in the delay in marketing of the same length of time and thus reduced the expected rate of return.

CHAPTER 9

PROMOTIONAL EXPENDITURES

INTRODUCTION

It is estimated that there are about 22,000 drugs available to doctors, though the number actually used on a regular basis is far less. The standard handbook of prescription drugs for doctors, *The Physicians' Desk Reference,* runs to over 1,500 triple-column pages. Moreover, the pharmaceutical industry is characterized by innovational competition which assures the continual appearance of new and improved drugs. Very few of today's leading drugs were known in the 1950s. Doctors are therefore faced with a formidable learning task if they are to familiarize themselves with an appropriate pharmaceutical armamentarium.

There is a great deal to learn about any drug in order to use it properly. To prescribe well, doctors must know what the appropriate drugs are and the correct dosages for each disease. They have to have information about the properties of the different drugs for patients, classified by various characteristics such as age, weight, liver condition, renal competence, and heart condition. The learning task would be hard enough if it only consisted of obtaining the information, but it must be retained as well. A doctor attending patients in a hospital emergency room usually does not have the time to look up a drug in a handbook to find out whether or not it will treat a specific infection or whether it is safe to prescribe for an elderly, debilitated alcoholic. Even under more relaxed conditions a doctor must be able to identify a drug to use a handbook. *The Physicians' Desk Reference* is a valuable working reference tool, but the doctor cannot come to it expecting it to tell him which drug to use for an indication. In addition, the handbook provides little basis for comparative judgments among drugs. The physician must know enough about the drugs he uses to make the judgments himself.

In order to persuade doctors to prescribe its product, a manufacturer provides both favorable and unfavorable information about its properties, for otherwise he risks the distrust of doctors who use it and suffer unpleasant surprises.

Marketing managers are human and will not always be faithful to this farsighted view of the benefits of completeness of information. Some will be too eager for sales to be able to refrain from excessive claims. But drug promotion must convey correct and reasonably complete information to be credible and thus effective.

This view runs contrary to the one which regards drug promotion as essentially misleading and uninformative. The latter view holds that drug promotion consists largely of numerous repetitious messages which tell little about each drug, contain outright lies, and avoid mention of any unpleasant side effects. Moreover, the story goes, what little information is conveyed to doctors is done inefficiently and entails enormous waste. The drug firms unload on doctors thousands of pieces of mail which provide the same message, and send around hundreds of detailmen who make the same pitch. The technique applied in drug promotion, according to this view, is the same one that is used in TV commercials; it belabors consumers with repetitious messages containing little or no information.

This negative view disregards the informational service provided by promotional activities in the drug industry. The present chapter explores the implications of the demand for information by doctors. The discussion here will depend heavily on the theory of information first introduced by Professor George Stigler and later developed by Professor Phillip Nelson with respect to information concerning the quality of goods.[1] We will go on to consider the evidence concerning the information provided by the industry to doctors.

We will test the implication that the more innovative firms will spend more on promotion than will other firms, since they have more new drugs about whose properties they must inform doctors. In addition, we examine some of the benefits of promotional efforts to patients, including the rapid diffusion of new drugs among doctors and the additional assurance of quality. We also examine the evidence that promotional expenditures have resulted in the overprescribing of drugs and therefore in an increase in the incidence of gram-negative bacteremia and in deaths from adverse drug reactions. Moreover, this chapter considers the ratio of advertising expenditures to total sales which has been used in economics as an index of advertising intensity. This ratio appears to be higher in the drug industry than in most other industries. We examine the sources of this high ratio and find that it is not due to intensive advertising campaigns in behalf of individual products. Finally, the hostility of economists and of others to promotional activities is discussed.

THE THEORY OF INFORMATION APPLIED TO DRUGS

Nelson's theory of information, which is presented briefly below, will be applied to the promotion of drugs. Nelson himself argues that advertising provides information concerning the quality of goods generally. The fact that a product is advertised in itself conveys important information. Manufacturers of goods whose quality is most difficult to appraise will advertise the most, and, among these, suppliers of the best "values" will advertise the most. Economists may remain skeptical of the validity of this argument when it is applied to consumer goods generally. The theory, however, has special relevance to drugs, since, as we have seen, a great deal of specific information is required by doctors in order to use drugs effectively. Thus we can apply Nelson's theory to drug promotion, although we need not at the same time subscribe to the validity of the argument in its more general application.

Nelson's theory of information distinguishes between "search" and "experience" goods. Consumers can readily appraise the quality of such search goods as ladies' dresses, hand tools, and fresh foods by inspecting them. In contrast, consumers must consume such experience goods as washing machines, canned foods, and liquor in order to appraise their quality directly. Accordingly, consumers depend on other sources of information concerning the quality of experience goods, including manufacturers' advertisements. This type of service becomes important when errors entail large costs.

Advertisers supply information by making specific claims which describe the attractive features of their products. Many advertisements therefore are filled with information concerning a product's uses and other characteristics. Not all claims are true, but an advertiser cannot expect to continue to fool many people, and those who expect to continue in business indefinitely cannot rely on false claims as a matter of policy.

An important element of Nelson's theory is that the return on advertising increases with the quality of goods for any given price. The audience usually includes many previous consumers of an advertised good. The more pleasant their experience has been, the more favorably consumers will respond to an advertisement and the more often they will buy the product. Displeased consumers, by contrast, may react negatively to any reminder of the product, and they may tell their friends of their dissatisfaction with the product.

When we apply information theory to drugs, we must modify it in one respect. The theory represents consumers as making their own choices among different products and basing their decisions on their own experience or on information which they obtain for themselves from a variety of sources. In the case of drugs, however, consumers rely on doctors to make the choice, and doctors must judge the quality of the products on the basis of their observation of the success of therapy and of side effects. It is doctors who must consult sources of information concerning the quality of drugs. This modification does not affect the validity of the general argument, as long as we can make the reasonable assumption that the doctor chooses for his patients drugs which he believes are the ones which provide the best therapy. It must also be assumed, of course, that the best therapy is judged not only on the basis of successful treatment but also on the nature of its side effects. Indeed, the substitution of doctors for consumers as the judges of quality increases the strength of the argument, for they are trained to evaluate the effects of drugs and to appraise information concerning these effects. Furthermore, doctors have the opportunity to observe the effects of drugs in many patients and are in a position to obtain information from their colleagues and other sources concerning these effects in a larger group of patients than they themselves can directly observe. In other words, they are in a better position to obtain and evaluate information concerning drugs than are the consumers relative to the many products.

Drugs fit the category of experience goods better than most goods; one can learn little about the quality of a tablet from its appearance, and since drugs have many quality dimensions, the quantity of useful information about each of them is large. A drug is a complex product, the effects of which may be numerous, and these effects vary among patients. To use a drug well, doctors must be able to anticipate these effects accurately. Hence the demand for information concerning the quality of drugs by doctors is much greater than the demand for information by consumers generally concerning the quality of other products. Doctors' prescriptions for a drug will therefore tend to increase with the quantity of information which they have about the drug for any given level of quality and price, and manufacturers will have an incentive to supply information.

Manufacturers will tend to advertise their better drugs more than those about which they have less confidence. The return on the investment in advertising will tend to increase with the quality of the drugs, given the price of the drugs and the size of the market for drugs providing therapy for the disease. The better the experience of their patients has been with the drug, and the more favorable the information about it from colleagues and other sources, the more favorably doctors will respond to an advertisement and the more often they will prescribe the drug. Those doctors whose observations have been unfavorable will react negatively to reminders by advertisements, and they will inform their colleagues of their observations more frequently when they are reminded than when they are not. Thus Nelson's argument that the return to advertising expenditures for consumer goods generally increases with the quality of the goods holds with greater force for drugs than for other goods.

Furthermore, companies will find that false claims persistently made over a period will not increase sales. Doctors prescribe drugs over long periods, and if they learn to distrust the statements of a particular company, the resulting loss in its reputation for honesty will lead doctors to be much more skeptical of later claims made by its detailmen. The resulting loss in sales may well exceed any temporary gains.

Not all claims are true, partly because marketing managers, who are no more altruistic or far-sighted than any other group of people, may be eager for sales. But manufacturers of highly advertised products who expect to continue in business indefinitely cannot rely on false claims as a matter of policy.

Companies will not advertise the advantages of competitors' products, and doctors thus receive partial rather than complete reports. It is the doctor's complex task, therefore, to appraise the rival claims for competitive drugs that provide similar therapy. He can be sure that if any scientific studies favor a single drug, its manufacturer will inform him of the good news quickly enough. He will also hear the bad news concerning any drug from the detailmen representing the manufacturers of competitive drugs, if not from its own detailmen. Much of the difficulty in this area, however, comes from the uncertainty associated with the use of drugs which is characteristic of medicine generally. We will consider the problems raised by uncertainty later.

OTHER SOURCES OF INFORMATION

Critics of the industry doubt the ability of doctors to balance the conflicting claims of manufacturers of competitive drugs and to make good prescribing decisions on the basis of detailmen's biased presentations. They have therefore urged doctors to use alternative sources of information, including articles in medical journals and the reports to colleagues. In addition, doctors have been urged to rely more on expert opinion such as that represented in the American Medical Association's Council on Drugs which published the handbook *AMA Drug Evaluations*. In fact, the suggestion has been made that a federal agency create such an expert group to advise doctors.

Medical journal articles are helpful. But it is unrealistic to expect many doctors to keep abreast of the large journal literature. Since 1970 an average of 1,700 articles on any *one* of the twenty-five leading drugs has been published per year in 325 journals of medicine, pharmacology, chemistry, and pharmacy.[2] This astonishingly large number underestimates the size of the world literature on each of the major drugs, since there are other journals not even counted in the estimate. Reading review articles by experts helps doctors conserve time, but they cannot depend on such articles exclusively, since the experts frequently disagree.

For example, some experts say that doctors have no reason to prescribe expensive minor tranquilizers such as Valium and Librium rather than phenobarbital, which in the proper dosage has the same effect and is much cheaper.[3] Some doctors suggest that phenobarbital is risky for suicidal patients, since it is easy for them to take an overdose of phenobarbital with fatal results.[4] Other doctors insist that patients, particularly those in nursing homes, have been over-sedated for long periods on barbituates with undesirable side effects on the skin and parts of the nervous system. For such patients Librium or Valium may be preferred.[5] Experts also disagree about the relative merits of aspirin and indomethacin for the treatment of arthritis.[6] The doctors who prefer aspirin question the validity of the clinical evidence presented in favor of indomethacin;

the evidence is difficult to interpret because of the cyclical nature of the symptoms of arthritis and the fact that indomethacin generally is used only after aspirin fails to provide relief. Any apparent relief that follows the use of indomethacin might have come without it. Other instances of disagreement among experts are described in Appendix B.

Disagreement is unavoidable for several reasons. First, there is the intrinsic imprecision of clinical drug evaluation. Neither the disease nor the action of the drug may be well understood. Judgments of efficacy, therefore, are based on direct observation of symptoms or on subjective judgments of patients, neither of which can be highly precise. Complicating the problem still more is the variability of response of patients to individual drugs. Reports of clinical tests evaluate drugs on the basis of their average performance in a group of patients, but a drug can provide relief for many patients even when it does not do so for a majority.

Second, doctors, as well as patients, differ in therapeutic objectives and in their aversion to particular risks. The balance of therapeutic benefit and risk is always, to a degree, a subjective and personal decision of the therapist and patient and therefore not really decidable by the general considerations of experts. In this connection, expert pharmacologists may prefer the risk of failing to recommend a beneficial drug over that of recommending a harmful drug; missed benefits apparently arouse less hostility and publicity than harmful side effects. This bias in evaluation is more likely when such experts are supported by public funds and are therefore subject to scrutiny by government agencies. A private practitioner need not share this risk preference. The private practitioner is more likely to give greater weight to the beneficial effects and less weight to a small risk of harmful effects than is a government expert who is not immediately involved with patients. This is true especially when the practitioner stands to lose patient referrals from other practitioners.

Third, the expert cannot take into account how individual circumstances alter the risk preferences of doctors and patients. Thus, debilitated older patients who are in pain may be willing to accept the side effect of drowsiness in exchange for some gain in comfort. A busy executive will be less willing to accept this side effect. An expert writing for doctors dealing with the population as a whole may not take this into account.

Fourth, the "correct" procedure depends on the facilities available to a doctor and on the promptness with which treatment has to be administered. The correct treatment for a doctor who can get test results quickly from the laboratory of a modern hospital may be inappropriate or impossible for another, especially when delay results in deterioration in the patient's condition. In such instances, a case can be made that a broad-spectrum drug is preferable to a highly specific and more powerful drug.

Fifth, the choice also depends on the degree of specialization of the doctor. A highly trained specialist who is certain of the diagnosis is more likely than a general practitioner to choose the specific drug in preference to the drug with a broad spectrum of activity.

Sixth, the choice of a powerful drug will depend on the ability of a doctor to monitor a patient's progress closely.

Scientific authorities' views on ideal prescribing tend to ignore these kinds of practical and individual considerations, and doctors, therefore, have long insisted on their right to practice medicine without outside interference. Thus, we cannot expect them closely to follow the advice of an authority set up specially for the purpose. Various critics of the promotional activities of drug companies have suggested government sponsorship of an impartial body of experts to recommend drugs to doctors. But the disagreements among experts and the particular problems arising in the choice of drugs for specific patients by individual doctors make it unlikely that such a group of experts would prove adequate. Since doctors cannot accept expert opinion uncritically, they want to hear for themselves the claims of manufacturers, particularly when these claims are made by individuals such as detailmen who are familiar with the circumstances of the doctors' practice and their therapeutic preferences.

An equally important consideration is the time saved by doctors. The detailman provides a succinct summary of his product's merits and risks, as do the advertisements in medical journals and the mail circulars. The elimination of all drug promotion would result in greater demands on doctors to spend time learning about the qualities of drugs and probably in a reduction in the information which they acquire. Busy practitioners, who are the ones who write a relatively large number of prescriptions, are unlikely to devote the required time to learning about drugs in the event of a reduction in promotional efforts.

SOME EVIDENCE

PROMOTION AND INFORMATION. For the purpose of evaluating the promotional activities of the industry, it is important to establish whether or not the efforts convey useful information to doctors and whether the resources devoted to these efforts are wastefully excessive from a social standpoint. Recognizing that this is one of the major issues, in 1966 the Sainsbury Committee of the United Kingdom conducted a survey of physicians to evaluate the industry's promotional activities as sources of information.[7] The committee reported that the large majority of physicians regarded detailmen either as a very good or a fairly good source of information about the existence of new products and that detailmen were selected as the best single source of information by more physicians than was any other source. The respondents were less enthusiastic about the value of industry sources of information concerning the efficacy of new products. They had more trust in articles in medical journals and in recommendations from consultants.

The Sainsbury Committee investigated the information physicians obtained on four new drugs before prescribing them.[8] A large proportion of doctors had used only a single source of information, and for three out of the four drugs, company sources were most frequently mentioned as the single source. It may be unnecessary to point out the inconsistency between this observation and the earlier one that a majority of doctors appear to have more faith in medical journal articles than in company sources as sources of information concerning efficacy. That the information provided by companies was of value to practitioners is indicated by the large proportion of doctors who had not heard of the one product among the four studied which had been commercially available for only a few months. As many as 24 percent of the respondents had not heard of Ultralanum at the time of the interview. The significance of this observation is better understood when we realize that among those who had heard of the drug as many as 43 percent had prescribed it.

The survey also inquired about the value of individual sources of information. The large majority of doctors said they received too much literature through the mail, and nearly two-thirds believed that usually the information in this literature was not sufficient to enable a physician to decide whether to use the drug. Yet, although many doctors felt that mail circulars were insufficient as a sole source of information, a surprisingly large number said that they would lose an important source of information were mail promotion abandoned. While half of the respondents said they could do without mail promotion, the other half disagreed.

We will have more to say later about the amount of mail received by doctors. The question in the survey referred to the total amount of mail received from all companies, which may be large owing to the large number of companies and products. The amount of mail concerning individual products may be quite modest. We will investigate this aspect of the problem in our discussion of the costs of promotion.

The survey also inquired about respondents' attitudes to detailmen. According to the report, 60 percent of the respondents valued the information provided by detailmen sufficiently to see all of the representatives who attempted to obtain interviews. The survey also found that nearly half of the respondents felt able to decide whether to use a product on the basis of information given to them by detailmen. On the other hand, about one-third of the physicians interviewed felt that very often detailmen claim more uses for a product than was clinically justified. But approximately the same percentage believed that this never happened. Impressions were also mixed about the adequacy of the knowledge of drugs displayed by detailmen and about the extent to which they minimize side effects.

These results demonstrate that a large fraction of physicians in the United Kingdom regard the industry's promotional activities as a valuable source of information about new products; many depend on industry sources exclusively. Many doctors, however, do not hear of a new product until some time has elapsed. This suggests that the promotional efforts of the manufacturer in question were not sufficiently large for prescribers to be informed immediately on the release of a product.

Although many of the doctors said that they preferred journal articles as a source of information about the efficacy of drugs presumably because they are more objective than industry sources, we do not know how many doctors actually read and are influenced by such articles.

LIST 9-1
Items Discussed in an Article in *Physicians'*
Desk Reference Dealing with a Brand of Ampicillin

1. The spectrum of bactericidal activity.
2. The available dosage forms and strengths.
3. Instructions concerning administration.
4. Stability in presence of gastric acid.
5. Absorption, diffusion, and excretion characteristics.
6. Tolerance by patients.
7. A list of gram-positive and gram-negative organisms which are sensitive to ampicillin.
8. Lack of effectiveness against penicillinase-producing organisms.
9. Test for estimating susceptibility of bacteria to ampicillin.
10. List of indications for which ampicillin is useful.
11. Contraindications.
12. Warning about patients with history of susceptibility to penicillin hypersensitivity reaction and procedure for treatment of reaction.
13. Warning about use in pregnancy.
14. Warning about possibility of superinfections and assessments of renal, hepatic, and hematopoietic functions.
15. List of adverse reactions.
16. Warning against use for treatment of mononucleosis.
17. Instructions concerning appropriate dosage for patients classified by weight suffering from different types of infections.
18. Length of time required for treatment.
19. Instructions concerning use of pediatric drops.

Source: *Physicians' Desk Reference to Pharmaceutical Specialties and Biologicals,* 27th ed. (Oradell, N.J.: Medical Economics Co., 1973).

The results of the study by the Sainsbury Committee point up the informational content of the promotional material which the pharmaceutical companies distribute. That the promotional material contains a great deal of information is shown by an illustrative example of the content of the description of the properties of a brand of ampicillin which appears in the *Physicians' Desk Reference.* The entry reproduces the content of the circular which the manufacturer distributes to doctors with samples. A list of the items described is shown in list 9-1, which indicates that a large amount of information is conveyed. The detailman also distributes reprints of articles which have been published in medical journals in which doctors describe how they have used drugs for the treatment of different types of cases. *The Physicians' Desk Reference* contains a great deal of information, but no single entry covers all of the possible problems that a doctor will encounter in the treatment of a disease. Thus, a detailman who is promoting the use of a combination antihypertensive-diuretic drug will distribute copies of articles dealing with the types of drugs which are available for the treatment of hypertension and their mechanisms of action. Detailmen promoting the use of antiarthritic drugs will distribute copies of articles dealing with the effectiveness of different classes of drugs for the different forms of arthritis at various stages. The articles will report experimental evidence of the effectiveness of different drugs.

The obvious fact is that doctors are professional prescribers who require a great deal of information about individual drugs. The companies cannot expect to persuade doctors to use their drugs through simple huckstering. They must provide a good deal of information.

INNOVATION AND PROMOTION. The theory of information when applied to the drug industry suggests that innovative firms will spend relatively more on promotion than will others. Firms want to transmit information about new drugs which are unfamiliar to doctors. They also wish to remind doctors of old drugs. It may be argued however, that the payoff from advertising a new drug will be greater.

The alternative hypothesis for explaining interfirm variation in promotional expenditures stresses firm size. The literature of advertising frequently makes the assertion that firms achieve and maintain their large size by spending large sums on advertising.

To test these hypotheses we will analyze the promotional expenditures in 1973 of fifty-eight pharmaceutical companies, using the following equation:

$$\ln Pr = a + b \ln S + c \ln N_s$$

where Pr = promotional expenditures in 1973 of fifty-eight companies. Expenditures for detailing, mail, and journal advertising from National Mail Audit, National Detailing Audit, and National Journal Audit, all IMS America Ltd. Detailing expenditures reported by these IMS sources multiplied by 1.3633. This factor based on a comparison of total expenditures on detailing by the industry as estimated by IMS with the estimate by professional Marketing Research (PMR).

S = ethical sales of each company in 1965, as estimated by IMS America, Ltd., *US Pharmaceutical Market, Drug Stores and Hospitals.*

N_s = number of new entities introduced in 1965–70, weighted by sales in 1972. See chapter 5, pp. 87–89 for discussion of list of new entities. Sales estimated by IMS America Ltd., *US Pharmaceutical Market, Drug Stores and Hospitals.*

PMR's estimate of total promotional expenditures in the industry is higher than the IMS estimate and appears to be closer to the true value. Since it is recent introductions which will be promoted, we limit the count of new single chemical entities (NCE's) to those of 1965–70. Sales provide a measure of the importance of drugs and, therefore, our weights. The measure of firm size is sales in the first year of the period in which the count of NCE's is made. Since sales of NCE's provide an increasing percentage of total sales, the selection of a later year for the measure of firm size would result in the effect of new products on promotion being captured by the size variable.

The relationship between expenditures and the sales-weighted number of new entities is assumed to be logarithmic rather than arithmetic. In other words, it is assumed that a 1 percent increase in the sales-weighted number of new entities will increase promotional expenditures by some constant percentage. The arithmetic model would assume that an increase in the independent variable of $1 would increase promotional expenditures by some constant dollar amount regardless of the initial level of either variable. The logarithmic relationship also appears to be appropriate for the other independent variable, which is total ethical sales. The linear logarithmic form also has the advantage over an arithmetic regression equation of reducing the heteroscedasticity of the data.

The results are as follows:

$$\ln \text{Pr} = 6.9827 + .1274 \ln S + .1132 \ln N_s \tag{9.1}$$

$$
\begin{array}{lll}
(t = 1.5720) & (t = 4.248) & R^2 = .30 \\
(SE = .0810) & (SE = .0264) & F = 12.796
\end{array}
$$

These results confirm the hypothesis that promotional expenditures increase with innovation; the regression coefficient associated with the measure of innovation is highly significant. The alternative hypothesis that it is size of firm which determines promotional expenditure is not confirmed; the regression coefficient associated with sales is not significant.[9]

True, the innovation hypothesis does not do very well. We cannot say that information about the number and importance of the innovations of a firm will provide a basis for an accurate prediction of its promotional expenditure. Only 30 percent of the interfirm variation in promotion expenditures is explained by innovations. Apparently there are other important elements in the determination of promotional expenditures which have not been taken into account.

A second test has been applied to the hypothesis that promotional expenditures increase with innovations. This one examines variation in promotional expenditures among products rather than among firms. If the hypothesis is correct, promotional expenditures will vary inversely with the age of the product.

Promotional expenditures for the newest products will be larger than for older products.

The results were as follows:

$$\ln P_p = 7.12966 + .20 \ln N_{rp} - .45 \ln A \qquad\qquad (9.2)$$

$$(t = 6.30) \quad (t = -3.09) \qquad\qquad R^2 = .50$$

$$(SE = .032) \quad (SE = .145) \qquad\qquad F = 24.129$$

where P_p = total promotional expenditures in 1973 for each of the fifty leading drugs by sales in 1972. Estimates of expenditures on detailing, mail, and journal advertisements obtained from National Detailing Audit, National Mail Audit, and National Journal Audit, all IMS America, Ltd. The estimate for detailing was multiplied by 1.3633 to adjust for the higher level estimated by Professional Market Research.

N_{rp} = number of new prescriptions of each product in 1972 obtained from the National Prescription Audit, IMS America Ltd., 1972.

A = age of product in 1973. Computed as difference between 1973 and year of introduction.

The variable N_{rp} was used to measure the size of the market. The relation between the dependent variable and this variable is assumed to be logarithmic for the same reasons as were given in the previous analysis. The effect of age is also seen as logarithmic. An increase of one year in the age of a product will have a smaller effect on the promotional effort exerted on behalf of an old product than on that of a new product. This relationship is implied by the innovation hypothesis, since it suggests that additions to information are especially important in connection with new products.[10]

The regression coefficient of *ln A* is significantly negative, as predicted by the hypothesis. Additional support is provided for the hypothesis by the coefficient of determination which indicates that the two variables, number of new prescriptions and age of products, explain half of the variance in promotional expenditures among the products.

THE INFLUENCE OF PROMOTION

Critics of the industry accuse pharmaceutical manufacturers of manipulating doctors into prescribing drugs. This proposition is difficult to evaluate, since pharmaceutical firms tend to promote their successful drugs more heavily than other drugs. Nevertheless, the evidence which shows that some promotional campaigns are unsuccessful suggests that a drug must have valid therapeutic claims in order to become a big seller; advertising alone is insufficient for the success of a product.

Several companies have spent large sums promoting a number of new drugs which appeared in 1965 or later and have failed to obtain large sales. Merck tried to develop a large market for Vivactil, an antidepressant, but failed to do so. Expenditures on promotion in a single year were as large as $3 million, but sales never exceeded $2½ million. It was disappointed also in the sales of a new potent diuretic, Edecrin. A.H. Robins spent more on the promotion of its new tranquilizer, Tybatran, than it obtained in sales. Wyeth had similar lack of success with its tranquilizer Solacen. Parke-Davis failed to develop large sales for its new analgesic Ponstel, which appeared in 1967. Each of these new single chemical entities was ranked by the FDA as "little or no gain" in therapeutic competence over previous drugs.

On the positive side, drugs which have won large sales have had strong therapeutic claims. The notable successes of the 1960s included Hoechst's product Lasix, which filled a need for a rapid-acting strong diuretic. The product achieved its large sales without the benefit of an especially large promotional campaign. Because of its speed and potency, a single dose of Lasix per day is sufficient to achieve effective diuresis. It is effective even in the face of decreased renal blood flow or severe electrolyte imbalance and works in some cases refractory to other types of diuretics.

Other leading diuretics include the first two thiazides, Diuril and Hydrodiuril, which were pioneers in the area and therefore have not been displaced by later thiazide diuretics which have no great advantage over the original ones. *Drugs of Choice* says of Diuril: "Despite the negative features listed [hyperuricemia, skin rashes, some blood dyscrasias, reduction of blood pressure, and hypopotassemia], because of its apparent advantages, chlorothiazide continues to be the oral diuretic of first choice."[11]

Librium and Valium owe their remarkable success to uniqueness at the time of their introduction. They were the first minor tranquilizers able to calm anxiety without causing excessive sedation and suppressing alertness. These drugs have relatively few side effects and are useful in treating not only neurotic anxiety but also the delirium of alcohol and the apprehension of surgery or labor; they find further use as mild, short-acting anticonvulsants. A subsequent product, Serax, is also a benzodiazepine, as are Librium and Valium, but it offers no clear therapeutic advantages over the others, and although it was introduced in 1965, it has achieved only 1/25 of the combined sales of the two better-known earlier products.

The leading drug in the antihypertensive market, Merck's Aldomet, has a strong basis for its acceptance by doctors. Ser-Ap-Es, a combination of two antihypertensives and a diuretic, is an effective product for the treatment of hypertension. Another popular antihypertensive is Aldoril, which combines two popular drugs: Aldomet and Diuril.

Lilly's cephalosporin products have taken a large share of the broad and medium spectrum antibiotic market. Again, the products have strong advantages over alternatives available. Both Keflin and Keflex are effective against penicillin-resistant organisms and some gram-negative organisms which are beyond the spectrum of penicillin. In addition, most patients allergic to penicillin can be treated with the cephalosporins, and the toxicity of these products is quite limited.

Thorazine was a breakthrough drug for the management of schizophrenia. Although it was the first one found, Thorazine is also one of the most effective antipsychotic agents available to date, a fact reflected by its successful sales.

Lasix, Diuril, Librium, Thorazine, Aldomet, and Keflin were all ranked as "significant [therapeutic] gains" by the FDA. On the other hand, Hydrodiuril, Valium, and Keflex were rated "no gain." The FDA apparently assigned this "no gain" rating to these later products because they did not represent the major medical breakthroughs that their predecessors did. Yet Keflex represented a very useful advance because it provided an orally active cephalosporin comparable to the previously available injectable Keflin. Hydrodiuril and Valium have been able to obtain larger sales than their predecessors apparently because doctors preferred them. In addition, Hydrodiuril is a stronger diuretic per unit dose than Diuril.

We can conclude that drug promotion, while informative, is unlikely to succeed in winning large sales for a drug unless the drug has strong independent therapeutic claims.

THE BENEFIT FROM THE DIFFUSION OF AN INNOVATION

There can be little question that the promotional activities of drug companies benefit patients, but we still have the problem of whether the cost of promotion exceeds the benefits. We have seen some evidence from the Sainsbury Report that promotional expenditures are not excessive, for a large number of doctors remain ignorant of the availability of a drug after a few months of its release. Nevertheless, this evidence alone may not persuade many people that the benefits of promotion are worth the costs. Let us consider further the benefits to patients from the information obtained by doctors. More precisely, if the potential benefits from additions to the present level of information exceed the resulting additional costs, then society would benefit from an increase in promotional expenditures.

The benefits of greater information include those of more appropriate use of both old and new drugs. Doctors may not use a drug for a disease because they do not know of it, because they are not sufficiently familiar with its properties, or because, if they have heard of it, they do not happen to recall the fact of its availability at the time when they see a patient. In such instances the patient suffers because the doctor does not use an available drug, and additional promotional effort by the manufacturer would have benefitted him.

Sam Peltzman examines the losses due to doctors' failure to adopt new drugs owing to lack of information. He suggests that large promotional efforts were responsible for the rapid diffusion of the Salk vaccine among physicians and the resulting quick decline in the number of paralytic cases due to poliomyelitis. He estimates that if the use of TB drugs had spread as quickly as that of polio vaccine, 80,600 lives would have been saved. Similar computations for major tranquilizers yield an estimated savings of 645 million patient days.[12] Such figures suggest that society would have benefited from larger expenditures by the drug companies on the promotion of the TB drugs and major tranquilizers. These estimates for only two drugs thus also suggest that the rapid adoption of drugs leads to large social benefits and that the social benefits of the promotion of drugs also are large.

The estimate of the reduction in the number of deaths resulting from additional promotion of TB drugs is open to the criticism that it was not a lack of knowledge of the existence of these drugs and their therapeutic effects that kept doctors from rushing to prescribe them, but rather a fear of possible harmful side effects. They may have preferred to rely on older, more familiar therapeutic approaches until more experience accumulated. Similar reasons may be given for the slow rate of diffusion of the major tranquilizers in the treatment of hospitalized mental patients. But even if only part of the delay in the diffusion of the drugs reflected lack of information rather than caution in the face of the unknown, the promotional expenditures probably still were inadequate. The cost of even half of 645 million patient days can pay for a great deal of promotion, probably more than the entire industry spends on the promotion of all drugs in several years.

There is no reason to believe that the promotional expenditures for other drugs is any more adequate. There is some evidence therefore that the drug companies may be open to criticism for not spending enough on promotion rather than for spending too much!

Much of the criticism of promotional expenditures assumes that all or most doctors obtain more than enough information to be able to use a drug soon after it is introduced. This may be true for specialists who diligently follow the news of new drug developments in their respective fields and who need only a small number of journal advertisements to remind them of the availability of a drug which they use. For them the expenditures on promotion may be excessive, and their patients therefore may pay excessive prices to cover the costs of the promotional efforts. But many doctors do not follow drug developments closely and need more than a few advertisements as well as several visits from a detailman to keep them informed of the availability and the characteristics of a drug. General practitioners and surgeons are likely to belong to this group, not out of lack of diligence on their part, but simply owing to the impossibility of following drug developments in several fields. Specialists who do not adhere closely to their specialty are also likely to need the service of drug companies' promotional efforts.

In addition, as Peltzman points out, companies cannot vary their prices among customers according to the benefits received. They cannot discriminate in price between the patients of well-informed doctors who receive little new information from the promotional activities on an individual drug and others whose treatment is significantly improved by the information made available to their doctors. Some patients are overpaying and others are underpaying, but there is no way of avoiding this problem.

The problem is not peculiar to drug promotion. It arises in connection with the payment for services supplied in other industries as well. For example, retail customers who do not want sales help or credit pay for the costs of such services to those who do want it. Domestic consumers of electricity in off-peak periods pay for peak-period customers; readers of newspapers who limit their attention to the sports section pay for the general news supplied to other readers.

QUALITY CONTROL AND BRAND NAMES

We have implicitly assumed so far that the only quality problem in the selection of drugs arises from differences between drugs in their chemical design. We have assumed that when a doctor chooses from among Aldomet, Ser-Ap-Es, Lasix, and other drugs in the treatment of hypertension, his choice is based on information about the effects of the intended chemical composition of each of the drugs. But differences in efficacy and in safety between drugs can arise from differences in quality which are the result of differing degrees of quality control in the manufacturing process as well as from differences in chemical design. Plants may fail to keep their products free of impurities; individual tablets may contain too little or too much of the active ingredient; the sterility of injectable solutions may not be maintained; grain size and compaction may vary among producers of a given type of pill with therapeutic consequences.

Prescribers thus must consider the risk of shortcomings in the actual manufacture of drugs. The FDA attempts to provide assurance of the quality of available drugs through a surveillance and enforcement program. Chapter 11 demonstrates, however, that for a variety of reasons the FDA fails to provide such assurance. Doctors therefore cannot rely on the FDA to protect their patients.

Under these conditions, promotion of the product provides some necessary assurance of the observance of good manufacturing practices. A report of a defective batch of a heavily promoted and widely used drug will attract much more attention than will a similar report concerning an unknown product, with the result that sales will drop off much more. The manufacturer who promotes his product is unlikely to risk a loss of reputation (which is what the promotional effort is intended to build) through permitting manufacturing practices to deteriorate and by not investing adequate funds in the control of quality. In addition, the manufacturer of a brand-name product is more likely to maintain high quality because it accepts full responsibility. The promotion of a brand name has as a byproduct the location of responsibility for quality. By contrast, the source of an unbranded generic product remains unknown. Doctors have trouble differentiating one generic product from others of the same generic class. There is little incentive therefore for a generic manufacturer to maintain high quality in the absence of effective FDA enforcement. True, the large manufacturers produce generic products as well as brand-name products, and since their company names are well known they accept responsibility for these products. And when a physician specifies the manufacturer of a generic product as well as its generic name, he is doing the equivalent of prescribing a brand name. The risk of poor quality is much greater in the case of generic products coming from small manufacturers whose names do not appear on the prescriptions (see chapters 10 and 11). The only incentive which they have to ensure high quality, apart from FDA enforcement, is the possibility of detection by pharmacists who know the sources of individual generic products. But pharmacists discover defective products only when they are reported by patients or doctors. The doctor who observes a failure of a patient to respond to a generic drug or who is faced with some other unexpected reaction may be reluctant to go to the trouble required to trace the source, especially when, as is often the case, the nature of a reaction is uncertain. Moreover, the absence in generic drugs of the unique identity which accompanies brand names prevents doctors from obtaining, either individually through their own direct observation or by hearsay from other doctors, an impression of the quality of the unknown manufacturer's product.[13]

Chapters 10 and 11 develop this argument at length and provide supporting evidence. The evidence shows that the large manufacturers which sell the brand name products have a better record of quality performance than do small manufacturers, which produce unpromoted generic products. The latter sell their products to pharmacists on the basis of price. Pharmacists use them to fill generic prescriptions which do not also specify the manufacturer. In most cases pharmacists fill such prescriptions with brand name products or generic products of well-known houses having a reputation for good quality. But the industry does contain many small manufacturers who do sell their products, and for some of these products the potential risk of poor quality is serious. Hence, the problems raised by the existence of small manufacturers cannot be dismissed as insignificant.

PROMOTION AND EXCESSIVE PRESCRIBING

Drug promotion has been attacked for encouraging doctors to use drugs excessively and inappropriately from a medical standpoint. One of the chief subjects of the discussion of promotion has been the alleged resulting overuse of antibiotics. Testimony presented before the Senate Subcommittee on Health[14] suggested that doctors frequently prescribe antibiotics when there is no evidence of bacterial infection or in incorrect amounts. More specifically, Drs. H. E.

Simmons and P. D. Stolley have said that the overuse of antibiotics has resulted in increases in the incidence of gram-negative bacteremia with the further consequence of an increase in mortality rates. They cite an estimate of 300,000 cases annually of gram-negative bacteremia and more than 100,000 fatalities.[15]

Data on causes of death collected from death certificates by the U.S. National Center for Health Statistics indicate, however, that these estimates are gross exaggerations. According to these data, in 1970 only 3,535 deaths resulted from all types of septicemia, including gram-positive as well as gram-negative, and of these fewer than 250 were due to gram-negative infections.[16] The data are not clear on whether or not the number of cases of gram-negative bacteremia has increased. The evidence which indicates an increase, reported by Drs. Simmons and Stolley, may well be due in large part to the increased number of blood cultures carried out.[17]

Furthermore, other sources of any actual increase in incidence of gram-negative infections are much more important than the overuse of antibiotics. These include changes in the patient population and more heroic surgical procedures.[18] Studies of the incidence of gram-negative septicemia blame the concentration in hospitals of patients with established infections, the surgical treatment of a large number of poor-risk patients, the increased number of cases of severe trauma, and the increased use of drugs other than antibiotics, which reduce bodily resistance, including steroids and immunosuppressive and anticancer agents.[19] The increase in the number of debilitated, elderly patients suffering from cancer, cirrhosis, and diabetes has been an important factor. In addition, the number of surgical procedures which permit entry of bacteria to genitourinary and gastrointestinal tracts has increased.

In addition, there is no strong evidence that the resistance of gram-negative bacteria to antibiotics has increased.[20] These organisms have never been sensitive to older forms of penicillin and tetracycline, and some of the gram-negative infections are difficult to treat even with the newer antibiotics, the spectrums of which are broader than their predecessors'. More importantly, various studies indicate that the resistance of gram-negative organisms to those antibiotics which are used in the treatment of gram-negative infections has not increased and in fact has decreased.[21]

The other major attack on the promotion of drugs on the grounds that it encourages poor medical practice alleges that adverse drug reactions are responsible for 60,000 and 140,000 deaths annually in the U.S.[22]

The estimates are extrapolations of observations of deaths from adverse drug reactions reported in two studies, the Caranasos Study at the University of Florida Medical School and the Boston Collaborative Drug Surveillance Project,[23] which were planned to monitor drug related effects on therapy in medical wards. The Caranasos study found that of the 6,063 patients in hospital medical wards which were studied over a three-year period, eleven patients, or .18 percent, died from adverse drug effects. The national estimate of 60,000 is based on this observation by multiplying the total hospital patient population in the U.S.—32 million—by .18 percent. The Boston Project observed twenty-seven deaths from adverse reactions in a sample of 6,199 medical inpatients, or .44 percent.[24] The estimate of 140,000 is the result of applying this factor of .44 percent to the entire hospital population.

These estimates erroneously assume that the basic samples are representative of the hospital population. The samples, however, were drawn from medical wards where the incidence of adverse reactions is much higher than in other sections of the hospital, because they contain a high proportion of severely debilitated patients who are more vulnerable to all types of complications, including drug reactions.

Thus, in the Boston Project, of the twenty-seven patients whose deaths were ascribed to adverse drug effects, five were considered to be terminally ill and fifteen of the other patients were described as severely ill. Apparently the severity of the illness was an important factor in the deaths. When adverse drug reactions are blamed on excessive or improper use of drugs, the implication is that correct use and correct dosages will not lead to adverse drug reactions. Evidently, however, even though the deaths in these studies were attributed to adverse drug reactions, they were the result of appropriate therapy but therapy which necessarily involved considerable risk.

Moreover, the deaths from adverse drug reactions involved reactions to exceptionally potent, toxic drugs which are not used to treat many patients. The adverse drug reactions did not involve the improper use of drugs which are not especially toxic. The drugs used included anticancer drugs, digitalis, and heparin, all of which are known to involve serious risks. Thus, for the vast majority of drugs, the studies exaggerate the risk from inappropriate prescribing.

Finally, the accusation that the deaths were the result of drugs used improperly because of excessive promotion is unfounded, because most of the drugs were not highly promoted. Even in the two cases involving diuretics, which are promoted, promotion cannot be held at fault. One case involved a terminal cancer patient of seventy-one years of age and the other was an eighty-six-year-old patient suffering from congestive heart failure.

Other statements accuse doctors of prescribing antibiotics for viral respiratory infections for which they are ineffective. But it is not clear that this usage is due to promotion. Doctors disagree about the appropriate treatment of viral respiratory infections. Those who use antibiotics say that a test for streptococci requires a delay of a day or two for the laboratory test results to come in; such a test is expensive and also requires an additional visit to the doctor. They also defend the practice as defensive strategy to prevent bacterial superinfections. Others respond to the accusation by saying that patients expect to obtain a drug. In any case, there appears to be little reason to blame the promotional activities of the drug companies for encouraging overprescribing of antibiotics.

THE COST OF PROMOTION

POSSIBLE SAVINGS FROM THE ELIMINATION OF PROMOTION. Various authors, including Drs. Silverman and Lee, accuse the industry of excessive spending on promotion and point to the large share of the total cost of drugs represented by drug advertising. They suggest that the share of the manufacturer's sales dollar spent on promotion is as much as 20 percent. The point is further highlighted by a comparison with the share of sales represented by expenditures on research which they say is only about 9 percent.[25]

The judgment of whether the cost of promotion is excessive depends on just what the cost is. We need a good estimate of the expenditures on promotion by the industry. The judgment also depends on alternatives available for transmitting the information and the possible savings in costs to consumers from resorting to such alternatives.

We estimate that in 1972 pharmaceutical manufacturers in the U.S. spent a total of $721.8 million on promotion. The components of this estimate are presented in table 9-1. The notes in this table describe the sources and the procedures used in arriving at the estimate.

The possible savings to consumers from the elimination of promotional activities, when expressed as a percentage of total purchases of drugs, is much less than the usual estimate suggested for two reasons. First, the estimate of promotional expenditures just given accounts for only 12.4 percent of total sales at the manufacturers' level, which amounted to $5,800 million in 1972.[26] That the estimate of 12.4 percent is close to the mark is supported by similar estimates for the U.K. by the Sainsbury Report. The report estimated that promotional costs represented 14.9 percent of manufacturers' sales in 1963, 14.1 percent in 1964, and 13.9 percent in 1965.[27] So even at this level the percentage saving which is possible from a reduction in promotional activities is not as large as is commonly supposed. Second, promotional expenditures are a much smaller percentage of consumer expenditures than of manufacturers' sales, because the manufacturer's price is about half of the retail price.

However, even though we have used the higher of the two publicly available estimates of promotional expenditures (table 9-1), we may still be underestimating total expenditures. The coverage of Professional Market Research survey of companies may not be complete, and the resulting error may bias the estimate downward.

Consequently, we must consider the possibility that the estimate of promotional expenditures cited by Silverman and Lee may be correct. If, as they suggest, promotional expenditures amount to 20 percent of sales, then total promotional expenditures in 1972 were $1,181 million. The possible saving to consumers from the complete elimination of promotional expenditures, however, is only 10 percent of what they spend. The figure of 20 percent represents

TABLE 9-1
Promotional Expenditures by the
Pharmaceutical Industry in the
United States, 1972
($ Millions)

Medium	Expenditures
Detailing time	$396.3
Detailing literature	31.6
Journal ad preparation	8.7
Journal ad space	101.6
Direct mail	40.3
Sample distribution	88.2
Conventions and exhibitions	9.3
Audio visual presentations	5.4
Miscellaneous expenses	40.4
Total	$721.8

Sources: Expenditures for journal ad space obtained from *National Journal Audit,* IMS America Ltd., 1972. For all other expenditure figures, Professional Market Research was relied on. In every case, I used the higher of the two available estimates in order to err on the side of overstatement rather than understatement of promotional costs.

the share of sales at the manufacturer's level which is devoted to promotional activities. Only about half of consumers' expenditures for drugs goes to manufacturers; the other half is retained by retailers. When we express promotional costs ($1,181 million) as a percentage of consumer expenditures, it is approximately 10 percent rather than 20 percent. Further, this 10 percent is only the potential savings to consumers if all of the promotional expenditures were eliminated, resulted in an equal absolute reduction in dollar-costs to retailers, and all of this absolute reduction were passed on to consumers. Chapter 12 estimates that retailers pass on to consumers between 44 and 60 percent of manufacturers' price cuts. Thus, the saving to consumers would be roughly half that of the total reduction in costs from the complete elimination of promotional costs, or 5 percent of consumer expenditures. The actual saving from any program to reduce promotional costs would be even smaller. No one would urge that all promotional effort is wasteful. The most ardent critics of promotional activities concede that the activities inform doctors; they only claim that the total amount of effort is excessive. The total potential savings to consumers thus is somewhat less than 5 percent of their drug bills.

THE SOURCES OF THE HIGH ADVERTISING INTENSITY. Although our estimate of the percentage of manufacturers' sales represented by promotional expenditures, 12.4 percent, is much lower than others' estimates, it is higher

TABLE 9-2
Advertising-Sales Ratios in Forty-one Consumer Goods Industries, 1954–57

	Advertising Sales Ratio (%)		Advertising Sales Ratio (%)
1) Soft drink	6.2	22) Furniture	1.5
2) Malt liquors	6.8	23) Screens and venetian blinds	1.6
3) Wines	5.2	24) Periodicals	0.2
4) Distilled liquors	2.1	25) Books	2.4
5) Meat	0.6	26) Drugs	9.9
6) Dairy	2.2	27) Soaps	9.2
7) Canning	2.9	28) Paints	1.5
8) Grain mill products	1.9	29) Perfumes	15.3
9) Cereals	10.3	30) Tires and tubes	1.4
10) Bakery products	2.9	31) Footwear	1.5
11) Sugar	0.2	32) Hand tools	4.2
12) Confectionary	3.5	33) Household and service	
13) Cigars	2.6	Machinery (not electrical)	1.9
14) Cigarettes	4.8	34) Electrical appliances	3.5
15) Knit goods	1.3	35) Radio, T.V., and phonograph	2.2
16) Carpets	2.0	36) Motorcycles and bicycles	1.1
17) Hats	2.2	37) Motor vehicles	0.6
18) Men's clothing	1.2	38) Instruments	2.0
19) Women's clothing	1.8	39) Clocks and watches	5.6
20) Millinery	0.8	40) Jewelry (precious metal)	3.2
21) Furs	1.0	41) Costume jewelry	4.0

Source: William Comanor and Thomas Wilson, "Advertising, Market Structure, and Performance," *The Review of Economics and Statistics* 49, no. 4 (November 1967): 423–40, esp. p. 439.

than corresponding estimates for other industries. We have not made our own estimates for other industries, and therefore we have to rely on other studies. Comanor and Wilson estimate that in 1954 the advertising sales ratio for the pharmaceutical industry, which they estimated from Internal Revenue data, was 9.9 percent, which placed it third in a list of forty-one industries after perfumes and cereals (table 9-2).[28]

The critics of the industry suggest that the explanation lies in the large expenditures by large firms to promote their brands. We have already suggested one alternative explanation: the special need by doctors for information concerning product characteristics. Additional factors contributing to the apparently high advertising intensity include the large number of firms in the industry, the large number of doctors, and the large number of products.

The industry includes several hundred firms, each of which engages in some promotional activity even though its sales may be small. A modest effort thus can lead to a high advertising intensity for the industry, because a modest effort by a firm from the standpoint of what is needed to inform all doctors may require an expenditure which is high in relation to total sales when the company's sales are small. In addition, the audience is large: it consists of more than 200,000 doctors, to say nothing of the 14,000 pharmacists and thousands of nurses.[29] The cost of some types of promotion—notably detailing and mail—increases proportionally with the number of appeals made to individual doctors, and detailing is an expensive form of promotion, accounting for 59 percent of the industry's promotional expenditures.

Furthermore, many drugs having small sales must be promoted in order to inform doctors of their existence and of their properties. A small promotional effort, but one large enough to reach a large proportion of all doctors, will result in a high percentage of sales being devoted to promotion for each of many drugs. Thus, the large number of drugs with small sales is an element in the high promotional intensity of this industry.

Thus, the apparently large promotional expenditures per doctor by the industry as a whole and the high ratio of advertising expenditures to sales are both misleading. They do not signify numerous detail calls to each doctor in behalf of individual products or other forms of high-pressure advertising campaigns.

THE NUMBER OF COMPANIES AND THE NUMBER OF DOCTORS. If the advertising expenditures were high because of heavy campaigns by individual companies, then we would expect to find that individual companies spend large sums and that their expenditures per doctor are large. We will examine the promotional spending by the eight leading firms. In view of the uncertainty of the estimates of promotional expenditures, we will use both a low estimate which is the one presented originally (table 9-1) and a high estimate which is based on the assumption that promotional expenditures constitute 20 percent of sales.

On the basis of the low estimate, in 1972 the eight leading companies spent a total of $240 million on promotion (table 9-3), which is equivalent to $1,200 per doctor. The average expenditures per company on promotion was $30.0 million. The amount spent per doctor per company was $150.

The same table shows that one of the factors contributing to the apparently high ratio of promotional expenditures to sales is the large number of doctors. The average sales per doctor of each of the eight leading companies, therefore is small. On the average each doctor writes prescriptions which yield only $1,403 in sales to each of the leading companies. This means that even when expenditures are kept to fairly modest amounts, the proportion of sales represented by such expenditures may seem excessive. Thus, the modest average expenditure of $150 per doctor by each of the eight leading companies amounts to as much as 10.7 percent of their sales. The fact of the matter is that if each company is to approach every doctor, little can be done to reduce total expenditures by any large amount.

The substitution of the high estimate of promotional expenditures for the

TABLE 9-3

Analysis of Sales and Promotional Expenditures by Industry and by Eight Leading Companies, 1972

	Industry		Eight leading companies			
	Total ($ million)	Per doctor ($000)	Total ($ million)	Per doctor ($000)	Per company ($ million)	Per doctor per company ($)
Sales	5,800	29	2,245	11	281	1,403
Promotional expenditures						
Low	722	3.6	240	1.2	30.0	150
High	1,160	5.9	387	1.9	48.4	242

Source: Sales from IMS. Low estimate of total promotional expenditures for industry from table 9-1. High estimate of total promotional expenditures based on assumption that they amount to 20 percent of sales. Other estimates based on estimates of shares of promotional expenditures by individual companies in *National Detailing Audits,* IMS America, Ltd., 1972 *National Journal Audits,* IMS America Ltd., 1972, *National Mail Audits,* IMS America Ltd., 1972.

Note: Eight leading companies chosen by sales, based on *U.S. Pharmaceutical Market, Drug Stores and Hospitals,* IMS America, Ltd., 1972.

low estimate does not alter our conclusion. It implies an average expenditure per doctor by each company of $242, which still is not large when one considers the number of drugs which have to be promoted, the amount of information which must be transmitted about each drug, and the consequences of lack of information.

The leading firms, moreover, spend a smaller share of their total revenue on promotional expenditures than does the rest of the industry. As table 9-4 reports, assuming the low estimate for the industry, the proportion for the eight leading firms in 1972 was 10.7 percent, compared to 13.6 percent for the rest of the industry. This difference in percentages is further evidence of the importance of the large number of firms in the share of sales in the industry as a whole represented by promotional costs. If the number of firms were smaller, and the average sales per firm were larger, then the share of sales per firm represented by promotional costs would be smaller. The fixed costs of promotion represented by a minimum promotional staff contribute to the relatively high costs of promotion of the small firms. Another factor probably is that the smaller firms are promoting their brands heavily in order to gain a larger share of the respective markets in competition with established brands.

DETAILING. One criticism of pharmaceutical promotion is that the calls of companies' detailmen take an excessive amount of doctors' time. Moreover, these calls are excessive for the purpose of simply conveying information. Hence the funds and resources spent on detailing are socially wasteful.

TABLE 9-4
Percentage of Sales and of Promotional Expenditures Accounted for by Eight Leading Companies and Percentage of Sales Accounted for by Promotional Expenditures in Industry and among Eight Leading Companies

	Industry	Eight leading companies	Rest of industry
Sales	100	39	61
Promotional expenditures	100	33	67
Promotional expenditures as percentage of sales	12.4	10.7	13.6

Sources: Promotional Expenditures: *National Detailing Audits*, IMS America, Ltd., 1973, *National Journal Audits*, IMS America Ltd., 1972, and *National Mail Audits*, IMS America Ltd., 1972: Professional Market Research.
Note: Eight leading companies determined by sales, *U.S. Pharmaceutical Market, Drug Stores and Hospitals*, IMS America Ltd., 1972.
The figure of 12.4 percent is what we call the low estimate in the text.

A careful examination of the data on detailing leads to quite different conclusions. The total number of calls by the industry in 1972, for example, is quite impressive: 17.4 million. When we break it down, however, into the number of calls on each doctor in an average week by detailmen from all companies, it comes to only 1.7 (table 9-5). It bears repetition that this is the total number of calls by all detailmen taken together regardless of which companies they represent.

The number of calls by individual companies on each doctor thus is miniscule: all of the eight leading companies taken together make only one call on each doctor every other week. The data show that each of the leading companies call on each doctor an average of less than once per quarter (3.2 calls per year).

MAIL PROMOTION. Examination of the data for mail promotion yields a similar conclusion. The analysis provided by table 9-6 shows that the industry as a whole sends an average number of sixteen pieces of mail per week to every doctor. The eight leading firms together send an average of 8.4 pieces of mail weekly to each doctor.

EXPENDITURES BY THERAPEUTIC FIELDS. Sometimes it is suggested that doctors overprescribe antibiotics, tranquilizers, and other drugs because the industry spends large sums promoting drugs within each of these categories. The promotional expenditures per doctor for each of the ten leading therapeutic

TABLE 9-5
Number of Detail Calls per Doctor by Industry, by
Eight Leading Companies, and Average Number of
Calls per Doctor per Company, 1972

	Calls
Industry	
Total number made annually (millions)	17.4
Average per doctor	
Annually	87
Weekly	1.7
Eight Leading Companies	
Total number made annually (millions)	5.2
Average per doctor	
Annually	26
Weekly	.5
Average per doctor per company,	
annually	3.2

Source: Based on *National Detailing Audits,* IMS America Ltd., 1972.

Note: Eight leading companies determined by sales, based on *U.S. Pharmaceutical Market, Drug Stores and Hospitals,* IMS America Ltd., 1972.

TABLE 9-6
Estimates of Number of Pieces of Mail per Doctor by
Industry, by Eight Leading Companies, 1972

	Pieces of mail
Industry	
Total to all doctors	
Annually	170,794,000
Average per doctor	
Annually	859
Weekly	16
Eight Leading Companies	
Percent of all mail by industry	51.2
Total to all doctors	
Annually	87,468,000
Average per doctor	
Annually	437
Weekly	8.4
Average per doctor per company	
Annually	55
Weekly	1.1

Source: *National Mail Audits,* IMS America Ltd., 1973.
Note: Eight leading companies determined by sales, based on *U.S. Pharmaceutical Market, Drug Stores and Hospitals,* IMS America Ltd., 1973.

fields are shown in table 9-7. The expenditures for antibiotics are the highest of any class—$227 per doctor. This estimate is not so large as to convey the impression of overwhelming pressure.

EXPENDITURES PER PRODUCT. Much of the discussion of promotion suggests that promotional expenditures per product are excessive, that the present level of promotion is socially wasteful, and that it subjects doctors to an undue influence in their prescribing. The argument is also made that doctors prescribe individual drugs because of the influence of advertising—an argument which suggests that there were large promotional expenditures for each of the leading fifty products in 1973. Yet the average expenditure for each product in this group was about $2 million,[30] which comes to about $10 per doctor. This amount does not appear large enough to warrant charges of promotion having an unduly large influence on doctors.

HOSTILITY TO PROMOTION

The attack by many economists on the promotion of drugs is an aspect of their general hostility to advertising, an attitude which originates in the condemnation of the content of advertising as consisting mostly of false and misleading claims.

TABLE 9-7
Promotional Expenditures per Doctor by Entire Drug Industry in Leading
Ten Therapeutic Fields, 1972

Therapeutic Field	Dollars	Therapeutic Field	Dollars
Broad- and medium-spectrum antibiotics	$227	Plain corticoids	81
Ataractics/tranquilizers	176	Diuretics	70
Non-narcotic analgesics	108	Antispasmodics	70
Penicillins	102	Plain antacids	61
Oral cold preparations	86	Hypotensives	60

Sources: Estimates based on National Detailing Audits, IMS America, Ltd., 1972; National Journal Audits, IMS America, Ltd., 1972; National Mail Audits, IMS America, Ltd., 1972.

Furthermore, this view of advertising, as expressed, for example, by J. K. Galbraith,[31] condemns advertising for manipulating and deceiving consumers into choosing defective and socially harmful products, such as non-nutritious foods and speedy cars which consume excessive amounts of gasoline, in preference to intrinsically more desirable but unpromoted goods and services, such as housing and education. This objection does not originate within economics; rather, it is an expression of hostility to the hedonistic values which advertising expresses and to the hucksterism in advertising.

The condemnation which originates in economics itself is an interesting consequence of a theoretical model of perfect competition which is based on several assumptions designed to simplify the analysis of the effects of various changes, such as those in taxes, wage rates, and incomes, on prices. The model assumes that the market contains many sellers and buyers, that all potential buyers and sellers know the prices at which transactions have been conducted, and that there are no barriers to entry.

One assumption which has had a dominant influence in the discussion of promotion is that the product sold by different firms is homogeneous. It simplifies the analysis of the competitive behavior of firms by excluding changes in physical characteristics. The analysis is thereby confined to changes in the single variable, price, rather than in several variables measuring quality as well as price, and it effectively avoids the problems of appraising changes in quality. The approach is adequate for the analysis of the effects of various environmental changes on prices over short periods when the major changes are likely to take the form of price changes in any case.

The form of the model has severely limited and in fact distorted the discussion of promotional activities. Since by assumption products are homogeneous and buyers are informed, advertising activities can convey no information about physical characteristics of goods, to say nothing about the assumption that all potential buyers and sellers possess full information concerning prices. There is no room for promotional activities.

Traditional economic theory admits promotional activities by the back door in the analysis of oligopoly behavior. It comes in as a device used by firms to avoid price competition, which remains the only form of competition formally recognized within the analysis as beneficial to consumers. The major purpose of oligopoly theory is to analyze price behavior, and the same assumptions are made concerning product characteristics and information as in the model of perfect competition. The conclusion is reached that oligopolists will avoid price competition, and the price therefore will be higher than under perfect competition. Promotion is introduced into the analysis as a device used by firms to expand sales without reducing prices. Differences in product characteristics are admitted to the analysis in the same way, as devices for seeking increases in sales without cutting prices. So essentially promotional activities are viewed as wasteful and misleading. Product changes are regarded with the same skepticism.

The discussion thus has emphasized the irrational appeals made, the apparently deceptive quality of much advertising, and the total cost of advertising. No attention has been given within the traditional framework to consumers' problems of choice among alternative products which differ in quality as well as in price and the service provided by advertising in supplying them with information. Thus, differences in advertising content among markets have been ignored, as has the question of determinants of the effectiveness of advertising within markets.

The condemnation of pharmaceutical promotion fits neatly into the pattern of the more general condemnation. The critics maintain that drugs within broad classes are essentially homogeneous. The differences are slight modifications designed to permit the entry of firms into markets supplied by patented products. Their promotional efforts are wasteful of resources and they are deceptive. In fact, the costs of promotional efforts include the very serious consequences of overprescribing drugs and inappropriate uses of dangerous drugs.

In other parts of the book we have seen that innovational competition has been the major form of competition in this industry, not because of an effort to avoid price competition in this industry, but for a variety of reasons, including the protection of established brands by patents. This pattern of competition has yielded valuable as well as unimportant drugs. From a social standpoint it may well have produced a performance superior to that of a system in which patents would have been weaker and firms competed more in price and less in innovation.

CONCLUSIONS

We have evaluated the case against the promotional activities of the industry. There is no basis for the argument that promotion has led to overprescribing and to harmful treatment of patients. Promotional efforts in this industry have provided essential informational service to doctors. We have also considered the cost of promotion, and have not found it excessive. The apparently high ratio of advertising expenditures to sales can be explained by the special need for information in this industry, and by the large number of companies, doctors, and products. We have also seen that from the standpoint of the benefits of information to doctors and patients, a reasonable case can be made for the position that the expenditures on promotion by the industry have been inadequate rather than excessive.

CHAPTER 10

THE QUALITY OF DRUGS
AND GENERIC PRESCRIBING:
GENERAL BACKGROUND

INTRODUCTION

Critics of the industry who view the leading firms as oligopolistic exploiters of consumers see a way to redress the balance in favor of consumers through generic prescribing. The major firms' market powers, according to one popular interpretation, can be traced to the repeated drumming of brand names into doctors' minds by detailmen and by intensive promotional efforts which are paid for by consumers in the form of higher drug prices. Consumers are thus doubly exploited. Prices are higher under oligopoly than under pure competition. Consumers foot the bill for the creation of an oligopolistic situation because it is caused by promotional expenditures. These expenditures create product differentiation which is not objectively there. The critics also assume that Brand A is just as good therapeutically as Brand B, and that both brands are no better than the generic version which can be sold without all the expensive promotion, thereby saving the consumer considerable money. Later, in chapter 11, we shall explore the assumptions underlying this description of competitive behavior in the drug market. Here, we simply note the description without exploring its credibility. In the belief, however, that the assumptions are correct, critics such as Senator Nelson urge (a) that doctors prescribe generically and that hospitals adopt formularies which substitute, where possible, generic equivalents for the highly promoted, more expensive brand names; (b) the repeal of state laws prohibiting pharmacists from substituting generic drugs for brands specified in prescriptions; (c) the purchase of generics by the Department of Defense, Veterans' Administration hospitals, and other public institutions.

The recent change in HEW rules relating to its reimbursements of patients' drug purchases under the Medicare and Medicaid programs is consistent with this line of thinking. Under the new Maximum Allowable Cost (MAC) regulation,

HEW will reimburse patients only up to the amount which is set as a ceiling for the generically equivalent drug which is generally available.[1]

The MAC regulation and proposals to encourage the use of generics raise a large number of issues. Here we deal with only one of them, namely the possibility of quality deterioration in the supply of drugs. The problem is that a doctor may impose a significantly greater risk on patients who may be given a drug which is less effective or even toxic when he prescribes a generic rather than a brand-name drug. The debate over the various proposals designed to promote the use of generics has given greater attention to one aspect of this general issue, the "bioavailability question," than to the other, the question of good manufacturing practices by manufacturers of generics. We restrict our attention to the latter question, because it is more amenable to economic analysis.

A word about bioavailability, however, is in order, in view of its prominence in the public discussion. Two products are generically equivalent when the active ingredient in each is described by the same chemical formula. Nevertheless, they may not be therapeutically equivalent because of differences in inert ingredients which constitute the major part of the total weight of the drug in most cases and in certain physical characteristics of the active ingredient, including solubility and crystalline structure. Differences in physical characteristics of the active ingredient may arise from differences in manufacturing methods. The testing procedures specified by the U.S. Pharmacopeia (USP) and the National Formulary (NF) provide for a number of physical as well as chemical tests, but in general they do not provide a test of bioavailability, which would require an expensive clinical test of blood levels reached or pharmacologic response within specified periods after a drug is administered. The FDA therefore does not require it for most drugs (though proposals for new regulations include such tests). The original drug in a generic group must be proved to be effective and safe, and numerous clinical tests are required for this purpose. Once the drug is well established, firms which manufacture successors must submit evidence of chemical equivalence of the active ingredient and certain physical tests specified in the USP, in order to obtain the FDA's approval of an Abbreviated New Drug Application (ANDA). Manufacturers of such drugs do not have to go through the full procedure which is required of original manufacturers who must obtain approval of New Drug Applications (NDA's). Descriptions of the manufacturing procedure are also required. But bioavailability tests or clinical tests of efficacy and safety generally have not been required. The general consensus now seems to be that generic equivalence does not imply therapeutic equivalence. What remains unresolved as yet is the importance of the cases of generic equivalence in which there is lack of therapeutic equivalence. The reason for the uncertainty is the fewness of the studies dealing with this question.

After this digression, let us return to consideration of good manufacturing practice (GMP). A manufacturer can ensure a high level of quality of product, as measured by the percentage of total production which is defective, by increasing the resources devoted to production and to quality control. The manufacturer can use more personnel at key points in production where errors may be made, more supervisory personnel, employees with better training and education, and more people in quality control. In addition, the company can reduce the risk of defectives by sampling more frequently from each batch while it is in production, and more tests can be performed. How much resources should be spent on the quality of the product is an economic judgment.

In the debate over generic prescribing, the FDA has steadfastly maintained that its surveillance of manufacturing effectively shields consumers from the poor quality arising from the lack of observance of GMP regulation. In any case, according to the FDA spokesmen (somewhat contradictorily), branded drugs are no more reliable than generic products, because, it is alleged, the frequency of recalls has been as great for large as for small manufacturers. We shall see that the FDA is wrong on both these counts.

The risk of poor quality may be increasing regardless of what HEW and other government agencies do. Despite the supposedly great mind-bending influence of drug advertising on doctors, they have increasingly been prescribing generics. The percentage of all prescriptions which are generics has increased from 6.4 percent in 1966 to 10.6 percent in 1973.[2] The final percentage may not appear to be high at a first glance, but it is a large part of the total number of prescriptions for multiple-source drugs. There is no point in prescribing generically for single-source drugs, which manufacturers promote under their brand names, so we can assume safely that all prescriptions for such drugs specify brand names. Of all prescriptions, about 44 percent are written for multiple source drugs.[3] Thus, the percentage of prescriptions for multiple-source drugs which are written generically is much higher than the 10.6 percent for all drugs. The observed increase in the proportion of all prescriptions which are written generically has been growing in recent years largely because the patents for some important drugs have expired or have been contested and they have become multiple-source drugs. These include such important and widely used drugs as ampicillin, meprobamate, tetracycline, erythromycin, and rauwolfia diuretics. This change has attracted little attention because the debate over public policy continues to assume that, for the most part, doctors are gullible and prescribe brand names under the spell of advertising. We have, however, in point of fact entered an era in which generic prescriptions have become increasingly important, and the trend is continuing. The new competition from generics may be welcomed by economists who value the benefits of price competition, but any resulting deterioration in the quality of drugs may lead to a net social loss.

The FDA has accelerated the shift to generics by assuring doctors that they can prescribe them freely without any special precautions. Whether or not the FDA can rightly claim to provide such assurance has been a matter of some concern, and the validity of the claim demands some examination.

This chapter approaches the issue in the broader context of an analysis of the economic forces affecting the quality of drugs. For the sake of simplicity, we will begin with a consideration of the determinants of quality in a hypothetical unregulated free market. Following this analysis, we will go on to a consideration of the effect of regulation on the quality of drugs and specifically of the success of the FDA's activities.

THE QUALITY OF DRUGS IN AN UNREGULATED MARKET

THE DEMAND FOR QUALITY. We will analyze the determination of the quality of drugs in each generic class. This limitation excludes from the analysis differences among drugs owing to different chemical formulas of the active ingredients and considers only differences between generically equivalent drugs. Generically equivalent drugs may differ in therapeutic efficacy and in safety because of differences in potency and in physical characteristics of the drug which are not described by the chemical formula. These include disintegrability, solubility, and crystalline structure. The chemical formula describes only the active ingredient, which usually constitutes a small part of the weight of a drug; the remainder includes materials such as binders, flavorants, and coating agents. FDA regulations require that manufacturers of drugs which appear in the monographs of the USP and NF conform to standards set out in these compendia. The compendia not only provide the chemical formula, but also specify the allowed range of potency and certain chemical and physical tests which measure its efficacy and safety. A drug may fail to meet compendial standards because of poor manufacturing practices. In addition, even meeting the compendial specifications may not satisfy a doctor's demand for high quality, for, as we shall see, the prescribed tests in many cases are crude and incomplete. A doctor may therefore want more assurance of high quality than is provided by these tests.

We begin with the analysis of the demand for a drug. We expect the number of prescriptions for a good drug to exceed that of inferior drugs within the same generic class. The tendency for sales to increase among drugs with quality, however, may not be very strong. Not all doctors will insist on prescribing the "best" drug. Even though medical tradition generally is heedless of costs, some doctors will dismiss quality differences as unimportant when they see large price differences, and others may simply be unaware of them.

Nevertheless, we can assume that doctors will tend to prescribe well-manufactured drugs unless their prices are excessive. Accordingly, the demand equation for a drug can be written as follows:

$$n_1 = f(q_1, q_2, \ldots, q_m; p_1, p_2, \ldots, p_m) \qquad (10.1)$$

where n_1 = number of prescriptions for drug 1; q_1 = quality of drug 1; $q_2, \ldots,$ q_m = quality of other drugs in same generic class; p_1 = price of drug 1; and $p_2, \ldots, p_m$ are interpreted analogously.

The equation may not describe doctors' behavior very well if, as appears to be the case, they have little information concerning the quality of drugs. This lack of information has some interesting consequences. Doctors will engage in some search, and they will make as much use of their limited information as possible. Thus, they will make broad inferences. If they learn that drug X of company A has been found to be subpotent, then all of company A's products are likely to become suspect. Such inferences are likely to extend over time as well as over products, and the injury to a company's reputation may persist even though the problem is temporary. This tendency of doctors to generalize from scattered bits of information is reinforced by the limits on their time, and by the fact that the quality of drugs is not the only matter which requires their well-informed judgment.

Another consequence of the demands on the time and effort of doctors is that they will prescribe a small number of drugs for each disease.[4] It follows that a doctor must be persuaded of the good quality of a drug for it to obtain and retain a place in his armamentarium.

The competition among drugs for a favorable place in the memories of doctors has further implications, owing to the fact that they cannot directly perceive the quality of drugs.[5] Information relating to the quality of drugs will reflect their therapeutic or harmful effects, and doctors' attention is likely to be drawn to differences in the manufacturing quality (as distinguished from differences in efficacy which are attributable to the chemical formula) by reports of harmful effects which are traced to defects in manufacturing practices. The maintenance of manufacturing quality, thus, will prevent declines in sales due to bad news of harmful effects.

Such news spreads to doctors by word of mouth from colleagues, by articles in journals and trade magazines, and by the reports of detailmen of rival companies. The number of doctors who learn of a single incident within any specified period depends on the gravity of the harm done and on the number of prescribers of the drug. If a given proportion of doctors who directly observe a harmful effect inform other doctors, and a given proportion of these in turn inform still others, and so on, the number who hear the news is proportional to the number of doctors involved in the first place, which is proportional to the number of prescribers. But the number of doctors who hear the news in a given period will be more than proportional to the number of prescribers, because in the first and subsequent relays the number who are interested in and therefore pass the news on will also increase proportionally with the number of prescribers. Indeed, even nonprescribers will be interested in news about popular drugs and will pass it on. This tendency for the number of doctors who know of the harmful effects of a drug to grow more than proportionally with the sales of that drug will be reinforced by the greater interest of medical media in such drugs than in inconspicuous drugs.

This analysis can be summarized as follows: Let A = the total number of doctors who know of a poor quality batch of output from a company within a specified period; p = the number of doctors who actually observe the effects of this batch; a = the fraction of p who tell other doctors the news; b = the fraction of those who hear the news who repeat it; c = the fraction of those who hear the news in the second relay and who repeat it in the next relay; and so on. Now if $a = b = c \ldots$, then

$$A = p + ap + a^2p + \ldots + a^np.$$

We can assume that p is proportional to firm size. A increases more than proportionally with firm size if a increases with firm size. The argument suggests that a does increase with firm size.

A word about prices, which are included in the demand equation, is appropriate here. Price has an effect on the demand for drugs, especially when a drug has generic equivalents, for these are close substitutes for the drug in question. A generically different drug, by contrast, is less likely to be a good substitute for an established brand. Thus, the price of Miltown, which competes against other products within its own generic class, the meprobamates, will have a strong influence on the quantity of Miltown sold. The price of Valium, which is still under patent and therefore is the only product in its generic class, diazepam, will have some influence on its sales, although not as large. The minor tranquilizers include several different drugs with similar effects, all of which are to some degree substitutes for Valium. The price of Valium, therefore, has some effect on the quantity of Valium sold but not a great influence.

Let us consider the determinants of profits. Total profits equal total revenue minus total costs:

$$\pi = TR - TC.$$

We have established that the quantity of a drug sold, and therefore *TR*, will increase with quality over time. We can extend the analysis further. Total revenue equals the product of price and quantity.

$$TR = pq$$

where p = price and q = quantity sold. We can break q down into the number of doctors who prescribe the drug and the average quantity prescribed by each doctor:

$$TR = pN \cdot \frac{q}{N},$$

where N = the number of doctors prescribing the drug, and q/N = average quantity of the drug prescribed by each doctor.

We bring out the relationship between total sales and the number of doctors prescribing a drug, because the revenue which a firm gains from improvements in the quality of its product increases with the number of prescribers (if the average per prescriber remains the same). We have already suggested that the number of doctors who learn of a harmful effect of a drug increases more than proportionally with the number of prescribers and that the sales of a company's other products will also be reduced by such an incident. The important result of this analysis is that the loss in revenue resulting from the discovery of a given defect in quality increases more than proportionally with the sales of the drug in question.

THE COST OF QUALITY CONTROL. We turn next to the other component of the profit equation, namely Total Cost, or TC. In this connection, we have to consider whether large plants benefit from economies of scale in the control of quality (here "control of quality" is broadly defined to include manufacturing procedures designed to ensure a high level of quality as well as quality control procedures which are separately administered by a Quality Control organization). Such economies may originate from large overhead costs which do not vary with output and from the need to employ highly specialized skills which would be incompletely utilized by firms which produced a small quantity of drugs. If there are such economies, then small firms may not be able to provide adequate assurance of quality because the cost per unit of output will be excessive.

The regulations defining Good Manufacturing Practice which are issued by the FDA provide some clues to the relation between the cost of ensuring good quality and the size of output. The GMP regulations seek to prevent errors in manufacturing, such as mixups of materials intended for different products and mislabeling of final products. They also attempt to ensure that products have the specified potency and are free of contamination. In addition, they are designed to ensure that errors are discovered before a shipment enters the market, and if discovery takes place later, that the manufacturer will quickly be able to locate and recall the defective products.

To prevent mixups of materials and products and to permit the subsequent tracing of defective products, output is divided into batches or lots. This is not the only reason for the division of output into batches, but it is an important one. A continuous record of the identity, source, date of receipt, weights of the materials used in manufacture, and stages of processing and testing through which materials have passed is kept for each batch. The integrity of a batch is maintained from the time the materials are weighed out in the area of a plant known as the "pharmacy" through all of the stages of production. And each container is marked with a lot number, so that even after a lot is in the market the items can be identified. Within the plant, the materials that are used to make a lot are moved together from one stage of the process to the next. The manufacturing processes for oral products include the weighing of materials in the pharmacy, granulation, blending, tableting (or encapsulating), and coating. After an operation is completed, the equipment used is cleaned and washed thoroughly so that residues do not contaminate the next batch, whether or not the same drug is to be processed. The cleaning operation takes a good deal of time, and machines are idle until they have been cleaned and are ready for the next batch.

The larger plants have adopted the modular organization: the materials constituting a batch are moved together as a unit on pallets from one production process to the next, and each operation is separately located in a fully enclosed room. The drums of all components which are used to make up a lot are moved into the room and are kept there until the operation is completed and the product is tested. The drums containing the product then are moved as a unit to the room where the next operation is performed. This procedure not only prevents mixups of drums of materials intended for different batches, such as might occur when different batches are being processed on an undivided common floor area, but it also prevents the dust produced by the machine processing one batch from contaminating another batch on another machine. Air currents can pick up the dust which settles on nearby walls and floors, and on drums located in the vicinity, and so could contaminate other products, despite careful cleaning of machines and precautions in the moving of materials. When operations are conducted in closed and separately ventilated rooms and the walls and floors as well as the equipment are thoroughly cleaned and washed after each operation, the risk of contamination is reduced considerably. Since the modular organization requires large fixed costs for space, it results in economies of scale over a large range of output. Many large batches must be run through the plant to utilize a large space economically. GMP regulations do not require a modular organization. Nevertheless, they do insist on buildings which provide adequate space for "Orderly placement of equipment and materials to minimize any risk of mixups between different drugs, drug components, in-process materials, packaging materials, or labeling, and to minimize the possibility of contamination." The space must also be adequate for "the receipt and storage of components awaiting sampling and testing prior to release by the materials approval unit for manufacturing or packaging," "for manufacturing and processing operations," "storage of finished products," and "control and production-laboratory operations."[6] Even this statement suggests that a small firm will not be able to undertake the necessary space costs to minimize problems of quality control.

In addition, a substantial investment is required to set up the production and quality control procedures for each product. A quality control system for a product requires preparing an elaborate set of specifications for all the components of the product. The specifications include the methods for determining the identity, purity, strength, physical characteristics, uniformity, and quality not only of the final product but at each stage of production. The specifications also provide for packages, including glass containers, bottle closures, and cap liners. The manufacturing process is described on master formulation cards, and the components of each batch are traceable from the lot number of the final package. Approval by Quality Control is given and the product is released when all of the specifications are met and the records are complete. Firms have instituted control systems which utilize computers for the entry of results of tests and the production of batch records. The product release unit of the Quality Control Division can keep track of the progress of each batch and release the batch to the market when the computer record is complete and the specifications have been met. Since the high costs of these procedures are largely independent of the size of a plant, they are a source of economies of scale. In addition, the cost of setting up and maintaining records for each batch is fixed regardless of the size of the batch, so the larger the batch the lower the unit cost of record-keeping. This is another source of economies of scale.

The cost of operating the quality control laboratory also is likely to generate significant economies of scale over a considerable range of sizes. We have no estimate of the fraction of total manufacturing cost represented by the cost of quality control, but judging from the number of employees in the quality control laboratory of one large plant in relation to the total number of employees, it is large. Out of a total of 1,100 employees, this plant has 200 in the quality control department.

Economies of scale also originate in the number of persons of the appropriate training and experience required for the direction and operation of a plant and for quality control. The GMP regulations are vague on this matter, but they do suggest the importance of an adequate number of trained persons. Dr. A. Kirshbaum more specifically states that the quality control laboratory of a plant producing antibiotics requires a microbiologist, an analytical chemist, a pharmacist and helpers to perform routine tasks and clean up.[7] Whatever the required number is, it is safe to conclude that it will not increase proportionally with the output of a plant at least in the smaller size range of plants. In addition, economies of scale stem from the fact that the required training of such persons will not increase proportionally with the output of a plant. As we shall see later, many plants which manufacture drugs appear to be too small to support the needed managerial and quality control personnel, and in such plants therefore the control of quality is not performed adequately. The fact that they exist and produce drugs suggests that drugs of poor quality may be entering the market.

The cost per unit of output of sampling and testing by the quality control laboratory declines with increases in batch size. The batch is the unit for sampling of products after the completion of a stage of production, and the size of a sample necessary to provide a specified level of reliability does not increase with batch size. The unit cost of quality control is also reduced with increases in batch size by the fixed cost per batch of set-ups for the different tests. Thus, economies of scale in production associated with the control of quality originate in the costs which are fixed with respect to batch size.

The growth in output of a plant consists of growth in the average size of batches as well as in the number of batches, and growth in the average size of batches reduces the unit cost of those quality control operations for which the basic unit is the batch. One popular formula for optimum batch size in dollars— or, as it is usually known, Economic Order Quantity—is as follows:

$$Q = \sqrt{\frac{2as}{i}}$$

where a = annual output in dollars, s = set-up cost per batch, i = cost of carrying inventory for one year. Thus optimum batch size increases proportionally with the square root of plant size (measured by a), or less than proportionally with plant size.

Manufacturers' customer complaint departments and detailmen speed up the discovery and recall of defective products when these are not discovered until after they have been distributed. The costs of the customer complaint department and of detailing increase less than proportionally with sales.

Finally, there is the need of a back-up group of skilled, experienced people who are ready to step into key positions when the need arises and to act as troubleshooters whenever quality problems arise. The cost of maintaining such a group is unlikely to increase proportionally with output.

The analysis we have just gone through suggests a long-run average cost curve for quality control having the shape shown in figure 10-1. The long-run average cost curve (LRAC) is drawn so that there is a minimum efficient size (MES) of plant with respect to output. Thus, the curve shows a sharp drop in average cost of quality control over a range of sizes up to MES and then is flat beyond that size. Such a flat portion may not exist; the LRAC may continue to decline over a range extending up to the size of the largest plants, in which case only the largest plants would gain the full benefits of the economies of scale in quality control. The data are inadequate to establish the exact shape of the curve, and the preceding analysis only indicates economies of scale over some range.

FIG. 10-1
Long-run Average Cost Curve

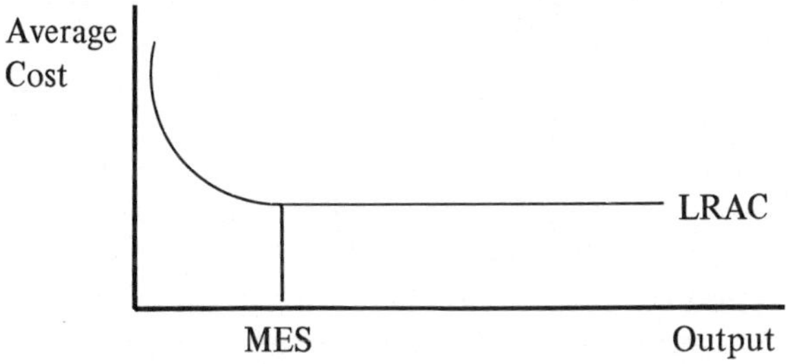

That there are many firms in the size range below MES is strongly suggested by the large number of very small establishments by almost any standard, according to the Bureau of Census's reports for the Pharmaceutical Preparations Industry (SIC 2834). In 1967 this industry contained 875 establishments. The distribution of these establishments among the employment size classes is reported in table 1-3 of chapter 1. In this table it can be seen that 43 percent of all establishments had four or fewer employees, and the average sales of these establishments was only $38,800. The point at which a plant is large enough to maintain adequate control over quality without accepting an impossibly large unit cost is unknown. But certainly in view of the earlier discussion, plants with fewer than nineteen employees are unlikely to be able to manage it, and such plants represent as much as 64 percent of all plants.[8] True, these plants make up an astonishingly small percentage of total sales—1.4 percent. One might conclude that so small a fraction of total output cannot present a substantial risk of ineffective and dangerous drugs to the public. This is a dangerous inference, however, because these plants have a much larger share of output of certain drugs. Their output is concentrated in drugs whose patents have expired and, more particularly, in drugs which the FDA classifies as "old drugs" which do not require the approval of NDA's. In some localities the risk may be much larger than the average, because small plants produce a large proportion of the drugs consumed. In addition, the number of plants in which quality control is less than adequate may be much larger than those having fewer than nineteen employees. If economic forces are insufficient to ensure adequate quality control until a much larger size is reached, then the risk is much greater.

A good theoretical case can thus be made for the propositions that (1) large firms have more to gain in revenues from maintaining a given level of quality in the manufacture of drugs than do small firms, and (2) the cost, per unit of output, of maintaining a given level of quality declines as firm size increases. The evidence will not be presented until the next chapter, but the theory alone is persuasive. Our analysis suggests that in order to minimize the risks of ineffective or of unsafe drugs, doctors should prescribe only brand-name products or generic products of large firms. We can have confidence in the quality of the generic products manufactured by large firms, but a doctor does not know the source of a drug when he prescribes it generically unless he also specifies a particular manufacturer, and this is tantamount to prescribing by brand name. Nor can he count on pharmacists to choose only reliable suppliers; in large cities he does not know which pharmacists his patients patronize. Moreover, the individual pharmacist has neither the time nor the resources to inspect suppliers' plants and to test samples. True, many pharmacists minimize the risk of poor quality by filling generic prescriptions with standard brands, even though the fact that a prescription is generic suggests the use of an off-brand product; but others are more attracted by the low prices at which generic products are offered by small manufacturers, the benefits of which they may retain for themselves rather than passing them on to consumers. Nevertheless, in spite of these dangers, many doctors prescribe generically when they think that there is some point to doing so, as when multiple-source drugs are available and it seems possible to save the patient some money on his drug bill.

Why do doctors prescribe generically? Our theory helps us understand why doctors do not prescribe only brand names. One reason is that the information which bears on relative risks is not clear, because the quality problems of large firms attract a great deal of attention while the quality problems of small firms are ignored. Moreover, no matter how large the resources devoted to quality control, the procedures are not always foolproof, especially when firms are under pressure. A firm may expand too rapidly for its control procedures and organization to keep pace; a plant may get too crowded unless its capacity expands rapidly; and the responsibilities of key people may become excessive. In addition, certain problems are very difficult, even when considerable resources are devoted to quality control. These problems include the maintenance of sterility when it is required and the prevention of penicillin cross-contamination. When large firms have encountered difficulties with these problems, they have made headlines. Thus, when doctors restrict their prescriptions to brand-name drugs, they can only reduce their patients' risks—they cannot eliminate the risks entirely. But doctors generally do not analyze the news reports of product defects to determine the relative risks of brands versus generics. Indeed, they cannot, since the defects of generics are not widely reported. And, many doctors may interpret the reports of incidents involving large companies to signify that they cannot trust their drugs any more than those of small companies. We shall examine the error of this assumption later.

THE EFFECT OF REGULATION

The FDA, the federal regulatory agency which is charged with assuring the quality of drugs, has frequently stated publicly that it is no safer for patients to use brand name drugs than to use generics. As evidence of the truth of this statement, agency spokesmen have pointed to the large number of recalls of brands. Dr. Henry E. Simmons, then Director of the Bureau of Drugs of the FDA, in an address before the California Council of Hospital Pharmacists, San Diego, on September 30, 1972, said: "Fortunately, in general, drug manufacturers, large or small, generic and brand, have accepted their responsibility and are taking appropriate steps to fulfill it." He also emphasized that it was the FDA's responsibility "to do everything within its power to assure that *all* [emphasis in original] drugs, generic and brand, made by big and small manufacturers marketed in this country are not only safe but effective; that they are honestly labeled and of the quality necessary to produce the intended effect; and that we maintain a surveillance system which will assure this quality continues once attained." In the same speech, Dr. Simmons pointed out that "in fiscal year 1972, we had a total of 638 drug recalls. Of this total, 291 were brand name and 347 generic products. Again the defects were encountered in big companies, small companies, brand and generic products."

Prescribers of generics entrust their patients' welfare to the FDA, which, after all, is charged with ensuring the efficacy and safety of drugs. The very existence of this agency implicitly guarantees the quality of drugs in the market, and when a governmental agency inspects plants of manufacturers for the observance of GMP, certifies batches of some drugs, tests samples of other drugs, and in other ways checks claims of manufacturers for the efficacy and safety of drugs, doctors are likely to be reassured. In addition, the FDA explicitly claims to provide adequate enforcement of GMP.[9] Finally, prescribers may share the natural inclination of many people to look to laws and to government to provide guarantees where the market mechanism is considered inadequate to protect consumers.

The effect of government guarantees is double-edged. They may provide some security, but they also reduce the precautions which people provide for themselves. Private safeguards may be inadequate, too costly, and perhaps even dangerous, and therefore the government should intervene. Protection against crime, fire, and attack by foreign powers thus are generally accepted examples of appropriate areas for public intervention: in these cases public intervention does not increase the risk which it is intended to ensure against. The case for governmental surveillance and enforcement activities in the manufacture and distribution of drugs is less obvious. Clearly the government's imprimatur encourages doctors to risk prescribing generics when they would otherwise be unwilling to do so. Thus, the FDA permits small generic producers to survive and so increases the risk of poor quality drugs.

Advocates of generic prescribing point to the successful use of generic products by large hospitals and by the military services. If these institutions can use them, they suggest, then doctors also can generally prescribe generics safely. The military procurement agencies, however, take the precaution of investigating potential suppliers of drugs, and they also perform their own tests of quality. In other words, they do not rely on the FDA guarantees. Large hospitals which purchase generics also investigate suppliers, and at the very least they buy only from large suppliers whose quality they trust. The doctor in private practice, on the other hand, cannot obtain the same assurance when he prescribes generically.

Is the FDA guarantee likely to be adequate? The agency's surveillance program includes the inspection of plants, the testing prior to marketing of samples of all batches of insulin, antibiotics, digoxin, and digitoxin, infrequent tests of samples of selected products by the National Center for Drug Analysis, and tests of products by district laboratories when problems are suspected. The burden of inspecting the large number of plants in the industry has been excessive; the FDA has not been able to meet the legal requirement of biennial inspection of all drug producers. Further, it is evident that the inspections usually are provoked by problems rather than being part of a systematic effort; and they are hurried rather than thorough.

The FDA does test all batches of antibiotics, insulin, digoxin, and digitoxin before marketing, because of difficulties in manufacturing and because of the vital importance to patients of the assurance of efficacy and safety. The FDA also tests samples of other products, either as part of a survey of the quality of production of a product by all manufacturers or when quality problems are suspected. These tests of final products are not, however, a substitute for quality control by the manufacturer. A test cannot detect an unspecified foreign substance. Only when a test is constructed specifically to detect a substance is one discovered. The FDA does specify penicillin as a contaminant in tests of other drugs because of the potentially serious risk of allergic reactions. And penicillin contamination has led to many recalls. But contamination is not limited to penicillin, and we must therefore depend on strict observance of GMP to ensure purity. Moreover, analysis at the time of manufacture cannot ensure that the product will be stable and retain its effectiveness. The tests of finished products may only be applied to the products shortly after they are manufactured and they therefore miss degradation of potency. A manufacturer must maintain samples of lots which have been distributed and test representative lots periodically to ensure that they still are effective.

A regulatory agency can provide society with a high level of protection against defective drugs, but the cost may be excessive. The cost, per unit of output, of this external governmental system of quality control is large, simply because the output of many firms is small. The agency must devote a large share of its total expenditures for the control of quality to the surveillance of plants which account for a small share of total output. The disproportion between the cost and the return is increased by the fact that these small plants are less likely to control the quality of their output than are large plants. Further, the agency cannot easily economize by limiting its sampling and inspection to a few small plants, since the observance of GMP is likely to be poor in many plants.

CHAPTER 11

THE QUALITY OF DRUGS AND GENERIC PRESCRIBING: EMPIRICAL STUDIES AND POLICY PRESCRIPTIONS

INTRODUCTION

The preceding chapter argued that the incentives for large firms to control quality were greater than those for small firms. The return on investment in quality control increases directly with sales because reports of product defects affect sales not merely directly through doctors who have used the defective drug but also indirectly through the communications network of the medical profession. Moreover, a "tainted" product may call into question the reliability of a producer's whole line, not just the single product. Thus, the adverse sales effect may spread far beyond the immediate impact. There is also an indirect link through promotion between sales and return on investment in quality control. Promotional efforts increase sales and hence up to a point also increase the return on the investment. The return on investment in quality control also increases with firm size because large firms enjoy economies of scale in quality control activities. The chapter also argued that the FDA fails to provide adequate enforcement of quality control through inspection of plants and tests of finished products. It cannot assure high quality even with much larger resources, because there are no precise standards and an adequate science base for the specification of standards does not exist.

In this chapter we continue the discussion by examining some empirical studies of the effectiveness of the surveillance and enforcement activities of the FDA and of the relative performance of large and small firms. We shall conclude this discussion with a consideration of public policy in this area.

226

THE EFFECTIVENESS OF THE FDA

This section reports and evaluates the results of various studies of the effectiveness of the FDA in enforcing GMP regulations. We will first consider two studies which were sponsored by the FDA itself.

THE FDA POTENCY STUDY. In 1966 the FDA tested for potency 4,573 samples of drugs produced by 245 manufacturers. Samples were classified as outside the limits of potency if the results were outside official USP limits or NDA specifications, or if (for other drugs) they were not within 80 to 110 percent of their label declarations. A total of 371 samples, or 8.1 percent, were found to be outside these potency limits.[1] This result indicates an excessively high rate of defective output. The FDA has interpreted this result to signify inadequate performance by the industry and in particular by large firms. We deal only with the question of the performance of the industry. And we postpone the discussion of the relative performance by large firms until later.

The results imply not only that the industry has an unacceptably high rate of defective products but also that the FDA's surveillance activities have not been adequate to the task of assuring safety and efficacy.

The more general survey of drugs made by Dr. Steers[2] for the National Center for Drug Analysis suggests that for most drugs an upper limit of 1 percent is acceptable. For drugs for which precision in potency is very important, even a limit for 1 percent may be excessive. In any case, this standard suggests that the rate of defective output is excessive.

It is difficult to evaluate these results. No detail was provided so that these results could be better evaluated. In addition, Dr. Steers's study did not include samples of antibiotics and insulin, presumably because the FDA certification of these products guaranteed the potency would be within allowed limits. Thus, we do not know how the drugs in particular therapeutic classes performed.

The validity of the result of the FDA study, moreover, has been questioned by the Pharmaceutical Manufacturers Association. A reanalysis of lots manufactured by PMA members, which the FDA survey contended was defective, revealed gross inaccuracies in the original study. According to the PMA, 102 products were reanalyzed, and of these the firms found that eighty-four were satisfactory. In other words, only eighteen of the original 102 that FDA found to be outside the acceptable potency limits were, on reanalysis, also found to be so.[3]

According to Dr. Goddard, at the time of his report to the Senate Subcommittee, thirty-eight manufacturers requested additional information, and in sixteen instances the manufacturer reported different results within the acceptable potency range. In six samples involving five firms, the FDA concluded that the original findings were in error. In three of these samples involving two firms, the FDA had incorrectly tabulated the NDA potency limits. In the remaining three samples, the FDA had not followed the prescribed methodology.

The reports of errors, some of which were acknowledged by the FDA, throw doubt on the validity of the study.[4] Hence, we cannot conclude that this study reveals inadequate quality assurance either by the industry or the FDA. The inadequacy of the study itself, of course, suggests that FDA's procedures for testing potency have been unreliable.

THE STEERS STUDY. The FDA set up the test program of the National Center for Drug Analysis in 1967 as part of its effort to ensure effective and safe drugs. Prior to that, FDA district laboratories analyzed as many as 30,000 drug samples per year, but since many of them were collected only as problems arose, the samples did not provide statistically reliable data on the quality of drugs available in the market. The plan was to provide information on selected categories of prescription drugs which were widely prescribed or therapeutically important and were produced by numerous manufacturers. The limiting factor was the capacity of the NCDA.

Steers reported that the NCDA employed forty-six staff members and the expansion plans call for 150 eventually. The drug monitoring branch which has actual responsibility for the assaying of the samples includes two laboratories, each with only about ten chemists or technicians.

The NCDA first undertook a program in which the samples were collected from retail pharmacists. This retail-based program did not ensure coverage of all products in the study; products with small sales were excluded.[5] In addition, the program could not cover drugs mailed for direct sales to physicians and those distributed to specialty hospitals and clinics. Many small manufacturers rely on direct selling by mail to doctors, since this method requires very little resources for promotion and distribution. The estimate of the proportion of defective drugs in the market may therefore have understated the true proportion owing to the exclusion of the products of small manufacturers.

Table 11-1 shows the summary of the results of the retail-based studies. Dr. Steers himself suggests that if more than 1 percent of the samples are defective, then it is a matter of some concern. The worst performers were reserpine, with 9.4 percent defective; oxytocics, with 5.9 percent; anticoagulants, 3.9 percent; nitroglycerin, 3.4 percent; and adrenocorticosteriods, 2.0 percent. According to Steers, most of the problems have to do with potency. Problems are most likely to arise when the ratio of the toxic to the inefficacious potency is low and the permissible range therefore may be too small for easy control by the manufacturer. Alternatively, problems arise because of special difficulties in manufacturing, as in connection with anticoagulants, cardiac glycosides, and nitroglycerine.

Steers's comments suggest that serious manufacturing problems are encoun-

TABLE 11-1
Summary of Retail-Based Studies

Study	Identification	Samples Analyzed	Defective Samples Number	Percent	Date Initiated	Date Terminated
001	Anticoagulants	1454	57	3.9	03 01 67	11 30 67
002	Tranquilizers	1411	5	0.4	03 01 67	11 02 67
003	Adrenocorticosteroids	2009	41	2.0	07 17 67	08 02 68
X07	Reserpine[a]	245	23	9.4	09 25 67	10 13 67
004	Hypoglycemics	997	1	0.1	12 01 67	05 24 68
005	Cardiac Glycosides	1677	23	1.4	01 15 68	10 29 68
006	Sulfonamides	1146	14	1.2	05 02 68	01 23 69
007	Amphetamines	1030	14	1.4	05 02 68	12 26 68
008	Barbiturates	1192	7	0.6	07 26 68	02 03 69
009	Antihistamines	926	4	0.4	08 01 68	01 31 69
010	Nitroglycerin	1343	45	3.4	08 01 68	03 11 69
799	Reserpine[a]	968	35	3.6	01 24 69	04 15 69
013	Oxytocics	188	11	5.9	03 01 69	04 18 69
014	Nonsteroid estrogens	1024	8	0.8	05 19 69	10 30 69
015	Thiazide diuretics	1161	14	1.2	03 01 69	09 03 69
016	Anticonvulsants	1087	6	0.5	04 15 69	10 30 69
017	Cardiac antiarrhythmics	973	3	0.3	04 01 69	09 03 69
018	Skeletal muscle relaxants	845	6	0.7	08 01 69	12 31 69
019	Skeletal muscle relaxants	816	3	0.4	08 01 69	12 31 69
020	Tuberculostatics	582	2	0.3	10 01 69	01 31 70

Source: Taken from Arthur W. Steers, "The Test Program of the National Center for Drug Analysis," in *Quality Control in the Pharmaceutical Industry,* ed. Murray S. Cooper (New York: Academic Press, 1972), vol. 2. p. 71.
[a]Samples collected at formulator.

tered in many plants. The high percentage of defectives among the anti-coagulants was the result of deficiencies in the manufacturing process and in the USP monograph providing the specifications. Because it is a low-dosage and unstable drug, nitroglycerin has an unusually wide USP potency limit. Nevertheless, the potency of different samples ranged all the way from 45.0 percent to 119.4 percent of declared potency, and twenty-one samples were outside the allowed limits. In addition, twenty-one of the samples (of the total of 1,343) failed to meet the test for weight variation.

Steers goes on to say that the USP monograph for nitroglycerin did not include the test for content uniformity. An individual tablet assay confirmed that there was excessive variation within individual lots. The range in one sample was 50.2 percent to 99.4 percent of declared potency.

In addition, the study found that samples of one firm's nitroglycerin tablets were manufactured over a period of as many as twelve years. A sample from another manufacturer was produced in 1953 and showed only 74.5 percent of declared potency. (The product has since been deleted from the manufacturer's line.)

The high level of defective samples in the original reserpine survey resulted in another survey being conducted after followup action by the FDA district offices. The latter survey showed a considerable improvement; the percentage of all samples which were defective fell from 9.4 percent to 2.6 percent.

The retail-based program was abandoned in favor of one based on formulators, or manufacturers, because the original program required substantial expenditures of inspection time, did not cover the output of all manufacturers, gave uneven coverage of lots, and problem areas were revealed only after distribution of the drug. The formulator-based program collected samples from formulators, branch warehouses, or major accounts.

Table 11-2 presents the results of the formulator-based studies reported by Steers. If we apply the same standard to these studies as Steers applied to retail-based studies, then of the fourteen studies shown in the table, nine showed excessive rates of defective products, and in these studies, as much as 2 percent or more of the batches analyzed were defective.

The percentage of batches which were found to be defective (25.9 percent) was especially startling in the case of digoxin (cardiac glycosides). As a result of this problem, the FDA advised all firms producing this drug that unreliable mixing methods were being used; the results indicated failure to perform individual tablet assays or the use of improper individual tablet assay methods. The FDA advised the firms to quarantine and discontinue distribution of all digoxin tablets for which they did not have total assurance of compliance with USP assay requirements. As a result of these problems, the FDA has subsequently required batch certification of digoxin and digitoxin before distribution, as with insulin and antibiotics.

THE RITTS REPORT. In May 1971 the FDA Ad Hoc Science Advisory Committee evaluated the performance of the Bureau of Drugs and made a report to the commissioner of FDA. The chairman of this committee was Dr. Roy E. Ritts, Professor of Microbiology and Immunology, of the Mayo Graduate School of Medicine, University of Minnesota.[6]

The committee concluded that the FDA was not adequately monitoring marketed drugs for uniform and accurate dosage forms, absence of contaminants, and disintegration characteristics of tablets or capsules. The report states that "data have been collected showing that an appreciable number of marketed drugs are substandard; selected studies have indicated about 25 percent for some drug groups."[7] According to the committee, the FDA's budget is inadequate for the purpose, and the methods of surveillance are too laborious.

FDA INTENSIFIED DRUG INSPECTION PROGRAM. In recognition of the inadequacy of its inspection program, in 1968 the FDA initiated what it called the Intensified Drug Inspection Program (IDIP), in which each of the selected plants was subjected to a detailed inspection of all aspects of its facilities and

TABLE 11-2
Summary of Formulator-Based Studies

Study	Identification	Batches Analyzed	Outside of Limits[a]		Subsamples Analyzed	Outside of Limits		Total Assays[b]	Date Initiated	Date Completed
			No.	Percent		No.	Percent			
222	Adrenocorticosteroids	348	18	5.2	2086	71	3.4	9404	12 04 69	08 21 70
223	Oxytocics	17	0	0.0	102	00	0.0	246	03 23 70	09 11 70
224	Adrenergics	142	3	2.1	823	16	1.9	1478	06 01 70	10 22 70
225	Major tranquilizers	24	0	0.0	144	00	0.0	800	09 14 70	02 03 71
226	Major tranquilizers	25	1	4.0	150	05	3.3	1072	08 17 70	02 03 71
227	Urinary antibacterials	42	1	2.4	252	06	2.4	1496	01 26 70	04 06 70
228	Androgenic hormones	133	7	5.3	798	14	1.8	3009	02 02 70	10 02 70
229	Diuretics	39	0	0.0	234	0	0.0	1200	12 10 70	06 11 71
230	CNS depressants	45	1	2.2	270	03	1.1	300	04 14 70	10 02 70
231	Antithyroids	31	0	0.0	190	00	0.0	1177	08 17 70	03 15 71
232	Cardiac glycosides	193	50	25.9	1158	235	20.3	16039	04 14 70	02 04 71
233	Coronary vasodilators	93	2	2.2	531	12	2.3	3329	04 23 70	11 05 70
234	Anticoagulants	43	0	0.0	258	00	0.0	1352	06 15 70	12 02 70
235	Antimalarials	92	4	4.3	547	18	3.3	4368	01 27 71	07 09 71

Source: Same as table 11-1, p. 74.
[a]Batches with one or more subsamples outside limits.
[b]Does not include disintegration, weight variation, and so on.

procedures by one or more inspectors over a prolonged period. Because of the costs of such inspections, only a small fraction of all plants were selected. The FDA reported to the House Appropriations Committee in 1972 that the program was intended to cover 323 manufacturers and associated commercial testing laboratories. The FDA selected larger plants for the program. At the time of the FDA report to the committee, 308 IDIPs had been completed. The IDIPs resulted in legal action being taken by the FDA against twenty of the firms, and thirty-one other firms had to give up the manufacture of prescription drugs because of their inability to comply with GMP regulations.[8] Taken together, these fifty-one firms constituted 17 percent of the total number of firms inspected. The proportion of firms in the industry as a whole which fail to comply is larger than 17 percent. The study sample contained a larger than proportional representation of large plants in the industry, and a greater proportion of large plants than of small plants in the sample was found to be in compliance. All or nearly all of the members of PMA, which represents large manufacturers, were included in the sample, and none of them were among these against whom action was taken or who were forced out of business.

The proportion of sales of drugs represented by firms which are not in compliance is unknown, but it is less than 5 percent, since PMA members account for 95 percent of sales and none of its members was found to be violating GMP regulations. Even this upper limit, however, represents an unacceptable risk, and in some types of drugs the share of sales accounted for by firms that are not complying with GMP regulations may be higher.

These studies by the FDA itself indicate that the resources of the agency and its inspection methods have been insufficient to provide adequate assurance of quality in the drug supplied.

DEFENSE PRE-AWARD SURVEYS OF MANUFACTURERS. Other evidence that the FDA fails to maintain adequate standards of quality in the supply of drugs has been advanced by the Defense Personnel Support Center, which purchases drugs for the armed services.[9] Despite the surveillance activities of the FDA, the DPSC has found it necessary to maintain its own staff of inspectors to check the conditions in plants of bidders for drug contracts prior to making awards. This procurement agency reports that a large proportion of bidders surveyed fail to qualify for awards because of poor quality control and poor housekeeping.

The DPSC does not survey all bidders; it surveys a potential contractor who has not previously supplied the item being procured when (a) there is some doubt as to the adequacy of quality control and housekeeping procedures; (b) there is a possible inadequacy of capacity of the prospective contractor; or (c) the item is to be furnished from a plant other than that of the bidder.

The results of the surveys suggest that a large number of plants fail to meet the DPSC quality assurance standards. In 1969 the DPSC conducted 149 pre-award surveys of domestic manufacturers, of which forty-eight resulted in disqualification of the potential contractor on the grounds of either poor quality control or poor housekeeping. Thus, thirty-two percent of all the surveys resulted in disqualifications. Since some plants were surveyed more than once, a smaller percentage of bidders was disqualified. A survey might be made when a bid was submitted for one specific product even though the bidder may have been surveyed previously for another product. For this reason, the observed percentage of surveys resulting in disqualification overstates the percentage of all drug producing plants which would not qualify.

Another source of overstatement is the fact that one of the criteria for the selection of a plant to be surveyed is the suspicion that the plant in question does not adequately meet the DPSC quality assurance standards. The effect of this bias in the selection of plants to be surveyed may be partly offset by the fact that surveys are made only when companies submit their plants for inspection by applying for contracts. Those companies whose plants are lacking in adequate quality control procedures are less likely to apply for contracts than are other companies. Nevertheless, the data suggest that the FDA surveillance and compliance procedures have permitted the continued operation of a large number of plants producing drugs which either lack satisfactory quality controls or maintain poor housekeeping.

Further evidence along the same lines was presented by Mr. Max Feinberg of the DPSC in 1972.[10] Mr. Feinberg reported that in 1971 the DPSC performed 138 pre-award surveys and that fifty-eight of these, or forty-two percent, resulted in disqualifications.

Senator Nelson has refused to accept the inference that consumers of drugs in the U.S. run a significant risk of inefficacy or toxicity. In a statement which was made on March 5, 1974, before the Senate Monopoly Subcommittee of the Small Business Committee, he pointed out that Mr. Feinberg had failed to report that the DPSC surveys only about 10 percent of its prospective contractors and that the DPSC does not inspect those suppliers who are expected to be able to perform satisfactorily. Accordingly, Senator Nelson said that the rejection rate of all prospective contractors is 4.5 percent, rather than 45 percent as suggested by Mr. Feinberg's estimate.[11] In addition, Senator Nelson presented statements by the FDA which suggested that the violations of good manufacturing practices found by the DPSC were trivial.

It may well be that Mr. Feinberg's evidence exaggerates the risk of poor quality of generic drugs sold in the U.S. Nevertheless, even when appropriate corrections are made, it still appears that there is an excessive number of products on the market which fail to meet reasonable standards of quality. Even though the fraction of all potential contractors who are inspected is only 10 percent, those failing to qualify constitute a significant fraction of the total population of potential contractors. The criteria used by the DPSC in determining which plants it will survey suggest that most of those chosen are plants producing generic products, and that most of these plants are small. (We will postpone consideration of the question of the effect of size of plant on risk of poor quality until later.) Accordingly, the data indicate that the risk of poor quality from the purchase of generic products exceeds the 4.5 percent figure. We cannot estimate the risk more accurately, but it does appear to be substantial.

On Senator Nelson's other point, it is difficult to know whether DPSC's standards are unreasonable and result in trivial grounds for rejection. One would have to go through the records of the DPSC in order to come to some conclusion on this matter. In the absence of other evidence, however, there is no reason to suppose that the DPSC standards are excessively high. Moreover, the agency is under some pressure by Senator Nelson, among others, to accept potential contractors who are small, and there is probably little or no pressure in the opposite direction. One must not forget that these discussions took place at hearings of a subcommittee of the Senate Committee on Small Business.

GAO EVALUATION OF FDA COMPLIANCE PROGRAM. A recent (1973) report by the General Accounting Office provides an evaluation of the FDA's performance in enforcing compliance with good manufacturing practices in the drug industry.[12] The GAO report indicates that the problem of inspection of the drug industry is enormous and that the FDA's budget for this purpose is probably inadequate. According to the GAO, the FDA has the task of inspecting each of 6,400 drug producers (see chapter 10, note 8) at least once every two years. The inspections are required to determine whether sound methods and adequate facilities and controls are used in all phases of drug manufacture and distribution. The inspections cover equipment, finished and unfinished materials, containers, manufacturing records, and laboratory controls. Further, the FDA devoted only about $5 million to the inspection of drug producers, an amount clearly too small for the inspection of over six thousand establishments.

The GAO based its evaluation of FDA's performance on the inspection and enforcement program in three FDA districts in which 1,300 drug producers were located. One of the major questions dealt with in the evaluation was whether or not FDA had inspected all the drug producers at least once in two years, as required by the FD&C Act. The GAO found that at least 213, and perhaps as many as 336, had not been inspected during the two-year period, April 1969 through March 1971. The GAO report mentions that FDA officials acknowledged in May 1971 hearings before the Subcommittee on Intergovernmental Relations, House Committee on Government Operations, that 26 percent of registered pharmaceutical manufacturers were not inspected during the thirty-two-month period, July 31, 1968 through March 31, 1971.

The report attributes the failure to inspect producers to weaknesses in the inspection scheduling process, the priority given to reinspecting producers who had a history of deviating from GMP's, the diversion of manpower to crisis situations and headquarters-directed work, and the lack of available manpower.

The GAO randomly selected inspection records for seventy-four of the 213 producers who were not inspected during the preceding two year period in order to determine the size of the firm, kinds of products and past inspection history. Many of these producers manufactured nonprescription drugs. Nearly all of them were small producers. Thus, thirty-nine had annual sales of less than $10,000. Only five had annual sales of over $1,000,000. Previous inspections of these plants had found errors in labeling. Other deviations included failure to prepare control records, to establish production and control procedures, and to code finished products. There were also inadequate laboratory controls to insure that components and finished product conformed to appropriate standards of identity, strength, quality, and purity. Despite their poor history, these plants were among those which were not inspected in the two-year period of April 1969 to March 1971.

The lack of observance of GMP procedures is illustrated by the GAO in a report concerning one of the seventy-four uninspected producers—one which manufactures high-purity laboratory chemicals and solvents and, on special order, a drug for peptic ulcers, for which sales are estimated annually at $45,000. The inspection for June 1970 did not take place, nor did the inspection rescheduled for March 1971. The Defense Supply Agency inspected the producer in June 1971 and found inadequate control of raw materials and the possibility of contamination from other products in the manufacturing operations. Equipment was not routinely inspected and cleaned before and after each use, positive identification of material was not maintained during processing, the plant was not clean and orderly, and windows and doors in the plant were not screened to prevent the entrance of insects and other pests. The Defense Supply Agency notified the FDA of these findings by letter in July 1971, but by April 1972 the FDA had still not reinspected the producer.

The report also found that compliance with GMP by many of the drug producers which were inspected had not been enforced. During fiscal year 1971 the agency made 7,124 inspections, of which nearly 4,000 were follow-ups where deviations from GMP had previously been found. In 2,174 of the following inspections, the producers still were not complying with GMP.

On the whole, the GAO report concluded that the FDA failed to enforce adequately the regulations governing good manufacturing practices. The GAO attributed the failure to the inadequate budget of the FDA, but whatever the explanation, the GAO report does not permit the acceptance of the claim by the FDA that it provides adequate assurance of the quality of drugs.

DRUG BIOEQUIVALENCE STUDY PANEL. The most important of the studies concerning the state of manufacturing practice in the industry appeared as recently as July 1974. This study was prompted by the concern over drug bioequivalency aroused by the prospect of enactment of the Weinberger, or Maximum Allowable Cost (MAC), proposal for new regulations covering the reimbursement of drug costs. These regulations, which have since been enacted, imply that generic drugs are satisfactorily substitutable for each other and for brand-name drugs. The choice of drug should therefore be made solely on consideration of comparative prices. This makes sense only if generic equivalence is accepted as providing therapeutic equivalence.[13] The report of the Drug Bioequivalence Study Panel was addressed to the general question of bioequivalency, which includes the question of differences in the bioavailability of drugs which, although generically equivalent, differ in their efficacy or in their safety because of differences in the choice of excipients, manufacturing processes, and in standards of quality control. The report also appraised the enforcement of good manufacturing practice by the FDA.

In general, Senator Nelson and others who maintain that the FDA provides adequate assurance of good quality rely on evidence of conformity to USP or NF standards, which together can be referred to as compendial standards. Much of the discussion of drug quality assumes the adequacy of these standards. However, the report finds that in many instances the compendial standards contained in the USP and NF are "inaccurate, insensitive and nondiscriminating." In particular, the compendial tests for identity, purity, and potency which form the legal basis for the determination of compliance with FDA regulations are inadequate. The deficiencies are traced to the reliance of the compendia on tests which are so simple that they can be performed in retail establishments by pharmacists who do not have the required instrumentation or analytical skill to perform more sensitive assays. The standards remain inadequate despite the fact that physical tests and assay procedures have been developed which are of much greater sensitivity.

The report also attributes the backwardness of the compendial standards to the fact that there are insufficient funds to support the scientific staffs needed by the USP and the NF to examine suspected problems. In addition, revisions are too infrequent to keep up with technological changes. Partly for these reasons, FDA guidelines for good manufacturing practice, which are based primarily on compendial standards, lack precision and are subject to different interpretations.

The report is also critical of the compendia for not specifying standards or tests for certain excipients and so permitting manufacturers to set their own standards. The absence of such standards can lead to variation in the therapeutic properties of drugs.

One of the more important issues in the field of the regulation of the quality of manufacturing of drugs is the question of the possibility of controlling quality through final-product tests only. The FDA bases its enforcement of quality standards on tests of final products specified by the official compendia, which the FDA and the organizations responsible for the compendia have long defended. Spokesmen for some larger pharmaceutical manufacturers, on the other hand, have stated at Congressional hearings that final-product tests alone are inadequate. Quality tests, according to these spokesmen, must be part of a total quality assurance program which includes many raw-material and in-process tests, approved manufacturing procedures, and other final-product tests, which are not required by the official compendia. This issue has arisen as a result of the suggestion by the large companies that consumers of generic drugs whose source is not known to prescribers risk poor quality even though the products may meet compendial standards. Representatives of the FDA and of the organizations responsible for the compendia have maintained, on the contrary, that the risk is small, especially in relation to products which are certified. The study panel's conclusions concerning the deficiencies in the compendial standards therefore are particularly important.

The study panel maintains that the compendial monographs are deficient in not describing the processes of manufacture. Hence the report suggests that the official tests are inadequate for the control of quality because they do not assure the exclusion of substances which they cannot detect. In addition, the results of the disintegration and dissolution tests are unsuitable for use in the control of manufacturing. The dissolution tests may produce different results depending on the choice of equipment or dissolution medium, which are not specified. The monographs, according to the report, should specify the precompression mixture as a means of assuring content uniformity and dissolution properties, but they fail to include such specifications.

One of the more surprising deficiencies in the compendia is in the rules for the acceptance of batches after sampling. The probability of a batch with a high proportion of defectives being accepted is unacceptably high. According to the report, batches of which 20 percent are defective with respect to the disintegration standards would pass the specified test as frequently as 39 percent of the time; a batch with 20 percent defective units with respect to the dissolution test will be accepted 58 percent of the time; a batch having 25 percent defective units with respect to content uniformity will be accepted 25 percent of the time.

The description of FDA standards by the study panel indicates that the consumers of brand-name products on the whole receive more protection than the consumers of generic products. Most brand-name products are original products, and their manufacturing processes and methods of quality control must conform to the specifications of the NDA governing their production. The NDA is prepared by the original manufacturer but must be approved by the FDA prior to marketing, and unlike the corresponding USP or NF monograph, it specifies details of the production process. The manufacturer of a generic product and of other duplicate products which are sold under brand names receives approval of an Abbreviated New Drug Application (ANDA), which specifies only the official compendial standards for controlling the quality of the final products. The raw materials can be used after an identity test by the supplier of the raw materials. Excipients which are not covered in a compendia do not have to meet any specifications at all.

Even if the FDA's standards, tests, and sampling procedures were satisfactory, it still would not provide adequate quality assurance to consumers owing to its inadequate inspection program. According to the study panel, the National Center for Drug Analysis of the FDA can test only a few thousand batches of drugs per year, which is inadequate for 800 plants (the panel's estimate) and the large number of products. The panel also states that the plant inspection program is inadequate, and, in view of the large number of plants and products, it doubts whether the present system of inspection can establish assurance of quality. Furthermore, in those regions where there are too few plants to justify full-time inspectors for pharmaceutical plants, the inspectors also inspect food plants. In addition, in the panel's opinion, the training of FDA inspectors is inadequate for pharmaceutical work. Moreover, the report is pessimistic about the FDA's ability to provide quality assurance within the present limits on its budget.

The recommendations of the report stress the need for specifying standards for materials and manufacturing processes in addition to those required for final products. The report recommends certain types of tests for bulk active ingredients and suggests the specification of particle size, crystalline form, compressibility, and rate of dissolution. Such tests may be important when changes in processes or starting materials are made, and they are particularly useful for insoluble active ingredients, because of the difficulty of applying dissolution tests to the final products.

The report recommends that dissolution tests be included in the specifications of final products. The tests should be specific to the particular drug and should take into account possible interactions with gastrointestinal fluids. The apparatus currently in use is not readily adaptable to such changes of solvent. Because regulations for the certification of antibiotics do not presently include dissolution tests, problems of bioavailability of certain antibiotics may have been due to the absence of standards of dissolution.

Concerning statistical procedures, the report recommends certain changes directed to the detection of batches containing a high proportion of defective products. It advises changes in sample sizes, in the use of sequential sampling, and in inspection procedure, and recommends that acceptance or rejection should be based on the totality of tests and on all important characteristics rather than on the basis of individual tests.

A basic general recommendation of great importance would require individualized specifications for each manufacturer as well as for each product, rather than (as now is the case for generic products) standards which are set only with respect to products. The panel states that such individualization for manufacturers is required by differences in manufacturing processes and excipients among plants. The quality assurance program would be designed by the manufacturer and approved by the FDA. The plan would take into account the individual features of the plant rather than follow a standard format, and it would be modified with changes in technology or whenever it was otherwise appropriate.

More frequent inspection of plants by the FDA is also urged. It suggests that the FDA should have the authority to obtain companies' records for the determination of compliance. The greater inspection burden which would result would require substantial increases in the number and in the capability of inspectors.

The report's recommendation of individual standards which would be designed by the manufacturers themselves is perhaps the most significant. The agency's role in the provision of quality assurance would be limited to approving and enforcing these standards, but the change would place greater demands on the inspection staff, for it would require that inspectors enforce individualized rather than standard regulations. Each plant would be regarded as a separate problem. In addition, it would require the FDA to work with individual manufacturers to develop new tests and standards to keep pace with changes in technology. For the program to be at all feasible, the changes would require that the FDA and the industry work together in a cooperative manner rather than as adversaries.

The report's comment on the need for revisions in standards as technology changes provides a partial explanation of the lack of precision in the description of GMP on which the FDA bases its regulation. Other difficulties for regulatory and enforcement activities are raised by the fact that there is more than one way to assure quality even under the best current technology. The description of GMP is open to different interpretations, and unless the violation is very obvious, little can be done to enforce the regulations. The study panel's proposal to individualize standards is intended to deal with this problem.

We have seen that the report agrees with representatives of the large firms who have insisted that to assure high quality in the manufacture of drugs, plants must maintain close control throughout the manufacturing process and intermediate products must be inspected; the assurance of high quality cannot depend on final-product testing alone.

Implicitly, the report suggests that an adequate quality assurance program requires the limitation of output to larger firms, since small firms do not have the resources to maintain control over all stages of production and to design their own quality controls. We do not have enough information to be able to estimate the cut-off point, which may vary among products. But clearly the preparation of plans for quality assurance and the numerous intermediate tests which would be required by the report's recommendation would be difficult for small firms to support.

THE RELATIVE PERFORMANCE OF LARGE AND SMALL FIRMS

The earlier discussion of size of firm in relation to quality control suggested that the quality of drugs produced by large firms would be better than that of small firms. Following our own analysis of data on recalls, we shall review some studies related to firm size and quality control.

ANALYSIS OF RECALLS BY SIZE OF FIRM 1973. Table 11-3 reports the results of an analysis of recalls in 1973, as listed in the FDC reports (the "Pink Sheets").[14] For purposes of the analysis, firms were divided into three group sizes: over $50 million in sales, $5–$50 million in sales, and less than $5 million in sales. The measure of performance is the ratio of the number of recalls in a size class to millions of dollars of sales in that class. This is the measure of the relative risk of poor quality in drugs purchased from firms. According to this measure, the risk of poor quality when one buys a drug from a medium-sized firm is 3.7 times as large as the risk from a drug from a large firm (.0286 ÷ .0078). When one shifts from a large firm to one in the smallest size class, the risk goes up to nearly 28 times (.2153 ÷ .0078). The analysis confirms the hypothesis that the quality of drugs improves with the size of the manufacturer.

These figures overstate the relative riskiness associated with the use of drugs from smaller firms to the degree that individual recalls by large firms involve larger sales. Another possible source of bias is the relative frequency of inspection, but this is unlikely to be serious since most inspections appear to be the result of reports of defects by pharmacists or other troubles.

A possibly important bias toward overstating the risk of poor quality from the purchase of drugs of large firms arises from voluntary recalls. Many recalls are voluntary in the sense that the manufacturer discovers a product defect and initiates a recall, rather than ignoring it in the hope that the FDA will fail to become aware of it. The data do not distinguish voluntary from FDA-initiated recalls, since officially nearly all recalls are "voluntary" even when they are the result of FDA's surveillance activities. But if our theory is correct about the relative importance to large firms of the maintenance of good quality, then the bias in the data resulting from voluntary recalls is unfavorable to the hypothesis that the quality of drugs produced by large firms is better than that of small firms.

We will consider the relative outputs involved in individual recalls by large and medium-size firms first. If the problem involves several products rather than

TABLE 11-3
Number of Drug Recalls per Million Dollars in
Sales by Size of Firm, 1973

Firm Size Class ($ million)	Number of Recalls	Total Sales ($ million)	Number of Recalls (per Sales in $ million)
Less than $5	59	274	.2153
$5–$50	21	735	.0286
$50+	32	4,097	.0078

Source: FDC Reports—"The Pink Sheet": Drugs and Cosmetics, F.D.C. Reports, Inc. Washington, D.C., (weekly), 1973.
Note: List excludes vitamins, drugs removed as a result of withdrawal of NDA, or of class action.

a single product, it will show up as several recalls. A recall usually involves only one batch of a product, so we shall ignore the possibility that a recall involves more than a single batch of any product. We have estimated on the basis of data on recalls that the risk of a consumer purchasing a drug of poor quality from a medium-size firm is 3.7 times as large as from a large firm. This risk may be offset by a difference in the size of batch: if the average batch of a large manufacturer is 3.7 times larger then the average batch of a medium-size manufacturer, then there will be no difference in risk. That this is quite possible is suggested by the large range of blender capacity; the larger blenders are ten times the size of the smallest. We have seen that blender capacity is an upper limit to batch size.[15] Consequently, the comparison of recalls of products of the larger firms with those of medium-size firms is inconclusive with respect to the relative risk of poor quality.

The comparison of the largest firms with the smallest firms is more decisive. The average batch in the largest firm-size group is unlikely to be as much as 27.6 times as large as in the smallest firm-size group, since the largest blenders are not 27.6 times as large as the smallest blenders. The formula for economic order quantity suggests that batches in the largest firms will be more than 27.6 times as large as those in the smallest firms when the sales of the product are more than 761 times as large. Since the sales of individual firms in the smallest size class frequently can be measured in the tens of thousands of dollars, this is quite possible. But the range of blender sizes then is the determining factor.

Another comparison can be made between the size classes of firms described in table 11-3. It was suggested earlier than we could expect small firms in this industry to require a larger fraction of the total resources devoted to surveillance and compliance activities by the FDA than was warranted by their proportion of total sales. We see that this has been the case. The largest firms account for as much as 80.2 percent of total sales, but their percentage of total recalls in 1973 was only 28.6 percent. Since recalls indicate problems with quality control and the FDA assigns its inspectors and other personnel involved in enforcement activities to deal with problems as they are reported, it is evident that the largest firms utilize a much smaller proportion of the FDA's resources than their share of total sales warrants. Medium-size firms evidently utilize a somewhat larger proportion of total FDA resources than would be warranted by their sales. A more striking lack of balance is observed for the smallest firms. Although they only account for 5.4 percent of total sales, their share of recalls is as much as 50.7 percent. This large percentage of recalls suggests that a disproportionally large fraction of FDA's resources was devoted to the surveillance of the quality of product of the smallest firms.

DEFENSE PRE-AWARD SURVEYS. We have already referred to the analysis of 149 defense pre-award surveys. An analysis of the results by size of firm which Mr. Ahart provided in his testimony to the Nelson subcommittee[16] shows that proportionally more small firms failed to observe GMP than large firms. A total of thirty-nine of ninety surveys of small firms, or 43 percent, resulted in disqualifications on GMP grounds. By contrast, only 15 percent of surveys of large firms resulted in disqualifications on these grounds (nine disqualifications on GMP grounds out of fifty-nine surveys).

The only objection which might be raised against the validity of these results is that inspectors may have been biased against small firms and therefore disqualified them when similar deviations of a minor character in large firms would not have resulted in disqualification. There is no evidence for the existence of this bias. It is improbable because, as we have already mentioned, the political pressures are in favor of making awards to small business. Colonel A. J. Snyder, the Chief of the Medical Procurement Division of the Directorate of Procurement and Production of the DPSC testified directly on this matter, and he said that the agency seeks to give small business a certain percentage of total purchases, but that it is very difficult to reach this percentage in drugs despite a great deal of time and effort. He attributed the difficulty to the nature of the industry and particularly to the difficulty which a small firm has in supporting a substantial staff for quality control.[17]

The percentage of surveys of small firms resulting in disqualification on GMP grounds, in fact, understates the extent to which small firms generally would be found to be in compliance with DPSC requirements. The percentage of disqualifications would have been higher if the definition of small business did not include many firms which are large when compared to the average size of firm in this industry, even though they may be small by the standards of other industries. Thus, the DPSC defines a small firm as one which has fewer than 750 employees. As table 1-3 shows, a plant that has 500 employees is above the 95th percentile in the size distribution of plants in the drug industry. In addition, the DPSC concentrated its purchases of drugs from small firms among those at the upper end of the small-firm size range. The bulk of sales of such drugs by so-called smaller firms were by A. H. Robins, Travenol (part of Baxter Laboratories), William Rorer, Chase, Strong-Cobb-Arner, and McGaw, which together accounted for 79 percent of the total sales of combination drugs by smaller companies.[18] By the standards of the drug industry, the first three of these six companies are large companies. The DPSC thus minimized the risk of poor quality by favoring the larger of the "small" companies. Further, and more to the point, the percentage of surveys resulting in disqualifications understates the proportion of small companies in the industry which would fail to meet DPSC standards because the surveys presumably also were concentrated in the upper range of sizes among "small" companies. A more representative sample would have resulted in a higher rate of disqualification.

INTENSIFIED DRUG INSPECTION PROGRAM. We have already discussed the results of the IDIP in relation to the performance of the FDA in assuring the quality of drugs produced by the industry as a whole. These results are amenable to analysis by size of firm as well. We can assume that the program resulted in the inspection of plants of all or of nearly all PMA members, since one of the criteria for selection was size of plant, and PMA includes the firms with the larger plants. At the time of the report by the FDA to the House Appropriations Committee, 308 IDIP's had been completed, and fifty-one of these had resulted in legal action or in the firm going out of business. If 100 of PMA's approximately 110 members had plants inspected under the program, then 208 other plants were also inspected. Thus we can say that a measure of the performance of smaller firms is provided by the proportion of this number constituted by the 51 which the FDA found in default—that is, 25 percent; and this can be compared to 0 percent for the larger or PMA firms.[19] The performance of large plants was much better than that of small plants.

GUMBHIR SURVEY OF PHARMACISTS. In 1972 Dr. Ashok Gumbhir of the College of Pharmacy, Ohio State University, surveyed pharmacists on the quality of generic and brand name drugs.[20] One of the questions simply asked pharmacists to compare the quality of brand-drugs as a group with that of generics. Of the responding pharmacists, 73.3 percent judged the quality of brand-name drugs to be superior. This judgment was backed up by the responses to a question which related specifically to observable quality differences traceable to the extent of compliance with GMP. The question asked about the frequency of broken or chipped tablets, tablets of unequal size, open capsules, and so forth. As many as 85 percent of the pharmacists reported that they rarely or never had any bad experiences of this type with brand-name drugs. The same report was given by 50 percent of pharmacists for generic drugs. Apparently, the frequency of defective products among generic drugs is relatively greater than among brand name drugs.

Other responses were consistent with these results. Apparently the quality of brand-name drugs was high regardless of price, for only 17 percent of pharmacists said that the quality of such drugs was related to price. The same thing apparently was not true of generic drugs, for 73 percent said that among such drugs quality did increase with price. Along the same lines, most pharmacists did not require the assurance of the reputation of the manufacturer for brand-name drugs, but it was of utmost importance for a majority in relation to generic products: only 20 percent said that the manufacturers' reputation was important in their decision to purchase brand-name products compared to 57 percent for generic products.

The emphasis in the questions was on what is called pharmaceutical elegance, which refers to the physical appearance of drugs. The responses to the open-ended question concerning quality probably also emphasized pharmaceutical elegance, since this is what pharmacists can observe directly. They are less likely to learn about the more important properties of efficacy and safety. This consideration diminishes the significance of the Gumbhir Survey. Nevertheless, the results are consistent with what we expect and thus serve as additional confirmation of the general validity of our theory.

THE FITELSON LABORATORIES STUDY. The discussion of the relative performance of large and small firms up to this point has depended on studies of plant inspection, of drug recalls, and a survey of pharmacists. The remainder of the discussion concerns studies of tests of final products. The Fitelson Laboratories, an independent testing laboratory, studied three products for the *Medical Letter*. The products were meprobamate, prednisone, and the antihistamine known as chlorpheniramine maleate.[21]

The laboratory tested twenty samples of tablets from twenty different manufacturers of the antihistamine product and applied USP standards. The required tests concerned the identity of the drug, disintegration time, weight per tablet, and a chemical assay test. All of the twenty samples met USP standards.

The same tests were applied to the meprobamate products of nineteen different manufacturers. Again, all of the samples fulfilled the specifications of the USP.

Since prednisone is a particularly potent drug, the USP requires the four tests listed earlier and two additional ones: a chemical assay to determine the amount of foreign steroids present in the drug and a test of the uniformity of the content of each tablet. The Fitelson Laboratories found that all twenty-two manufacturers of prednisone met the USP standards.

These results indicate that the risk of poor quality is negligible regardless of source in the purchase of three drugs tested. The results of the Fitelson Laboratories study thus contradict the results of the other studies which we have examined. As has already been suggested, the difference may be due to the fact that this study depended only on tests of final products rather than on plant inspections or on drug recalls.

RESERPINE STUDY. Ciba manufactures Serpasil, which is the leading brand of reserpine. The company commissioned Hazelton Laboratory to buy as many generic reserpine products in the market as they could, as well as its own brand and the brands manufactured by Upjohn, Lilly, Squibb, and Wyeth, and to perform the tests specified by the USP. The Hazelton Laboratory purchased seventy-seven samples of the products of sixty-nine manufacturers. It reported that seventeen of the samples failed to meet USP standards. All six of Ciba's own products met the USP standards. Ciba did not ask the Hazelton Laboratory to decode the products of other manufacturers, so it could not report on the performance of manufacturers of other brands.

Mr. Charles T. Silloway, the president of Ciba, who reported the results to the Nelson subcommittee stated that he believed that the other large manufacturers' products probably met the USP standards and that all of the defective samples came from the small manufacturers of generics. In support of this interpretation, Mr. Silloway said that the main problem in the manufacture of this product was the maintenance of uniformity in reserpine content among tablets, because it constitutes a small percentage of the total content of the tablet. The quarter-milligram strength tablet has one part in 600 of the active material; the one-tenth-milligram strength tablet has one part in 1,500 of the active material. To disperse evenly a tiny amount of active ingredient through millions of tablets is difficult and requires sophisticated techniques. A company which produces reserpine in small quantities, and this only occasionally, is likely to have variation in the content among tablets and even among lots.[22] These results suggest that the quality of generic reserpine products which come from small companies could well be unreliable.

CONJUGATED ESTROGEN TABLETS. Ayerst Laboratories analyzed twenty-three samples of conjugated estrogen tablets manufactured by eighteen manufacturers, not including Ayerst itself. The purpose of the study was to determine whether the manufacturers of generic estrogen tablets met compendial standards, as is generally assumed by people recommending generic prescribing. The results were that 61 percent of the samples tested were below the minimum potency specified by USP; 96 percent were outside the specified limits for sodium estrone sulphate; 100 percent failed identity test B.[23] Dr. Cavallito, who reported the results, did not say so, but presumably Ayerst, which manufactures the leading brand, succeeds in meeting the standard, and this assumption was not challenged by Senator Nelson and other critics of leading firms who heard the testimony.

When, in the course of the testimony reporting these results, Senator Kennedy asked Commissioner Schmidt of the FDA questions directly concerning products which do not meet USP standards, the commissioner stated that he was not surprised to hear about drugs not meeting USP standards, in view of the number of firms engaged in the production of drugs and the complexities of manufacturing.[24] This evidence also suggests that the quality of drugs produced by small generic manufacturers is probably unreliable.

FDA POTENCY STUDY. The FDA potency study of 1966, which was referred to earlier, found that of the samples of brand name products, 8.2 percent were outside acceptable potency limits, compared to 7.7 percent for generic products. These results have been frequently quoted to deny the generalization that brands are superior to generic products.

As the previous discussion of this study indicated, serious questions have been raised about the validity of the results. We cannot therefore accept the validity of the study with respect to the relative performance of brand and generic products.

DIGOXIN. In 1972 Dr. Simmons broke down the results of the NCDA study of digoxin by brand-name (Lanoxin) and generic products.[25] No defectives were found for the major manufacturer (Burroughs Wellcome), which, according to Dr. Simmons, accounted for 86 percent of the market; in contrast, there was a 37 percent rate of defectives for the remaining manufacturers.[26] Again, we see evidence of relatively poor quality associated with small manufacturers.

VETERANS' ADMINISTRATION. The Veterans' Administration has the products of new contractors tested by the FDA. A compilation of the reports for 784 tests in 1970 shows a total twenty-nine of rejections, representing 3.7 percent. None of the 254 tests of brand name products resulted in rejections. All rejections were of generic products, which represented 530 tests.[27] The conclusion thus is similar to that reached in connection with most of the other studies.

DISCUSSION

The review of studies dealing with the relative quality performance of large and small firms leads to the striking observation that those studies which are based on laboratory tests of final products yield mixed results, while the others which rely on the analyses of drug recalls, results of plant inspections, and the survey of pharmacists' judgments are uniformly unfavorable to small firms. (For the present purpose, brands are considered the products of large firms and generics of small firms.) Although the results of most of the studies which depended on final-product tests were unfavorable to small firms, one study, that of the Fitelson Laboratories, found no difference between large and small firms. All samples passed the tests. This one study is responsible for the conclusion that the results of final-product tests are mixed.

Why this difference between the two sets of results? The studies of drug recalls and of plant inspections reveal risks of poor quality which studies based on laboratory tests of samples are likely to miss. The frequency of mislabelling, broken tablets, open capsules, and other product defects does not appear to be so large as to have been discovered by the small samples taken from retailers for the Fitelson study. Further laboratory tests of final products are not designed to discover unspecified foreign contaminants, so the products of plants which do not maintain good housekeeping will pass laboratory tests even though they may have become contaminated.

In addition, as the Bioequivalence Study concluded, the USP and NF tests are not sufficiently sensitive to detect certain kinds of defects. These can be discovered only by tests performed during the manufacturing process. The report also pointed out that the probability of a defective batch passing the prescribed tests was unacceptably high under the USP and NF sampling procedures.

The results of the studies based on laboratory tests are also mixed because of the differences in the difficulty of manufacturing different products. The Fitelson study turned up results which appeared to indicate that generic products were no worse than brand-name products; but apparently the three products covered by the study were not very difficult to manufacture. The studies dealing with reserpine, digoxin, and estrogen tablets were very unfavorable to generic products. Apparently it is difficult to maintain the potency of reserpine and digoxin within the acceptable range, and the manufacture of the ingredients of estrogen tablets appears to be no easy problem. The similar results of the Veterans' Administration study may be also due to the difficulty of manufacturing some products. It is unlike the Fitelson study in that it is not restricted to just three products, and the list may have included some that were difficult to manufacture.

The evidence of the relative quality performance of large and small firms confirms the earlier arguments that there are economies of scale in the control of quality and that large firms have a greater incentive to invest in such control. Moreover, it supports the view that the FDA cannot be depended on to provide such assurance for small firms.

The weight of the evidence thus conclusively supports the earlier theoretical conclusion that the quality of drugs will increase with size of firm. The different studies are not unanimous, and we have tried to account for the differences, but there is no question concerning the thrust of the evidence. Consumers do risk purchasing a poor quality drug when they purchase a generic drug of which the source is unknown. The FDA program of surveillance of GMP is inadequate, and prescribers and the public are misled if they think that they can rely on this program to guarantee quality in the drugs they purchase.

Drug consumers cannot depend on the FDA to provide a guarantee of the quality of drugs based on tests of finished products. For at least some products the standards are inadequate and the tests are insensitive. The FDA must rely on the inspection of plants as well as on final-product tests.

Even inspection by the FDA, however, cannot provide adequate quality assurance unless manufacturers follow manufacturing procedures designed with the goal of maintaining a high level of quality and apply numerous tests of raw and in-process materials as well as of final products. Such extensive quality assurance programs by manufacturers are a condition of adequate quality assurance.

Firms should therefore be required by FDA regulations to submit individual plans for manufacturing procedures and for tests of each of their products for approval before they can initiate production or continue the production of drugs. The FDA would approve or disapprove such plans. In addition, the FDA should inspect plants with sufficient frequency to ensure that firms are in compliance. Firms would be free to change the plans as the need arises subject to approval by the FDA. This proposal is the same as the one advanced by the Drug Bioequivalence Study Panel.

Small firms are unlikely to be able to develop adequate quality assurance programs, since they do not have the required resources to undertake them. Policymakers who are concerned with the problem of the quality of drugs must therefore be prepared to accept the elimination of small firms from the industry as a result of regulations which are intended to provide quality assurance. The elimination of small firms will not reduce significantly the extent of competition, because such firms do not compete with the larger firms in the supply of quality-assured products. They compete by offering drugs, the quality of which is doubtful, at low prices. In any case, the number of firms which would survive would be large.

We do not recommend that government regulation be abandoned and that the market be left to regulate the quality of drugs. The market does provide incentives to the largest firms to maintain high-quality products, but it cannot be depended on to work perfectly, and the pharmaceutical market presents a special problem. Physicians frequently find it difficult to know the source of the lack of efficacy of a drug; the patient's condition rather than a defect in the drug may be responsible. Similarly, what may appear to be a side effect may come from other sources. The collection and distribution of information about the effects of individual drugs by a drug monitoring agency can improve the working of the market in this respect, but it may be very difficult to interpret data on effects of drugs, even with the assistance of detailed studies. In addition, not even all of the large firms will always adhere strictly to a quality assurance program. Various pressures—perhaps including those arising from expansion and the consequent failure of a quality control organization to keep pace and also the resulting limits of plant space—may lead to product defects. A regulatory authority therefore can serve a useful function in the assurance of the quality of drugs.

Public policy should at the same time make use of the incentives provided by the market. From the standpoint of quality assurance, consumers would be better off than they are now if output were concentrated among a few firms and only promoted brand-name products were sold. If a company chooses to promote its own name and encourages physicians to specify its name along with a generic title on a prescription, then the consumer will receive equal protection whether a "branded" generic or a brand-name drug is purchased.

On the other hand, we cannot depend on the FDA or some other regulatory agency exclusively. Unless the industry has the required resources and incentives, the FDA cannot perform its task. Distrust of large firms has led their critics to call for greater reliance on the FDA as a guarantor of the quality of drugs in the industry including those of small firms. And the drive to reduce prices of drugs through the wider use of generic products has led to similar demands for greater governmental control over quality. The FDA itself has encouraged such demands, and at the same time (inconsistently) has claimed that its surveillance and enforcement activities provide adequate quality assurance. This claim is excessive. The FDA alone cannot provide the required assurance.

Just as there is risk associated with exclusive dependence on the market place as a regulator of quality, dependence on a government regulatory agency also has its risks. An agency's regulation may be nominal rather than effective because the regulation may be poorly conceived and misguided. The proper tools may not be available for regulation without the cooperation of the industry and in the absence of specific manufacturing and quality-control procedures. To depend on the FDA to provide the equivalent of a *Good Housekeeping* seal of approval on the basis of finished-product tests overrates the available tests. In addition, the agency may not develop an effective plan because the assurance of quality is not its sole objective. Among other things, it seeks its own survival, which is at the mercy of members of Congressional committees and other Congressmen, who are acutely sensitive to the related political issue of Big Business vs. Small Business. Those members of Congress who have been interested in the drug industry are hostile to the suggestion that the use of generic products entails risks of poor quality. They may also be hostile to new regulations intended to provide quality assurance which threaten the survival of small drug manufacturers.

We therefore cannot endorse the new MAC regulations which assume that the FDA provides adequate quality assurance for most multiple-source drugs. A minimum prerequisite to the enactment of any plans to encourage wider use of generic products is the adoption of better quality assurance programs by all potential suppliers of generic products.

Furthermore, to rely on the suppliers of generic products to provide quality assurance even with a stepped up FDA enforcement program is risky, since they lack the market incentives which may be necessary for adequate quality assurance. The threat of penalties resulting from FDA enforcement efforts alone may be an insufficient incentive. This threat in the past has not prevented firms from producing and selling drugs which violated the regulations, and to judge from comments by the GAO, such violations have been numerous. The threat of more severe penalties may, of course, improve performance. At the same time, however, the requirement that companies develop detailed plans in cooperation with the FDA is likely to complicate enforcement, for the FDA may then be held accountable for the plans along with the firms. The incentives which firms have to maintain high quality are compromised when they are shared with a government agency. The FDA itself may be inclined to disown responsibility when it is shared with private firms. In short, we are forced to rely on market incentives as well as on FDA enforcement. It is not clear, however, that an increase in the FDA's responsibility for the development and enforcement of GMP regulations will improve the performance of the industry. The issues are sufficiently complex that we cannot be certain that larger resources devoted to surveillance and enforcement activities will result in better quality. In our view, an improvement is more likely to result from greater accountability for quality by manufacturers. Currently the manufacturers are liable for damages to patients resulting either from inefficacy of drugs or from side effects. The effectiveness of such liability suits in enforcing the observance of good manufacturing practices depends on the ability of plaintiffs to identify faulty drugs and to establish that manufacturers were negligent.

If we are to depend on market incentives, then, it becomes difficult to approve the marketing of unpromoted generic products which are not associated closely with the name of a company. In fact, unless a company is well known to doctors, its assurance is doubtful. Even well-known companies cannot be expected to have spotless records, but our confidence can increase with the reputation of a company. This conclusion may be distasteful to economists and others who would like to be able to purchase drugs much as grain mills buy wheat without regard to the identity of sellers, as in the model of perfect competition. But drugs are not wheat, and safety and efficacy demand that prescribers know the source of the drugs which their patients consume.[28]

CHAPTER 12

PRICE COMPETITION

INTRODUCTION

This chapter reports that in the 1960s and early 1970s major drug manufacturers of antibiotics engaged in active price competition. After patents of large-selling drugs expired, major manufacturers entered with competitive generic versions, offering them at lower prices, and the original producers cut their prices after suffering large losses in market shares. The pattern was not uniform among drug markets. In some cases entry and price competition took place before patents expired, and in other cases the original producers cut prices without waiting for entry. But the pattern which we have described appears to have been the general one in antibiotics markets, and the deviations were unimportant from the standpoint of the results for prices. Antibiotics became a jungle, with prices falling to levels which were well below those at the beginning of the 1960s. Price competition in other drug markets, where it was not as severe, is also described in this chapter.

The models of oligopolistic behavior which have influenced much of the discussion about competition in the drug industry have been wrong, at least when applied to this industry. Such models predict that oligopolists will collude to maintain prices and at the very least simply refrain from price competition. Obviously if they manage to maintain prices, they stand to earn higher profits than if they cut each other's prices. The appeal of the model's rationality is almost irresistible. A price cutter cannot expect to increase its share of the market in the face of certain retaliation by rivals. The only result will be a loss of profits both for itself and for other firms. This model is so persuasive that for many economists a high degree of concentration in a market is presumptive evidence of restraint on price competition. This is why the measurement of concentration ratios has become a major activity among economists engaged in industry studies. Yet, as we will see, the conditions of competition in the drug industry are more complex than the model anticipates, and there has been a great deal of price competition.

Walker[1] and others have suggested that the reluctance of drug manufacturers to cut prices is reinforced by the lack of interest of doctors in the differences in prices among drugs. Why cut prices if the number of prescriptions written for a brand is inelastic with respect to the price of the brand and with respect to the prices of other brands? Those who propose this reason for drug manufacturers refraining from price competition do not notice its inconsistency with the argument based on oligopolistic restraint arising from fear of retaliation. Oligopolists need not fear retaliation if buyers (in this case prescribers) are unaware of prices. The two arguments may be presented as alternative explanations of any observed reluctance to cut prices, but not as parts of the same explanation. In any case, the present chapter considers both arguments.

We will be concerned only with those drugs which have become multiple-source drugs. We will not attempt to assess the extent of price competition between drugs which are generically distinct and therefore are described usually as single-source drugs. Multiple-source drugs include all drugs for which the patents have expired, for invariably small manufacturers will imitate them. The technology of duplicating a drug is not difficult and does not require large quantities of capital. Nor does the FDA make large demands on the producers of duplicates for proof of safety and efficacy. Multiple-source drugs also include drugs which are produced by more than one manufacturer even though the patent has not expired. The patent holder may license others to produce and sell the drug, or it may not be able to enforce the patent against infringement. During the 1960s and early 1970s manufacturers of large-selling multiple-source drugs engaged in severe price competition, especially in antibiotics. We will analyze and describe this price competition. We do not wish to suggest that price competition is absent among manufacturers of single-source drugs. But the extent of such competition is more difficult to determine than that among the manufacturers of rival drugs within a generic class. And in general it is probably weaker, since closer substitutions can be made between drugs within the same generic class than can be made between drugs in two different generic classes, even though the latter may be within the same therapeutic class and thus offer similar therapy. The chemical differences between drugs, and their different generic titles, may be sufficient to prevent doctors from prescribing one rather than the other because of price differences. In addition, pharmacists are unlikely to use generically different drugs as substitutes for brands which are specified in prescriptions.

Let us return to the consideration of the oligopoly model of price competition. The wide divergence between the prediction of the model and the actual behavior of drug manufacturers suggests that the model ignores certain forces which promote price competition in drug markets. These forces are very powerful. A firm which cuts its price will do so for a single product and not for its entire range of products, and the sales of this product will represent a small share of its own total sales. The firm need only obtain a price which is barely above the marginal cost of production in order for the product to contribute to overhead costs. Furthermore, the new product with its reduced price will have a small share of the sales of its generic class, and it must compete against the original product which is familiar to doctors. The firm can expand the sales of this product, which is merely an imitation, only by cutting its price. It is the seller of the original brand which does not want to cut its price. Thus, we see that the interests of different sellers are not symmetrical, contrary to the assumptions of the model of oligopolistic behavior. It is this assymmetry which leads to price competition. The model of oligopoly is plausible only because it explicitly or implicitly assumes that oligopolists in each market have exactly the same interests. Occasionally, discussions of the model recognize that differences in market shares and in costs lead to disagreements among oligopolists and to price competition. The importance of such disagreements is never evaluated, and the popularity of the oligopoly model which predicts restraint on price competition suggests that such disagreements are viewed as rare. But there is no evidence to support this view. In any case, it is clear that in the drug industry the interests of sellers diverge greatly.

Thus, we must analyze the conditions in the drug industry which encourage price competition. The examination will cover the conditions of entry and the effects of entry on prices. We deal separately with the entry of small and of large firms, since the effects of small firms on prices are much less than those of large firms. As we will see, the original firm may not cut its own prices to match price cuts by small firms, even after it has lost a large share of the market, but price cuts by other large firms are another matter. The original firm generally does not maintain its own price in the face of price competition from other large competitors. We will analyze the decision of a large firm to imitate an established drug. We will see that it must forecast large sales to expect a reasonable return on investment. Thus, the large firms do not enter into the production of all drugs no longer protected by patents.

A very important and little-noticed aspect of competition in this industry is the relationship between the marginal cost of a drug and the fully allocated average cost. This characteristic of the industry induces price competition of the most disastrous kind. The effect of the excess of average over marginal cost is exacerbated by the differences between companies in the distribution of sales among products. Firms are induced to set prices which are below average cost when the product represents a small fraction of total sales, and overhead and other costs can be borne by other products. Their mutual interest in avoiding price competition thus is not sufficiently powerful to prevent large firms from cutting their prices.

The industry is beset by other conditions which promote price competition. Thus, despite assertions to the contrary, a large proportion of prescriptions of multiple-source drugs are generic. Such prescriptions open the door wide to price competition, for pharmacists can and do fill such prescriptions with low-price drugs. It makes no difference whether prescriptions for single-source drugs are written generically or by brand name, since there is only a single drug. Where it matters, doctors do write many generic prescriptions. Nor need all of them write such prescriptions for price competition to be effective. The elasticity of demand with respect to price may be high even when only a substantial fraction of prescriptions for a drug are written generically. Another factor which increases the price elasticity of demand for a product is the extent of brand substitution by pharmacists. The more pharmacists who substitute generic and other low-price drugs for those specified in prescriptions, the higher will be the price elasticity of demand. The extent of such substitution turns out to be surprisingly large. Doctors thus need not be aware of prices for manufacturers to feel the effects of competitors' price cuts on the sales of their products.

A description of price competition in antibiotics follows this analysis. Special attention is given to tetracycline, erythromycin, ampicillin, and penicillin VK. We will see that large firms entered these markets and cut prices despite the prospect of poor sales. We will also see that the Squibb Company was an especially aggressive price cutter.

The analysis of the decision to enter suggests that companies cannot expect entry to be profitable, especially if they must make deep price cuts, unless they forecast large sales. The entry of some of the firms into a large number of fields despite their knowledge of the small sales of previous entrants suggests that they were desperately seeking opportunities to increase sales. As a matter of fact, the most active firms were not among the leaders in the innovational race, so their hopes of profits from innovations were relatively dim.

Other therapeutic fields did not witness as vigorous price competition as the antibiotics for a variety of reasons. In some cases, the sales of a drug were too small to attract the entry of large firms following patent expiration. In other cases the drugs were old, and numerous small firms produced and sold them at prices which were low at the outset of the 1960s. In the case of some drugs, it is still too soon after the expiration of patents for the large firms which have entered to attract substantial sales, even at prices well below those of the market leaders. The price competition in antibiotics cannot be considered to be peculiar in any way, and as patents on more large-selling drugs expire, we can expect the price competition observed in the antibiotics to be repeated.

The analysis of price behavior which precedes the descriptions in this chapter attempts to construct some generalizations. These generalizations are not always accurate descriptions of the actual behavior. Thus, SmithKline, the original producer of chlorpromazine, cut its price before entry took place; Lederle refused to reduce the price of tetracycline before it had lost a large part of its sales; and there are other divergences. The generalizations thus are not good predictors of the details of actual behavior. But the generalizations provide a useful rough approximation of the behavior of major manufacturers. The differences in detail between the model which we have constructed and the actual behavior are unimportant for most purposes of the analysis of drug prices. And without an attempt at constructing some generalizations, it would be impossible to make any sense out of the behavior.

THE CONDITIONS OF COMPETITION

THE ENTRY OF SMALL FIRMS. When a patent on a drug expires, many companies will enter into the production and sale of the product, as table 12-1 shows. The table lists drugs on which the patents expired in the years 1966 and 1967, and the sales of each of these products in 1966. We can see that, despite the small sales of the original products, many companies entered.

Evidently, entry barriers for duplicates, unlike new chemical entities, are virtually nonexistent. The manufacture of a new chemical entity must meet the FDA's onerous demands for evidence of efficacy and safety. The approval of a duplicate drug, by contrast, is much easier to obtain. The Abbreviated New Drug Application must describe only the manufacturing procedures and chemical and physical tests of quality; clinical tests are required only occasionally.

Nor are entry costs large for the ANDA. The firm may already own a pharmaceutical plant, and usually it can purchase bulk ingredients. The machinery required for blending ingredients, tableting, encapsulating, coating, and bottling can be used for many different drugs, and a plant may have excess capacity. In addition, plant expansion is easily financed. The manufacture of a drug, in many cases, is not much more complicated than what used to be done by retail pharmacists, and the minimum requirements for quality control, as described by the FDA in its GMP regulations, can be met without large capital expenditures. Small firms thus can and do enter the industry.

TABLE 12-1
New Manufacturers in 1969 of Drugs on Which the Patents Expired in 1966 or 1967

Brand Name	Generic Name	Sales of Brand(s) in 1966 ($ million)	Number of New Companies in 1969
Dramamine	Dimenhydrinate	4.8	11
Chlortrimeton	Chlorpheniramine maleate	5.8	48
Hydrocortone Cortef	Hydrocortisone	2.1	69
Meticorten Deltasone	Prednisone	2.0	63

Sources: Number of new companies in 1969 based on a count of manufacturers announcing prices in *Drug Topics' Red Book,* 1970, New York. Sales data from *U.S. Pharmaceutical Market, Drug Stores and Hospitals,* IMS America, Ltd.

Further, the small generic producer does not have to finance a large promotional campaign. The firm neither expects nor requires a large share of the sales of a generic class. Its appeal is based on price; it need only notify distributors who send circulars to retail and hospital pharmacists, and occasionally to physicians.

Manufacturers of duplicate products, whether they are large or small, have an important advantage over the original producer which permits them to undercut the latter's price. For duplicate manufacturers, the sales of the duplicate are a small source of profits, so they can sell their product at a price which barely covers their marginal costs. They can choose not to charge the product with a share of the costs of administrative overhead, R & D, and other charges not directly attributable to the product. Such a decision is possible for a firm when a product does not account for a large share of its total sales. The larger this share is, the more difficult it is for companies not to allocate part of the overhead costs to a product. The original producer, however, does not usually have this option, since even the largest companies do not have more than a few large-selling brand-name products.

This consideration is important for the analysis of competitive behavior in the drug industry for two reasons: (1) overhead costs make up a large fraction of total costs; and (2) the share of total sales accounted for by a product varies among companies. Direct manufacturing costs, which include only the cost of materials, direct labor, and fuel and power, are a small part of the total cost of drugs. But the overhead costs must be covered out of the revenues from the sales of some products. Thus, a company will persist in attempting to maintain the price of one of its major products even in the face of price-cutting by other firms, and other firms will find it very attractive to cut the price on that product in order to increase their sales so long as the price is above the marginal cost.

A small manufacturer of a new duplicate product will also undercut the price of the original product because its share of the market will be small, and its only appeal lies in a low price. The low price may not result in attracting large sales. Many small manufacturers distribute their products only through mail orders and do not promote their products extensively. Few pharmacists carry any one product of this type. Consequently there may be large differences in prices even among generic products.

Thus the lower prices at which the duplicate manufacturers offer their products need not win them a large part of the sales of their generic or therapeutic classes even after several years. Table 12-2 shows that as late as 1971 original brand-name products whose patents expired in 1966–67 retained a large part of the sales of their therapeutic classes. Of the six drugs shown in the table, three (Hydrocortone, Meticorten, and Cortef) saw large declines in market shares.

Under these conditions we cannot expect the original producers to reduce their prices. Table 12-3 shows that the manufacturers of the original drugs which

TABLE 12-2
Percentage of Therapeutic Market Retained by Original Products
after Patents Expired in 1966–67

Brand Name	Therapeutic Market	Percentage of Sales 1966	Percentage of Sales 1971
Dramamine	Antinauseant	21.5	16.9
Chlortrimeton	Antihistamines	21.2	21.1
Hydrocortone	Plain corticoids	1.7	.9
Cortef	Plain corticoids	1.0	.6
Meticorten (Sch.)	Plain corticoids	1.9	.4
Deltasone	Plain corticoids	.8	1.1

Source: Patent dates supplied by Pfizer, Inc. Sales from *U.S. Pharmaceutical Market, Drug Stores and Hospitals,* IMS America, Ltd.

retained their market shares maintained their prices. The manufacturers of the three products the shares of which dropped sharply did not react uniformly. The price of Cortef was maintained, while the prices of Hydrocortone and of Meticorten were reduced. It is worth noting that since 1971 the price of Meticorten has come down much more. It is currently about $2.40.

Thus the original manufacturers in some cases successfully met the competition of the small entrants who sold their products under their generic names. Doctors either had not heard of generic entrants into the market or they were

TABLE 12-3
Price Stability by Original Products after Patents Expired in 1966–67

Brand Name	Therapeutic Market	Price in 1966	Price in 1971
Dramamine (50 mg. 100 tabs)	Antinauseant	3.74	3.78
Chlortrimeton (12 mg., 100 tabs)	Antihistamines	4.77	5.54
Hydrocortone (10 mg, 100 tabs)	Corticoids	6.26	3.29
Cortef	Corticoids		
(20 mg, 1% top ointment)	2.92	2.92	3.22
(10 mg, 100 tabs)	2.78	2.78	3.33
Meticorten (Sch.) (5 mg, 100 tabs)	Corticoids	17.28	9.12
Deltasone (5 mg, 100 tabs)	Corticoids	2.30	2.14

Source: Patent dates supplied by patent department, Pfizer, Inc. Prices were average realized prices, *U.S. Pharmaceutical Market, Drug Stores,* IMS America Ltd., December 1966 and December 1971.

afraid to take the risk of poor-quality drugs by writing generic prescriptions; moreover, they may not have been sensitive to price differences.

Yet, there are small firms which successfully sell their products. Evidently some doctors write generic prescriptions and some pharmacists use the products of small generic firms to fill such prescriptions. In addition, as we will see later, some pharmacists substitute generic products for brand name products specified in prescriptions, and they do not necessarily obtain the permission of physicians to make the substitutions, even though this is illegal in most states. Still, the small firms may not provide a serious threat and thus do not necessarily provoke the original producers to price-cuts. The entry of major firms producing a generically similar drug and selling it at a lower price, on the other hand, will generally force the original firm to cut its own price.

The reasons for such a counter-action are not hard to ascertain. The major firms promote their branded generic products in medical journals and through detailmen, and in this way they persuade physicians to prescribe generically. Physicians come to believe that several reputable manufacturers supply essentially the same product and that pharmacists can supply a low-cost product of good quality. Generic prescribing, then, avoids the nuisance of a phone call from a pharmacist requesting permission to substitute another product when he is out of the one originally specified by the doctor. Prescribing generically also saves doctors the trouble of remembering several brand names. But when doctors prescribe generically, they neglect the possibility of the prescription being filled with an inferior product—or else they may trust the pharmacist's choice of supplier. But it must be emphasized that until major firms enter a market, the number of generic prescriptions usually remains small. Once the larger firms come in, the number of generic prescriptions rises, and with it, paradoxically, the opportunity for small generic firms to sell their products, for unless the doctor prescribes the brand (or specifies a manufacturer), the pharmacist legally can fill generic prescriptions with the product of any manufacturers, small or large. The entry of major firms into the sale of generic antibiotics in the late 1960s thus opened the gate for more small generic producers.

Several large manufacturers entered the manufacture of each of several antibiotics in the 1960s and early 1970s. By 1973 generic prescriptions accounted for nearly 40 percent of the total number of prescriptions for the major multiple-source antibiotics among the leading 200 drugs.[2] The practice of generic prescribing is not limited to multiple-source drugs which are manufactured by several large firms. Doctors have been accustomed to generically prescribing some old drugs, despite the fact that small, unknown manufacturers supply a large part of the total sales. In the case of digoxin and digitoxin, the practice has involved a serious risk of inefficacy and toxicity for the patient. The FDA recognized this risk when it required batch certification of these products.

The price of the original drug is unlikely to be cut after the entry of small generic producers. The manufacturer would cut its profits by reducing its price.

This can easily be seen. Suppose the manufacturer of the original product were to reduce its price by 5 percent. To maintain profits, the increase in the quantity sold would have to be more than 5 percent, because of the increase in direct costs resulting from the greater output. Since the small generic producers account for a small share of total sales in any given case, the manufacturer of the original product is unlikely to recoup in sales the loss of revenue resulting from a price cut.

Further, the loss in income from a price cut is immediate, while the reduction in quantity sold owing to new entry is gradual. A firm will base its price policy on the present value of its expected profit stream over a period of several years rather than on profits expected over, say, the next year, and profits in the distant future receive less weight in any decision than an immediate loss of the same dollar magnitude. A firm will be reluctant to cut its price for another reason: the future is always less certain than the present, and an immediate cut in price is certain to reduce revenues.

The consequences of refraining from a price cut and thus encouraging the entry of new competitors take a long time to work themselves out, and the eventual outcome for the firm is difficult to predict. The firm may prefer, therefore, to risk the consequences of competition from a new entry rather than cut its price. The entry of small firms thus may not influence the price decisions of the manufacturer of the original brand. As we will see in the case of meprobamate, the entry of small firms resulted in a marked deterioration of the market share of the original brands, but did not result in their prices being reduced.

THE ENTRY OF LARGE FIRMS. The most effective price competition comes from the entry of large firms. We turn, therefore, to the large firm's decision to duplicate a product on which the patent has just expired.

The management will use profit-and-loss analysis to determine the minimum required level of sales for entry to be profitable. The analysis, which forecasts the ratio of profits to sales, is based on estimates of the ratio of the cost of goods sold to sales, and on a predetermined level of promotional expenditures which is considered "necessary." The "cost of goods sold" has the usual meaning of manufacturing costs exclusive of R & D and central office costs. It includes depreciation on plant and equipment as well as materials, labor, and fuel costs. The following formula adopts this convention. It departs from the customary approach in only one respect: the formula allows explicity for nonplant over-head costs, which are expressed as a ratio to sales:

$$a = (1 - b - c) - P/S$$

where a = profits/sales, b = cost of goods sold/sales, c = nonplant overhead costs/sales, P = promotional costs, and S = sales. Thus:

$$S = P/(1 - a - b - c) \qquad (12.1)$$

To obtain the minimum required sales we need only substitute estimates of the required values on the right-hand side of equation 12.1. Note that profits, cost of goods sold, and overhead are represented by their ratios to sales, while promotional costs are represented by a dollar value. Further, although the values for a, b, c, and P are required minima for any firm, these minima will vary among firms depending on available opportunities and alternative business strategies. Nevertheless, the formula is useful for highlighting the considerations entering into entry decisions. It will be seen that the analysis suggests the large firms will consider entry worth the effort only if sales promise to be large in relation to the total sales of many drugs.

We need to amplify the point about interfirm differences in judgment about the required minima. The value of b may vary, because it is a percentage of sales and thus depends on a forecast of prices and quantities which will be sold, as well as cost estimates. Similarly, the value for c will vary. The minimum value will be relatively large when other opportunities for expansion promise a substantial contribution to overhead. A firm which has less attractive opportunities may require only a small contribution to overhead. Similar considerations influence the choice of the minimum profit margin, a.

In addition, the minimum expenditure contemplated for promotion, P, will vary. In part, this minimum depends on the company's views about the other required minima. If the firm is willing to accept a small profit margin, then its promotional expenditure will be small. Furthermore, the minimum promotional expenditure depends on the sales goal. Sales and promotional expenditures are not independent; a firm which seeks large sales must plan substantial promotional expenditures.

We can go through an illustrative series of calculations of the minimum sales required for a decision to enter. We will use estimates of a, b, c, and P which are realistic. Suppose a is set equal to the average before-tax profit margin on pharmaceutical products, which is approximately 0.3; b is set at 0.5; c is set at 0.1; and P at $1 million. Then S must be $10 million. In other words, when we adopt values which reflect roughly the experience of the industry, then minimum sales must be large.

If we eliminate the profit margin, a, and the overhead, c, and reduce promotional expenditure to $.5 million, the minimum S becomes $1 million. As we continue to reduce promotional expenditure, S approaches zero. Alternatively, we can anticipate that price competition will increase b (the ratio of the cost of goods sold to sales) to .7, so that the equation for S becomes:

$$S = .5/(1-.7) = \$1.67 \text{ million.}$$

We have suggested that the required sales have no lower limit. But, this ignores the administrative problems of handling another product. An additional product entails certain costs which are specific to it but which are treated as part of general overhead. Another product manager may be required, or a product manager who is already burdened with selling one or more products may have to cope with the problems associated with this additional product. Medical personnel must familiarize themselves with the properties of the new product and be prepared to deal with queries and complaints from prescribers. The volume of sales required to cover such specific costs cannot be ignored.

Major firms evidently have been persuaded by this type of analysis not to enter the manufacture of many products whose patents have expired. Hence, none of them entered into the manufacture of the products whose patents expired in 1966–67. Apparently the sales of these products were too small to attract the entry of large firms.

The major firms did, however, enter into the production of most of the drugs among the leading 200 which have become open to competition. Some of the drugs that have become multiple-source drugs have attracted at least eight or nine of the major companies; this is true of penicillin VK and V, ampicillin, tetracycline HCl, erythromycin, and reserpine and rauwolfia diuretics. We will analyze the pressures on firms to enter markets which have opened up during the 1960s and early 1970s. Table 12-4 shows the sales of these drugs in 1973. Except in a few instances, the major firms which entered the markets in these products failed to achieve large sales, as table 12-5 shows. Only 49 percent of branded generics, as they are called, achieved sales exceeding $500,000.

We saw earlier that a profit-and-loss analysis would incline firms to expect large sales before they entered a market. Yet, they entered despite poor prospects for such sales, and some of them did so after they could observe that previous new entrants had failed to prosper. The entry of a large number of major firms into each of the various multiple-source drug markets thus suggests pressures on firms to compete in these markets. At least for some of the firms, the alternative opportunities available for the growth of sales were poor. We can see in table 12-6 that most of the major companies entered into the production

TABLE 12-4

1973 Drug Store and Hospital Purchases of Multiple-Source
Single Entity Drugs Selected from among the Leading 200 Drugs ($ Millions)

	Purchases		Purchases
Meprobamate, oral	$24.1	Propoxyphene hydrochloride[a]	$18.9
Penicillin G Potassium, oral	10.7	Erythromycin	69.6
Penicillin VK and V	42.8	Prednisone	4.1
Ampicillin, oral	65.4	Reserpine and rauwolfia diuretics	75.1
Tetracycline HCL	36.5	Chlorpromazine, oral	20.8
Conjugated estrogens	48.6		

Source: U.S. Pharmaceutical Market, Drug Stores and Hospitals, IMS America Ltd., 1973.

Note: Selection of drugs excludes older drugs as follows: PETN, thyroid, digoxin, codeine, chloral hydrate, paregoric, nitroglycerine, phenobarbital.

[a]Excludes combination drugs.

TABLE 12-5
Large Firms Engaged in the Production of Multiple-Source Drugs,
Their Sales and Promotional Expenditures in 1973, and Dates of Product Introductions

Generic class	Brand Name	Introduction Date	Sales ($000)	Promotion Expenditures ($000)
PETN	Peritrate*	1951	$15,033	609
	SK-PETN	1971	15	0
Meprobamate	Equanil*	1955	14,802	198
	Miltown*	1955	7,231	796
	Meprobamate (Parke Davis)	NA	11	0
	SK-Bamate	1971	113	6
Penicillin G Potassium	Pentids*	1951	8,058	506
	Pfizerpen	1968	1,895	200
	Penicillin (Lilly)	NA	24	0
	Penicillin (Parke Davis)	NA	4	0
	Penicillin (Upjohn)	NA	1	0
	Penicillin* (Wyeth)	1951	176	0
Penicillin VK and V	V-Cillin K*	1957	22,765	837
	Compocillin VK	1957	2,875	366
	Pen Vee-K	1958	7,736	717
	Pfizerpen VK	1971	1,110	204
	Penapar VK	1972	445	203
	SK-Penicillin VK	1971	569	156
	Ledercillin VK	1968	2,070	552
	Betapen VK	1970	678	340
	Uticillin VK	1970	911	79
	Robicillin VK	1971	1,446	474
Ampicillin, oral	Polycillin*	1963	23,086	1606
	Principen	1967	11,809	1488
	Omnipen	1966	10,263	1132
	Pen-A	1972	4,747	306
	Amcill	1968	6,291	337
	Penbritin	1964	6,170	373
	SK-Ampicillin	1971	3,326	357
	Alpen	1969	1,145	12
	Totacillin	1969	2,630	187
	Pensyn	1972	1,891	110
Thyroid	Cytomel*	1956	3,029	16
	Thyroid (Parke Davis)	NA	807	0
	Thyroid Tabs (Lilly)	NA	443	0
Tetracycline HCL	Panmycin*	1954	2,527	237
	Achromycin V	1957	8,331	477
	Bristocycline	1954	344	2
	Sumycin	1957	10,568	886
	Cyclopar	1970	421	117
	Tetracyn	1953	2,143	56
	SK-Tetracycline	1971	543	205
	Robitet	1971	1,943	534
	Tetracycline (Wyeth)	1973	21	0
	Dema	1972	16	1
Digoxin	Lanoxin*	1933	6,758	292
	Digoxin (Lederle)	1970	29	0
Codeine	Codeine (Lilly)	NA	1,785	0
	Codeine (Wyeth)	NA	743	0

TABLE 12-5 (continued)

Generic class	Brand Name	Introduction Date	Sales ($000)	Promotion Expenditures ($000)
	Codeine (MSD)	NA	3	0
	Codeine (Parke Davis)	NA	0	0
Chloral Hydrate	Noctec*	1952	2,148	13
	Somnos	NA	61	0
	Chloral Hydrate (Lilly)	NA	6	0
	Chloral Hydrate (Wyeth)	NA	34	0
	Chloral Hydrate (Parke Davis)	NA	27	0
	Chloral Hydrate (Abbott)	NA	11	0
Conjugated Estrogens	Premarin*	1942	48,155	4552
	Conestron	1945	57	7
Paregoric	Parepectalin	NA	1,643	417
	Paregoric (Lilly)	NA	185	0
	Paregoric (Wyeth)	NA	9	0
	Paregoric (Upjohn)	NA	1	0
	Paregoric (Parke Davis)	NA	123	0
Propoxyphene Hydrochloride	Darvon*	1957	17,369	265
	SK-65	1973	293	995
	Dolene	1973	169	263
Nitroglycerine	Nitrobid*	1965	6,926	1570
	Nitroglycerin (Lilly)	NA	1,722	0
	Nitrostat	1971	1,390	365
	Nitrospan	1967	995	28
Erythromycin	Ilosone	1958	25,163	1976
	Ilotycin	1952	866	74
	E-Mycin	1968	5,978	534
	Pfizer E	1973	1,389	276
	Erythrocin*	1954	25,287	2883
	Ethril	1972	1,137	419
	Erypar	1972	588	139
	SK-Erythromycin	1972	649	133
	Robimycin	1972	787	648
	Erythromycin Stearate	1954	188	0
Prednisone	Deltasone*	1955	1,903	201
	Panacort	1957	64	0
	Meticorten (Schering)	1955	154	1
	Servisone	1970	14	0
	Delta	1955	4	0
	Prednisone (USV)	1957	53	0
Phenobarbital	Phenobarbital (Lilly)	NA	876	0
	Phenobarbital (Abbott)	NA	60	0
	Phenobarbital (Parke Davis)	NA	471	0
	Phenobarbital (Wyeth)	NA	238	0
	Eskabarb	NA	328	0
	Stental Extentab	NA	51	3
	Phenobarbital (Upjohn)	NA	5	0
Reserpine	Serpasil*	1953	3,831	373
	Raused	1954	29	0
	Reserpoid	1954	74	0
	Eskaserp	1955	1	0

TABLE 12-5 (continued)

Generic class	Brand Name	Introduction Date	Sales ($000)	Promotion Expenditures ($000)
Rauwolfia-diuretics	Ser-Ap-Es/Ser-Ap-Es Esidrix	1960	24,323	2458
	Hydropres, Diupres*	1959	20,246	680
	Salutensin	NA	11,765	557
	Hydromox R	1965	588	7
	Regroton	1964	8,330	693
	Naquival	1962	509	1
	Extna-R	1965	117	0
Chlorpromazine	Thorazine*	1954	22,816	855
	Promaoar	1973	167	32
	Chlor PZ	1973	157	169
	Chlorpromazine (Wyeth)	1972	156	17

Source: U.S. Pharmaceutical Market, Drug Stores and Hospitals, National Journal Audit, National Detailing Audit, National Mail Audit, IMS America, Ltd.
Note: Where no introduction date is available, original drug is not shown.
*Original drug in class.
NA: Not available.

of most of the multiple source drugs. The table reveals that SmithKline, Wyeth, Parke Davis, and Upjohn have been especially active in entering newly opened therapeutic fields with branded generics.

Furthermore, it is evident that in order to obtain large sales, it is necessary for a firm to enter ahead of other major firms. From table 12-5 it is apparent that the large-selling drugs were among those that were the first to enter. Another condition for large sales in these markets has been large promotional expenditures. Table 12-5 shows that the firms with the leading branded generic spent considerably more promoting them than was spent on behalf of other branded generics.

We will see later that the companies which made large gains in sales also were leaders in price-cutting. The changes in sales thus cannot be attributed only, or even primarily, to large promotional expenditures.

MARGINAL AND AVERAGE COSTS. The difference between average and marginal costs encourages firms to imitate an established drug and to compete in price. This difference also encourages firms whose share of sales of a generic class of drugs is small to increase sales by reducing their price below the level of average cost. We will discuss more fully this aspect of the cost curves and the consequences for competitive behavior.

The other important element of the market structure which contributes to the tendency of firms to cut prices below fully allocated average cost is that overhead costs need not be allocated to an individual product or group of products. The companies do not have their sales evenly distributed over several

TABLE 12-6
Generic Classes and Dates of Introduction of Branded Generics Produced by Major Companies

Company	Generic Class	Drug	Date
SmithKline	Meprobamate	SK-Bamate	1971
	Penicillin VK, V	SK-Penicillin	1971
	Ampicillin	SK-Ampicillin	1971
	Tetracycline HCL	SK-Tetracycline	1971
	Proposyphene HCL	SK-65	1973
	Erythromycin	SK-Erythromycin	1972
	Phenobarbital	Eskabarb	NA
	"	Eskaphen b	NA
	Reserpine	Eskaserp	1955
Wyeth	Ampicillin	Omnipen	1966
	Penicillin VK,V	Pen-Vee-K	1958
	Tetracycline HCL	Tetracycline	1973
	Chloral Hydrate	Chloral Hydrate	NA
	Conjugated Estrogens	Conestron	1945
	Erythromycin	Erythromycin Stearate	1954
	Chlorpromazine	Chlorpromazine	1972
	Meprobamate	Equanil*	1955
Parke Davis	Meprobamate	Meprobamate	NA
	Penicillin G Potassium	Penicillin G	NA
	Penicillin VK and V	Penapar VK	1972
	Ampicillin	Amcill	1968
	Thyroid	Thyroid	NA
	Tetracycline HCL	Cyclopar	1970
	Codeine	Codeine	NA
	Chloral Hydrate	Chloral Hydrate	NA
	Paregoric	Paregoric	NA
	Nitroglycerine	Nitrostat	1971
	Erythromycin	Erypar	1972
	Prednisone	Paracort	1957
	Phenobarbital	Phenobarbital	NA
	Chlorpromazine	Promapar	1973
Squibb	Penicillin G Potassium	Pentids*	1951
	Ampicillin	Principen	1967
	Tetracycline HCL	Sumycin	1957
	Chloral Hydrate	Noctec	1952
	Erythromycin	Ethril	1972
	Reserpine	Raused	1954
Pfizer	Penicillin G Potassium	Pfizerpen	1968
	Penicillin VK and V	Pfizerpen VK	1971
	Ampicillin	Pen A	1972
	Tetracycline HCL	Tetracyn	1953
	Erythromycin	Pfizer-E	1973
Lilly	Penicillin G Potassium	Penicillin	NA
	Penicillin VK and V	V Cillin K*	1957
	Thyroid	Thyroid Tabs	NA
	Codeine	Codeine	NA
	Chloral Hydrate	Chloral Hydrate	NA
	Paregoric	Paregoric	NA
	Nitroglycerine	Nitroglycerine	NA
	Propoyphene Hydrochloride	Darvon*	1957
	Erythromycin	Ilosone	1958
	Phenobarbital	Phenobarbital	NA

TABLE 12-6 (continued)

Company	Generic Class	Drug	Date
Upjohn	Penicillin G Potassium	Penicillin	NA
	Penicillin VK and V	Uticillin VK	1970
	Tetracycline HCL	Panmycin*	1954
	Paregoric	Paregoric	NA
	Nitroglycerine	Nitroglycerine	NA
	Erythromycin	E-Mycin	1968
	Prednisone	Deltasone	1955
	Phenobarbital	Phenobarbital	NA
	Reserpine	Reserpoid	1954
Lederle	Penicillin VK and V	Ledercillin VK	1968
	Ampicillin	Alpen	1969
	Tetracycline HCL	Achromycin	1957
	Digoxin	Digoxin	1970
	Proposyphene Hydrochloride	Dolene	1973
	Prednisone	Servisone	1970
	Rauwolfia-Diuretics	Hydromox R	1965
Robins	Penicillin VK and V	Robicillin VK	1971
	Tetracycline HCL	Robitet	1971
	Erythromycin	Robimycin	1972
	Phenobarbital	Stental Extentab	NA
	Rauwolfia-Diuretics	Exna-R	1965
Bristol	Penicillin VK	Betapen VK	1970
	Ampicillin	Polycillin*	1963
	Tetracycline HCL	Bristalcycline	1954
	Rauwolfia-Diuretics	Salutension	NA
Beecham	Ampicillin	Totacillin	1969
USV	Tetracycline HCL	Dema	1972
	Nitroglycerine	Nitrospan	1967
	Prednisone	Prednisone	1957
	Rauwolfia-Diuretics	Regroton	1964
	Chlorpromazine	Chlor PZ	1973
Burroughs Wellcome	Digoxin	Lanoxin*	1933
Merck	Codeine	Codeine	NA
	Chloral Hydrate	Sominos	NA
	Nitroglycerine	Nitroglycerine	NA
	Prednisone	Deltra	1955
	Phenobarbital	Phenobarbital	NA
Abbott	Chloral Hydrate	Chloral Hydrate	NA
	Erythromycin	Erythrocin*	1954
	Phenobarbital	Phenobarbital	NA
Rorer	Paregoric	Paregoric	NA
Marian	Nitroglycerin	Nitrobid	1965
Schering	Prednisone	Meticorten	1955
	Rauwolfia	Naquival	1962
Ciba	Reserpine	Serpasil	1953
	Rauwolfia	Ser-Ap-Es	1960

Sources: U.S. Pharmaceutical Market, Drug Stores and Hospitals, IMS America, Ltd.;
Paul de Haen, *Nonproprietary Name Index,* various years.
   *Original brands.
   NA: Not available.

products. Even the major companies usually have very few big sellers plus a large number of drugs with small sales. In fact, the annual sales of many of the drugs sold by the major companies amount to less than $1 million. Each of the ten leading companies thus has a handful of drugs which account for 50 percent of total sales (see chapter 6). The remainder of its sales is distributed over a large number of products. This means that while a company will resist reducing the prices of its major products, it will not be reluctant to cut the prices of its other products. Furthermore, these same products generally have a small share of their respective therapeutic markets. If they are imitations of other drugs, the only way in which their sales can increase significantly is through price cuts to levels below those of the original drugs. But the sales of the original drugs generally contribute a large share of the sales of their manufacturers, and price cutting therefore will significantly influence their total profits.

Furthermore, the price elasticity of demand of a product which has a large share of a market is less than that of product having a small share. In the case of the latter, a price cut can double its share of the market. The same price cut is unlikely to have as large an effect on the share of the market of a product which already has a large share. Thus a price cut for a leading brand is much more likely to lead to a reduction in revenue than is the same price cut for a brand having a small share.

We have not considered the original prices of leading brand-name products, which, it must be remembered, begin as new products. The original prices are fixed on the basis of uncertain forecasts of sales and the prices of competitive products which may already be available. Much of the information concerning a product's advantages over its competitors comes in only after it is marketed. Doctors, moreover, hesitate to adopt a new product until they receive assurances from colleagues of its superiority over competitive products for some purposes and some patients. Most products never succeed in winning a large market. A company will expect small sales in the case of some drugs including those which treat rare diseases. But companies may refrain from demanding a price which fully covers the costs of such "service" drugs, because to do so would inflict economic hardship on patients.

In most cases, the ultimate size of sales cannot be predicted. It will depend on physicians' judgments of the relative merits of different drugs, which usually cannot be assessed without considerable experience in actual office and hospital use. Clinical trials provide an indication, but they are a good predictor only in rare cases. Under this uncertainty the firm cannot fix a price which is certain to cover fully allocated average cost. The firm therefore will fix the price at a level which is more or less equal to those of competitive products. If the product is to be one of several in the same therapeutic class, then the price may be somewhat lower than those of earlier products.

Under these conditions the leading products of a company are vulnerable to price competition when their patents either expire or are ineffective in preventing others from entering a market. These leading products have a large share of their respective therapeutic markets. Their properties are well known to doctors, and for many patients they are superior to other drugs in the same therapeutic market. A company which imitates one of these products shares in the benefits of the earlier developmental work and promotion. Since the imitation contributes a small share of its total sales, the company can fix a price below fully allocated average cost. Later imitators will come in at successively lower prices in order to obtain a share of the market. The earlier entrants with imitations will try to maintain or increase their respective shares by meeting the prices of later arrivals. The original company eventually is forced to match these prices.

GENERIC PRESCRIBING. It has been suggested by various observers that patent expiration does not lead to price competition, because most prescriptions call for a specific brand-name product and doctors may be indifferent to price considerations. But, even if only some prescriptions are generically written and some doctors consider price, price-cutting may be sufficiently effective to force the prices of original brands to be reduced. Moreover, pharmacists may substitute low-price drugs for expensive drugs, and the illegality of this practice in most states is widely ignored, as we shall see later. The fact of the matter is that price-cutters have increased their share of sales of multiple-source drugs and have forced other firms to reduce their prices. Such price competition has been especially marked in antibiotics. We will consider some of the sources.

The expiration of patents covering large-selling drugs has led to the entry of large, as well as many small, firms into the production of each of these drugs. In the case of some drugs, including ampicillin and tetracycline, entry did not await the expiration of patents. The effect of entry has been to encourage doctors to write generic prescriptions, with the result that the number of generic prescriptions has grown (table 12-7). Between 1966 and 1973, generic prescriptions grew from 6.4 percent of all prescriptions to 10.6 percent.[3] The growth in the generic fraction of prescriptions for multiple-source drugs has been especially rapid. Table 12-8 describes this growth.

TABLE 12-7
Generic Prescriptions as Percentage of All
Non-Compounded New Prescriptions

	Percentage		Percentage
1966	6.4	1970	9.0
1967	7.1	1971	9.2
1968	8.2	1972	9.7
1969	8.8	1973	10.6

Source: *National Prescription Audits*, IMS America, Ltd.

TABLE 12-8
Generic Prescriptions as a Percentage of New Prescriptions
for Leading Multiple-Source Drugs, 1966 and 1973

	Percentage in 1966	Percentage in 1973
Thyroid	28.4	33.2
Penicillin VK and V	0	14.2
Penicillin G Potassium, oral	27.2	35.8
Tetracycline HCL	29.8	40.7
Erythromycin	8.9	17.4
Ampicillin, oral	4.1	49.7
Barbiturates	22.1	30.1
Sedatives, nonbarbiturates	8.8	8.2
Digitalis preparations	37.5	39.5
Total	19.2%	30.7%

Source: National Prescription Audits, IMS America, Ltd.,
1966, 1973.

Generic prescribing encourages price competition by legally permitting pharmacists to fill a prescription with a drug for which they have to pay a low
wholesale price. Pharmacists will tend to use low-price drugs to fill such prescriptions, since they need not pass on all of the resulting savings to consumers. It is
true that pharmacists can, and some do, fill generic prescriptions with expensive
brand-name products. These pharmacists may not wish to take the risk of poor
quality associated with generic products, so they may keep only the most
popular brand-name products in stock. Limiting their stock in this way may also
reduce their inventory investment and costs of operation. But the effect of price
competition on market shares will be felt even if only a substantial number of
pharmacists use low-price drugs to fill generic prescriptions.

Some information on the share of generic prescriptions filled by low-priced
drugs is provided by the results of a survey conducted in 1973 by R_xOTC Inc.,
of Philadelphia, which sent comparison shoppers with generic prescriptions for
ampicillin or erythromycin to drug stores in twelve metropolitan areas. Table
12-9 summarizes the results.

These results demonstrate that pharmacists used low-price drugs for a large
proportion of generic prescriptions. Thus, "generic drugs or other brands" were
used for 43 percent of generic ampicillin prescriptions. "Other brands" signifies
those which are not specified in the list, including Alpen, Pensyn, and Ampen.
Drugstores purchase most of the generic products and other brands at lower
prices than they do Polycillin, the leading and original brand-name product.
Further, we can also see that Polycillin, which is the most expensive brand,
accounts for a smaller share even of generic prescriptions which are filled by
brand-name products than it does of all brand-name prescriptions. In 1972
Polycillin obtained 38.3 percent of all ampicillin prescriptions which specified

TABLE 12-9

Percentage Distribution among Brand Name and Generic Products Used
for Filling Generic Prescriptions for Ampicillin and Erythromycin, and
Effective Wholesale Prices of Brands, June 1973

	Percentage used for generic prescriptions	Prices (250 mg/20 caps)
Ampicillin		
Polycillin*	8	$2.66
SK-Ampicillin	9	2.25
Principen	9	1.65
Omnipen	3	1.97
Penbritin	5	1.84
Amcill	5	1.89
Totacillin	5	1.73
Pen A	13	1.42
Generic or other brands	43	
Total	100	
Erythromycin		
Ilosone	6	$3.90
Erythrocin*	17	2.58
E-Mycin	21	2.18
Bristamycin	4	1.79
SK-erythromycin	5	1.93
Erypar	6	1.76
Pfizer E	4	1.56
Ethril	5	1.79
Generic or other brands	31	
Total	100	

Source: Percentage of generic prescriptions from R$_x$OTC, Inc.,
Philadelphia; prices estimated from *U.S. Pharmaceutical Market, Drug
Stores,* IMS America, Ltd., June 1973.
*Original drug.

brand-name products.[4] By contrast, it accounted for 14 percent of all generic
prescriptions in the survey which were filled by brand-name products.[5] Thus,
when druggists have the opportunity, they tend to use the less costly products.

The results for erythromycin are similar. Pharmacists filled 31 percent of
generic prescriptions with "generic products or other brands." In addition, the
most expensive brand-name product, Ilosone, was used relatively little for
generic prescriptions, despite large sales and presumably, therefore, large stocks.
Thus, the most popular brands for filling generic prescriptions were E-mycin and
Erythrocin, which were considerably lower in price than Ilosone. The prices of
other brands were even lower, but pharmacists apparently did not maintain
sufficient stocks for any one of these brands to be used frequently. Nevertheless,
if we group these other brands, we can see that their low prices had the expected
effect. Thus, although as a group they accounted for only 19 percent of the total

number of prescriptions which were written for brand-name products,[6] their share of generic prescriptions filled by brand-name products was 35.4 percent.

BRAND SUBSTITUTION. Another source of price competition is brand substitution. A pharmacist can legally substitute another brand-name product or a generic product for the one specified in a prescription, providing he obtains permission from the prescriber. Only four states and the District of Columbia at present do not require such permission.[7] The R_xOTC, Inc. survey reveals that pharmacists make many substitutions, and by far the majority of them are made without permission, even in states where the practice is illegal. Table 12-10 reports that pharmacists substitute a generic product or another brand for the specified brand in 33 percent of ampicillin prescriptions, 30 percent of erythromycin prescriptions, and 26 percent of penicillin VK prescriptions. These are astonishingly large percentages. Physicians do not give permission for most of them, according to the survey. For example, 82 percent of the substitutions for Pfizer E, Pfizer's brand of erythromycin, lacked permission. The corresponding percentages for Pen A, Pfizer's brand of ampicillin, and for Pfizerpen VK, are 76 percent and 84 percent respectively.

The large influence of price is also seen in the substitutions for Polycillin, Erythrocin, and Ilosone. Inadequate stocks are unlikely to account for percentages as large as those shown in table 12-11, since these are the products with the largest sales.

Finally, the distribution of substitutions among products actually used shows that low-price products were favored. Table 12-12 shows the distribution of substitutions. Generics obtained a large percentage of the substitutions. Pharmacists did not use Polycillin in substitutions as much as physicians chose it in writing prescriptions. More generally, the low-price brands took a larger share of the substitutions than they did of the original prescriptions.

TABLE 12-10
Percentage of Prescriptions Specifying Brand Names for
Ampicillin, Erythromycin, and Penicillin VK, Filled as
Ordered, Substituted, or Refused, June 1973

	Percentage			
	Filled as Ordered	Substituted	Refused	Total
Ampicillin	52	33	15	100
Erythromycin	55	30	15	100
Penicillin VK	65	26	9	100

Source: R_xOTC, Inc., Philadelphia Survey, 1973.

TABLE 12-11

Wholesale Prices, and Percentage of Prescriptions Filled as Ordered, Substituted,
or Refused by Brands of Ampicillin and of Erythromycin, June 1973

Brand	Price per 250mg./20 caps	Percentage			
		Filled as ordered	Substituted	Refused	Total
Ampicillin					
Polycillin	$2.66	74	12	15	100
SK-Amp	2.25	41	43	16	100
Principen	1.65	64	26	12	100
Omnipen	1.97	63	32	5	100
Penbritin	1.84	64	27	9	100
Amcill	1.89	48	37	15	100
Totacillin	1.73	18	57	25	100
Pen A	1.42	39	38	23	100
Erythromycin					
Ilosone	3.90	84	10	6	100
Erythrocin	2.58	85	12	3	100
E-Mycin	2.18	87	10	3	100
Bristomycin	1.79	39	36	26	100
SK-erythromycin	1.93	30	51	19	100
Erypar	1.76	19	62	18	100
Pfizer E	1.56	52	25	23	100
Ethril	1.79	54	30	16	100

Source: Same as table 12-9.

TABLE 12-12

Percentage Distribution of Substitution for Brand-Name Drugs Specified in Prescriptions
among Products Used and Effective Wholesale Prices of Brands of Ampicillin and
Erythromycin, June 1973

Brand	Percentage	Price per 250mg./ 20 caps		Percentage	Price per 250mg./ 20 caps
Ampicillin			Erythromycin		
Polycillin	8	$2.66	Ilosone	6	$3.90
SK-Ampicillin	7	2.25	Erythrocin	22	2.58
Principen	12	1.65	E-Mycin	18	2.18
Omnipen	12	1.97	Bristomycin	4	1.79
Penbritin	8	1.84	SK-erythromycin	4	1.93
Amcill	4	1.89	Erypar	4	1.76
Totacillin	3	1.73	Pfizer E	8	1.56
Pen A	9	1.42	Ethril	6	1.79
Generics or other brands	38		Generic or other brands	29	
Total	100		Total	100	

Source: Same as table 12-9.

PRICE COMPETITION IN ANTIBIOTICS

Price competition has been vigorous in antibiotics. Despite therapeutic differences, the competition has extended across generic classes. Apparently, the overlap in uses among antibiotics is sufficient for price differences to influence the sale of products. That this is so is suggested by the name "broad- and medium-spectrum" antibiotics. Although broad and medium spectrum antibiotics are not good substitutes for all indications, they are sufficiently good substitutes for many indications, so that differences in prices can influence market shares, as we shall see.

The market for antibiotics is large enough to have attracted many of the large firms. Total antibiotic sales (including penicillin) amounted to $597.6 million in 1973.[8] The large firms which are in the market have sold duplicates of other manufacturers' products as well as their own patented sole-source products. In addition, competition in the 1960s was intensified by the introduction of several important new chemical entities, including ampicillin and the cephalosporins.

Toward the end of the 1960s the number of antibiotics marketed by major companies increased sharply. Some of the firms obtained licenses of production from Beecham, the original patentee of ampicillin, and others obtained sublicenses from Bristol, the first licensee. Others entered with generic versions of penicillin VK and erythromycin. Consequently, at the end of the 1960s the market shares differed sharply from those of 1960.

The years 1961 to 1963 saw the beginning of vigorous price competition in virtually all of the broad- and medium-spectrum antibiotics. Several important products in different generic classes had the same list price in 1961: $30.60 per bottle of 100 tablets. By 1963 their prices had declined by 28 percent to a level of about $22.00. The group included Achromycin V, Achromycin, Declomycin, Ilosone Terramycin, Signemycin, Tetrex, Erythromycin, and Sumycin. Other products whose prices fell by similar percentages included Achrocidin, TAO, Panalba, and Mysteclin F. The decline in the price of Panmycin HCl was larger, 41 percent; it fell from $35.70, which was above the standard of $30.60, to $21,00, which was under the new standard price. In the following year, this discrepancy was eliminated by a rise to $21.99.

Only the price of Chloromycetin remained constant over this period. The product had been under attack for exposing patients to a risk of aplastic anemia. Under the circumstances, doctors' decisions to prescribe this drug would not depend on its relative price, and Parke Davis, faced with declining demand, saw no advantage in reducing the price.

Between 1963 and 1966, price reductions were confined to tetracycline products and Terramycin, and the uniformity of prices therefore broke down, with the prices of Achromycin and Achromycin V, Achrocidin, Terrastatin, TAO, Tetracyn, Tetrex, Colymycin, and Panmycin, falling sharply. Further declines in the prices of most major products came in 1967 and 1968. Two exceptions were Erythrocin (Abbott) and Ilosone (Lilly), which are the leading products in the erythromycin group. The prices of tetracycline products continued to decline until 1972, when their prices were 85 percent below the 1960 level.

The above description of price movements is based on list prices reported in *Drug Topics' Red Book*. The effective prices computed from the reports of sales and quantities sold in IMS drug stores conformed to the same general pattern. For some products, notably Lederle's Achromycin and Achromycin V, effective prices declined sooner and more sharply than list prices. The fluctuations in effective prices associated with stable list prices reflected special deals, including free packages with each purchase of a certain minimum number of packages.

During the 1960s, Lilly's new cephalosporin products, Keflin and Keflex, were introduced and quickly took a large share of antibiotic sales; their share grew from zero in 1963 to 21.3 percent in 1973. Nevertheless, the effective price of Keflin declined from $5.00 per unit in 1964 to $2.85 in 1972. The novelty of the product and its popularity did not prevent a large decline in price. Another new product was Vibramycin, whose effective price rose between 1967 and 1969 and again in 1972. The analysis of the pricing of Vibramycin reveals an interesting aspect of the problem of the measurement of prices. On a tablet basis, the price was high. But for the patient it was the cost of a daily dose that was significant rather than the price per tablet. The usual prescription for an antibiotic calls for four doses daily, but one of the features of this product is that only a single dose is necessary. Thus, the daily dose cost is less than that of several other major products.

The causes of the decline in prices are difficult to assess. The price declines set in before the expiration of patents on tetracycline, erythromycin, and oxytetracycline. The patent on tetracycline expired as late as 1972, but litigation and licensing had limited its effectiveness throughout the 1960s. Many branded generic antibiotics which entered in the late 1960s contributed to the declines, as did the introduction of ampicillin and the cephalosporins. By the mid-1960s, then, there were several types of antibiotics, and sales of each generic type were shared by several competing brand-name products.

Furthermore, the familiarity of the products and the large number of major firms manufacturing antibiotics led to an increase in generic prescribing, especially of tetracycline and ampicillin. The practice was encouraged by the certification of antibiotics by the FDA, which seemed to give doctors some assurance of adequate quality, regardless of source. Certification does not, in fact, provide such a guarantee, as the discussion in chapter eleven indicates, but doctors may have felt reassured.

TETRACYCLINE. Tetracyline's patent, which expired in 1972,[9] was still in effect when price competition in the tetracycline market began in 1962. The brand-name products were limited to Achromycin and Achromycin V (Lederle),

Tetracyn (Pfizer), Panmycin (Upjohn), Sumycin (Squibb), and Tetrex (Bristol). Lederle had. the lion's share of the market in 1962, with 85 percent of total sales.[10] Generic products were also available, however, and as they took an increasing share of the market, Lederle's share fell from 85 percent to 72 percent between 1962 and 1964. Perhaps in response to this decline, price cuts were initiated by the major firms, including Lederle, and the prices of several brands of tetracycline fell from $26.01 to $22.00 between 1962 and 1964 (table 12-13).

As our analysis of price behavior suggests, even large firms which have a small share of the market will be induced to cut prices. Thus, in 1964, Squibb, which had a small share of the market, undertook the initiative and began to cut prices aggressively. Its average effective price in 1964 was $15.60 (table 12-14), which was less than the price of any of the other major firms' products. By 1968 its price had fallen to $3.91. Squibb's strategy won it insignificant increases in its share of the market until 1967, when its sales leaped to over 7 percent. The following year saw an increase to over 16 percent. Since then, Squibb's share has leveled off at about 20 percent. Squibb did not limit its attack to cutting prices. Over the same period (1964–68), its promotional expenditures for Sumycin are estimated to have grown from $14,000 to $200,000 per year.

The other companies were forced to retaliate. Between 1964 and 1968, Lederle's share of total sales dropped from 72 percent to 33 percent, and Pfizer's from 11 percent to 4 percent. In 1965 Lederle cut its price from $19.43 to $17.84 (table 12-14), and Pfizer's price cut was similar. Curiously, in that year Upjohn raised its price from $15.23 to $17.22. In 1966 Squibb cut its price from $14.28 to $12.35, and the other major manufacturers followed. Lederle reduced its price for Achromycin from $17.84 to $15.92, and Pfizer and Upjohn's reductions were similar. Then in 1967 Squibb slashed its price to $4.96. Although Lederle's response was substantial—a reduction to $11.59—its price remained over twice as high as Squibb's. Pfizer and Upjohn also reduced their prices—Pfizer to a level slightly below that of Lederle, and Upjohn to one which was somewhat higher. In 1968 Squibb reduced its price further to $3.91, and in that year Pfizer and Upjohn came down to prices in the same region— Pfizer to $4.93 and Upjohn to $4.77. Lederle did not follow suit and continued to maintain its price in 1969. After 1969 Squibb did not reduce its price further. Upjohn, on the other hand, cut its price below Squibb's in 1970 and made further cuts in 1971 and 1972. Pfizer followed with a similar price cut in 1971. Lederle finally tried to regain its share of the market by reducing its price to $7.72 in 1970 and to $4.65 in 1971.

Thus, our model of price competition fits the observed behavior reasonably well if not exactly. The model is correct in predicting that large firms with small market shares will cut prices. On the other hand, it is incorrect in describing Lederle's behavior over the entire period. Contrary to the model, Lederle, the company with the largest market share, reduced its price between 1962 and

TABLE 12-13

Red Book Prices of Leading Tetracyclines, 1960–72 (100 caps., 250 mg.)

Brand and Manufacturer		1960	1961	1962	1963	1964	1965	1966	1967	1968	1969	1970	1971	1972
Achromycin V	(Lederle)	$30.60	$30.60	$38.82	$22.00	$22.00	$17.60	$17.60	$14.69	$11.22	–	–	$11.22	$4.50
Achromycin	(Lederle)	30.60	30.60	38.82	22.00	22.00	17.60	17.60	14.69	11.22	–	–	11.22	N.A.
Terramycin	(Pfizer)	30.60	30.60	26.01	22.00	22.00	19.80	19.80	19.80	17.80	–	–	–	17.80
Terrastatin	(Pfizer)	N.A.	N.A.	28.96	23.92	–	–	–	23.92	21.52	–	–	–	21.52
Tetracyn	(Pfizer)	30.60	30.60	26.01	26.01	22.00	19.60	17.60	14.96	11.00	4.25	–	–	4.25
Tetrex	(Bristol)	30.60	30.60	25.88	22.00	22.00	17.74	–	17.74	14.95	–	14.95	13.09	13.09
Panmycin HCL	(Upjohn)	35.70	35.70	30.15	21.00	21.99	17.58	17.58	14.94	14.94	7.89	7.98	4.70	3.94
Sumycin	(Squibb)	30.60	30.60	26.00	22.00	22.00	22.57	22.57	17.04	4.25	–	–	–	4.25

Source: Drug Topics' Red Book, 1960–72.
N.A.: Not available.
–unchanged.

TABLE 12-14
Effective Prices of Tetracyclines, 1964–72 (100 caps., 250 mg.)

Brand and Manufacturer	1964	1965	1966	1967	1968	1969	1970	1971	1972
Achromycin V (Lederle)	$19.43	$17.84	$15.92	$11.59	$11.52	$11.47	$8.00	$4.65	$4.38
Achromycin (Lederle)	19.23	17.83	16.59	11.79	11.84	11.64	9.40	6.20	N.A.
Terramycin (Pfizer)	21.02	20.09	19.58	18.26	18.19	18.10	18.33	17.58	18.39
Terrastatin* (Pfizer)	12.15	12.33	11.77	10.98	11.01	10.89	10.97	11.09	10.99
Tetracyn (Pfizer)	19.19	17.82	16.52	11.26	4.93	4.37	4.31	3.53	3.47
Tetrex (Bristol)	19.32	17.35	15.95	14.83	14.78	13.98	14.41	14.37	13.88
Tetracycline (McKesson)	6.58	6.68	6.50	5.84	4.76	4.14	4.11	4.33	3.98
Panmycin (Upjohn)	15.23	17.22	16.48	12.37	4.77	4.45	3.63	3.43	3.23
Sumycin (Squibb)	15.64	14.28	12.35	4.96	3.91	3.94	3.84	3.96	3.97

Source: U.S. Pharmaceutical Market, Drug Stores, IMS America, Ltd., 1964–72.
*Fifty 250-mg. caps.

1964. But the model's predictions of Lederle's subsequent behavior are correct. Lederle did not respond to Squibb's drastic price cut in 1967 before 1970, and although the reduction in that year was large, the price did not approach Squibb's. Only in 1971, four years later, did Lederle's price come down to a similar level. Although Lederle eventually reduced its price sharply, it did so much later—after its share of the market had fallen to less than one third. The model is correct in predicting that as the leading firm's share of the market continues its decline, it will be forced to reduce its price. Thus, the final outcome of the price competition in tetracyclines conforms to the model.

ERYTHROMYCIN. The patent for erythromycin did not expire before 1970, but prices for erythromycin declined along with those of other antibiotics in 1962 and 1963. Evidently Abbott (Erythrocin) and Lilly (Ilosone), the two leading manufacturers of erythromycin, believed that price reductions for other antibiotic products would reduce their sales of erythromycin unless they matched the price cuts. They thus did not await the expiration of the patent and entry before cutting prices by one-third (table 12-15).

Until 1965 the prices were nearly the same. Lilly's product, however, lost a substantial part of the market to Abbott. In 1961 Ilosone had more than 70 percent of total sales, compared to Erythrocin's share of less than 20 percent. By 1965 Erythrocin had nearly half of total sales and passed Ilosone. Nevertheless, prices remained stable until 1970, except for Abbott's reduction of its effective price in 1966 through special deals (table 12-16) while keeping its list price constant; the effective price returned to its previous level in the following year.

In 1970, with the expiration of the patent on erythromycin, Upjohn (E-Mycin), which had entered in 1968 but still had only a small share of the market, cut its price, beginning the pattern of price competition which our model predicts would set in. As a result, Upjohn's market share increased rapidly, from under 2 percent to over 8 percent. Between 1970 and 1972 its effective price fell from $17.26 to $11.71 (32 percent) for 100 250-mg. capsules. Abbott responded with large price cuts, but Lilly's reductions were much smaller.

Upjohn may have been discontented with its prospects for profit generally as well as with its share of the erythromycin market. The company's total sales had been growing slowly in the preceding years. In 1970 the sales of its major product, Orinase, declined following the University Group Diabetes Program's unfavorable report which raised doubts about the long-term safety of oral antidiabetic drugs. In addition, Upjohn was forced to remove its large-selling drug, Panalba, from the market after litigation over the effectiveness of combination antibiotics. Upjohn's research program was very extensive, and many potential new chemical entities were being investigated. But the company had not introduced any large-selling new entity for several years. In addition, the

TABLE 12-15
Red Book Prices of Leading Erythromycins, 1960–1972 (100 caps., 250 mg.)

Brand and Manufacturer		1960	1961	1962	1963	1964	1965	1966	1967	1968	1969	1970	1971	1972
Ilosone	(Lilly)	$30.60	$30.60	$26.01	$21.99	–	–	–	–	–	–	–	–	$21.99
Pediamycin	(Ross)	N.A.	–	–	–	–	N.A.	18.00	–	–	–	–	–	18.00
E-Mycin	(Upjohn)	N.A.	–	–	–	–	–	–	–	N.A.	21.99	22.00	16.49	16.49
Erythrocin	(Abbott)	30.60	30.60	26.01	21.99	–	–	–	–	–	–	–	–	21.99

Source: Drug Topics' Red Book, 1960–72, suggested wholesale prices.
N.A.: Not available.
–unchanged.

TABLE 12-16
Effective Prices of Erythromycins, 1964–72 (100 caps., 250 mg.)

Brand and Manufacturer		1964	1965	1966	1967	1968	1969	1970	1971	1972
Ilosone	(Lilly)	$21.25	N.A.	$21.91	$21.87	$21.46	$21.76	$21.80	$21.23	$19.09
Pediamycin	(Ross)*	18.00	18.78	18.24	17.92	18.49	17.78	17.12	18.42	18.40
E-Mycin	(Upjohn)	N.A.	N.A.	N.A.	N.A.	21.77	22.05	17.26	14.77	11.71
Erythrocin	(Abbott)	22.04	22.21	18.24	22.21	22.35	22.19	22.25	20.23	14.71

Source: U.S. Pharmaceutical Market, Drug Stores, IMS America, Ltd., 1964–72; effective prices were obtained by dividing dollar sales values by units sold for various years.
N.A.: Not available.
*100 tabs, 250 mg.

prospect of new entrants to the erythromycin market with the expiration of the patent served as another spur.

As we have seen, Abbott and Lilly responded to Upjohn's price cuts with their own, notably in 1972. They reacted in this way even though the total market for erythromycin continued to grow in this period and their absolute sales continued to increase. It is likely that their sales in dollars would have grown even more had they not made the price cuts. Apparently they were responding to the threat of further growth in Upjohn's share rather than to the actual growth, for Upjohn's share was still small, even after the growth. In addition, they may have been reacting to the entry and the plans for entry of other firms. In 1971 Bristol entered, and in 1972 Parke Davis, Squibb, Smith-Kline, and Robins entered. Pfizer, McKesson and Phillips-Roxane followed suite in 1973.

AMPICILLIN. In 1963 Bristol-Myers (Polycillin), and American Home Products, through its subsidiary Ayerst (Penbritin), entered into the manufacture of ampicillin under a license from the discoverer, Beecham. Bristol granted sub-licenses, and by 1972 there were eleven major firms in this market. Each new entrant, with one exception (Parke Davis), adopted a low-price strategy and entered the market with its product priced lower than the leading product, Polycillin, and also lower than the products which had entered earlier (table 12-17).

In addition, several companies infringed on the patent. Most notable was a producer located in Italy which obtained FDA certification and supplied bulk ingredients to about 40 U.S. generic manufacturers. Bristol brought suit against

TABLE 12-17
New Entrants and Their Effective Prices at the Time of Entry Compared to the Price of Polycillin (Bristol) (100 caps., 250 mg.)

	1964	1966	1967	1968	1969	1972	1973
Polycillin (Bristol)	$26.85	$27.09	$25.88	$21.67	$21.54	$15.57	$13.80
Penbritin (Ayerst)	26.00						
Omnipen (Wyeth)		25.58					
Principen (Squibb)			19.20				
Amcill				21.12			
(Parke Davis)							
Alpen (Lederle)					19.21		
Totacillin					20.00		
(Beecham)							
Pensyn (Upjohn)						8.42	
SK-Ampicillin							11.61
Pen-A (Pfizer)							6.35

Source: Estimated from *U.S. Pharmaceutical Market, Drug Stores,* IMS America, Ltd., 1964–73.

these generic manufacturers, who responded in turn with suits against Bristol for violation of antitrust laws. The trial is still pending.

The consequence was that Bristol's share of the market dropped from 100 percent in 1963 to about one-quarter in 1973. The growth in total ampicillin sales permitted Bristol's sales, both in dollars and in units, to increase through 1969, but since then sales in dollars have declined, and sales in units have declined since 1971.

The two companies which had the greatest success in increasing their sales were Parke Davis (Amcill), and Squibb (Principen). Squibb has maintained the price of its product well below that of Polycillin, but above those of some of the other major firms (table 12-18). By contrast, Parke Davis priced its product at a higher level than all of the brands of major firms with the exception of Polycillin. Nevertheless, Parke Davis was able to sell large quantities. Only in 1970 did Parke Davis begin to cut its price aggressively. Despite the cuts, its sales declined in 1971.

The severe price competition has been associated with large promotional expenditures. Contrary to a frequent assertion, promotional expenditures have not been a substitute for price cuts. The promotional competition among the major sellers of ampicillin—including Bristol, Parke Davis, Squibb, as well as both divisions of American Home Products, Wyeth and Ayerst—has been severe. In 1969 Bristol's promotional expenditures in behalf of Polycillin reached nearly $5 million, and each of the others spent at least $2 million. Since then, promotional expenditures have declined.

Generic prescriptions have come to account for a large proportion of all prescriptions of ampicillin. Between 1966 and 1973, generic prescriptions have increased from 4 percent to 50 percent.

We will review the history of price competition in ampicillin. During the first four years following the introduction of Polycillin, prices on the whole were fairly stable (table 12-18). Ayerst offered its products, Penbritin, at a slightly lower price ($26.60) than that of Polycillin ($26.85). This strategy continued, and the differential increased over time.

In 1966 Wyeth, the other major pharmaceutical division of American Home Products, introduced Omnipen at a price of $25.65, which was below that of its affiliate, Ayerst ($25.88), while Polycillin's price was $27.09. As a result, in 1966 Polycillin's market share declined to less than three-quarters, although its absolute sales continued to increase dramatically. Bristol therefore kept its price to drug stores fairly firm in the fact of the new competition, but the average price to hospitals dropped from $25.21 in 1964 to $19.90 in 1966.

Competition became rough in 1967 with the entry of Squibb, which was to grow to be the second largest seller in the market, reaching nearly 20 percent of sales in 1971. Squibb employed the same strategy as it had employed earlier in the tetracycline market. Its prices were low, and it promoted its products among pharmacists and physicians. The range of prices for ampicillin prior to Squibb's

TABLE 12-18

Red Book and Effective Prices for Ampicillin, 1964–73 (100 caps., 250 mg.)

	1964	1965	1966	1967	1968	1969	1970	1971	1972	1973
					Red Book Prices					
Penbritin	$NA	$NA	$27.36	$27.36	$27.36	$21.82	$21.82	$21.82	$21.82	$21.82
Polycillin	NA	27.35	27.35	27.35	27.35	21.84	21.84	19.11	19.11	12.73
Principen				NA	NA	NA	19.00	19.00	19.00	12.67
Omnipen			NA	26.00	26.00	19.14	19.14	19.14	12.76	12.76
Amcill					NA	NA	21.60	21.60	19.14	12.76
					Effective Prices					
Penbritin	26.00	26.27	25.88	23.70	20.12	19.34	17.14	15.05	12.46	9.06
Polycillin	26.85	27.05	27.09	25.88	21.67	21.54	21.36	21.16	15.57	13.81
Principen			25.58	19.20	19.40	18.68	15.59	15.13	12.89	11.29
Omnipen				24.30	19.27	16.46	16.31	13.44	12.24	10.09
Amcill					21.12	21.14	16.41	13.19	11.66	8.84

Sources: *Drug Topics' Red Book, 1964–73,* and *U.S. Pharmaceutical Market, Drug Stores,* IMS America, Ltd., 1964–73.

entry had been from $26.00 to $27.00 per bottle. Squibb came in with a price close to $19.00 and the response was quick. Bristol reduced its price to less than $22.00, Ayerst to less than $21.00, and Wyeth to less than $20.00. At this time, Wyeth began to cut its price aggressively.

Despite its price cuts, Polycillin's market share contined to decline. One of the factors contributing to the decline was that by 1967 about 10 percent of new prescriptions were generic prescriptions, which were going to competitors.

In 1968, Parke Davis introduced Amcill. The price was higher than that of all brands except Polycillin, but the company's market share increased to over 12 percent of sales in 1971.

In 1969 the price difference between Polycillin and other brands widened. Earlier, the difference had rarely been more than $2.50, but by the end of 1969 the difference between the price of Omnipen (Wyeth) and Polycillin was more than $5.00. In addition, in the following year, sales of Polycillin began to decline. Nevertheless, Bristol held its prices during 1969.

In the same year, Wyeth cut its price further. In an apparent attempt to increase its market share, Wyeth cut its price from $19.25 to $17.00 in September. Squibb responded with a price cut to $17.86. In December Wyeth cut the price further to $16.17. Nevertheless, Wyeth continued to lose its market share, and in 1970 its sales actually declined.

In 1970 the growth of the market as a whole was smaller than it had been in previous years. Squibb's share continued to grow, and it became the second leading product. Parke Davis shifted its strategy to cutting prices and by the end of the year was selling at the second lowest price. Beecham and Lederle had entered the previous year, but in 1970 their sales were less than $2 million each.

Total sales of ampicillin declined in 1971, and by this year generics consti-tuted 34 percent of all new prescriptions. Bristol was suffering most from the growth in generic prescriptions, owing to its relatively high price. In spite of its low price, Parke Davis was unsuccessful in building sales. In 1971 SmithKline entered the market and broke the $10.00 floor.

The history of the ampicillin market bears out our expectations. Major firms with small market shares undertook aggressive price cutting in order to increase these shares. Squibb was highly successful and once it reached a large share of the market, it ceased to cut its prices aggressively. Other firms which then had small shares took the initiative. The market leader was reluctant to respond with price cuts until its sales actually declined, but eventually its prices did come down. We have also seen that the continued entry of large firms into this market encouraged doctors to prescribe generically. Pharmacists apparently filled the generic prescriptions largely with brands which were lower in price than that of the market leader.

PHENOXYMETHYL POTASSIUM PENICILLIN. Phenoxymethyl potassium penicillin, or penicillin VK, is an oral semisynthetic form of penicillin which is used to treat streptococcus, pneumococcus staphylococcus, and other infections. It has a high degree of substitutability with oral penicillin G. Penicillin VK has the advantages of greater stability than oral penicillin in the presence of digestive fluids, and a somewhat higher blood level of the active agent. There is no significant difference between penicillin VK and penicillin V (no potassium). Like other oral penicillins, penicillin VK is generally prescribed for a short course of therapy (10 days), and most (80 percent) prescriptions are new.

Total sales of oral penicillins (which include oral ampicillin) grew from $114.9 million in 1968 to $134.5 million in 1972. Sales of penicillin VK grew from $24.6 million in 1968 to $38.0 million in 1972. The rate of growth of 11.5 percent per year was faster than that of the total oral penicillin market of 4 percent per year. Penicillin VK increased its share of the "oral" penicillin market from 21.4 percent in 1968 to 28.3 percent in 1972.

The total penicillin therapeutic category is highly concentrated with a four-firm concentration of 75.1 percent in 1971, (eight-firm concentration ratio was 94.0 percent). There is some significant variation over time in the market shares of individual firms, if not in their relative positions. The concentration ratio of firms in the oral penicillin market is also high.

The examination of the penicillin VK market is divided into two phases, 1967–69 and 1970–72. The first phase, which brackets the expiration of the patent on July 31, 1968, was marked by severe price cuts by the market leaders (table 12-19). Effective prices declined from about $13.75 per 100 250-mg. tablets to about $8.90 per 100 250-mg. tablets. Lederle, the only new entrant during this period, entered in November 1968 with a price which was 25 percent below that of the leaders, but it did not respond to retaliatory cuts by the

TABLE 12-19
Red Book Prices of Phenoxymethyl Potassium Penicillin (100 caps., 250 mg.)

	1967	1968	1969	1970	1971	1972	1973
V-Cillin-K (Lilly)	$14.46	$11.55	$8.95	–	–	–	$8.95
Compocillin-VK (Abbott)	14.46	14.46	8.95	–	–	–	8.95
Pen-Vee-K (Wyeth)	14.62	14.00	8.90	–	–	–	8.90
Ledercillin-VK (Lederle)	–	NA	NA	7.34	–	–	7.34
Uticillin-VK (Upjohn)	–	–	–	NA	NA	6.48	6.48
Veetids (Squibb)	–	–	–	NA	NA	7.05	7.05
Betapen (Bristol)	–	–	–	NA	7.07	–	7.07
Pfizer-pen-VK (Pfizer)	–	–	–	–	NA	NA	7.00
Robicillin-VK (Robins)	–	–	–	–	NA	6.60	6.60
SK-Pen-VK (SmithKline)	–	–	–	–	NA	NA	NA
Kessor Pen-VK (McKesson)	–	–	–	–	–	6.25	6.25
Penapar-VK (Parke Davis)	–	–	–	–	–	NA	6.50

Source: Drug Topics' Red Book, 1967–73.
NA: Not available.
–No change.

market leaders. Ledercillin VK was able to achieve a market share of over 6 percent of penicillin VK sales during 1969.

The price chronology of the period is approximately as follows. In 1966–67, Wyeth, which was one of the market leaders, started to cut prices aggressively through special deals on its brand Pen-Vee-K (table 12-20). Lilly (V-Cillin-K) and Abbott (Compocillin-VK) responded with equally aggressive price cutting in 1967–68 which resulted in a 25 percent decline in prices before the patent expired in 1968. Then, as we just saw, Lederle entered and cut the price even more. The price erosion continued until 1969, when prices of the market leaders stabilized slightly below the new list prices of $8.90–$8.95. Lederle's price remained at $7.64. Price-cutting in 1966–68 cannot be ascribed to the new entry, which did not take place until November 1968. Yet price declines by the two market leaders was over 23 percent for the entire year.

Prices were stable in the early part of the second period. Eight additional sellers, all of whose prices were below those of the market leaders, entered.

As in the tetracycline and ampicillin markets, Squibb (Veetids) adopted an aggressive price policy. Squibb undercut the prices of the established brands by roughly $1.90 on the 100 tablet 250-mg. bottle. Squibb was able to maintain the lowest price per tablet to the retailer. In 1971 its price was $7.05 (list), compared to $8.95 for V-Cillin-K and $8.90 for Pen-Vee-K. In its first year it was able to achieve sales which amounted to over 5 percent of the market and its market share has not grown since then.

The market share of both Lilly and Abbott suffered as a result of the entry of the new firms. The sales and market share of Compocillin-VK declined. The sales of V-Cillin-K remained approximately constant despite the growth of the market. In 1972 Wyeth responded with price cuts, and Lilly went along. The price of Pen-Vee-K was cut to $7.44 and that of V-Cillin K to $8.31. In 1973 Pen-Vee-K's price was cut further to $6.81.

The development of this market clearly illustrates several points. Price cuts do occur prior to patent expiration and the entry of other firms. Wyeth, for example, cut its price during the early part of the period. Further, the "old" firms are more sensitive to each other's prices than to those of new entrants. Generic prescribing played a minor role. Generic drugs had little impact on the market in the four years subsequent to patent expiration. Total sales of Kesso-Pen (usually classified as a generic despite its own brand name) and the not otherwise specified category in 1972 totaled less than 0.3 percent of the market. Generic prescriptions were under 7 percent of those written in 1971; they did, however, rise to 14 percent in 1973. But, as we have seen, generic prescribing was not required for price competition.

Furthermore, the entry of new firms into a market may be delayed. The penicillin VK market was very attractive for many reasons: it was a large market; it was growing; and there were many firms in the wider oral penicillin market which were well situated for entry. Despite these enticements, only one of nine entrants entered in the year of patent expiration; three delayed two years; three

TABLE 12-20

Effective Drug Store Prices of Phenoxymethyl Potassium Penicillin (100 caps., 250 mg.)

	1965	1966	1967	1968	1969	1970	1971	1972
V-Cillin-K (Lilly)	$16.56	$14.38	$13.17	$10.05	$8.89	$8.91	$8.85	$8.55
Compocillin-VK (Abbott)	–	13.75	13.19	10.29	8.63	9.08	8.72	8.20
Pen-Vee-K (Wyeth)	15.00	11.29*	11.77	10.07	8.98	9.01	8.38	7.44
Ledercillin-VK (Lederle)	–	–	–	7.32	7.64	7.57	7.27	6.51
Uticillin-VK (Upjohn)	–	–	–	–	–	6.45	6.22	5.82
Veetids (Squibb)	–	–	–	–	–	7.12	7.07	6.65
Betapen-VK (Bristol)	–	–	–	–	–	7.83	7.73	6.39
Pfizer-Pen-VK (Pfizer)**	–	–	–	–	–	–	6.84	6.20
Robicillin-VK (Robins)	–	–	–	–	–	–	6.70	6.17
SK-Pen-VK (SmithKline)	–	–	–	–	–	–	4.88	5.75
Kesso-Pen-VK (McKesson)	–	–	–	–	–	–	–	5.83
Penapar-VK (Parke Davis)	–	–	–	–	–	–	–	5.51

Source: U.S. Pharmaceutical Market, Drug Stores, IMS America, Ltd., 1965–72.

Note: Price is equal to sales divided by unit.

*Based on very small number of observations.

**100 caps 400 mg.

entered three years after the expiration of the patent; and two entered four years later. The response of firms to a patent expiration is not certain or immediate. But, when their entry did occur, price competition became vigorous.

Finally, one cannot ignore the role of maverick firms. In this case, Squibb's policy of competing on price was an important factor in the decline of prices.

PRICE COMPETITION IN DRUGS OTHER THAN ANTIBIOTICS

So far there has been little price competition in multiple-source drugs other than antibiotics. Although patents no longer exclude entry, as yet there has been little entry to these markets by major firms. Small generic producers have entered in large numbers, and in some cases they have taken a large share of the market measured in number of units sold. But the original producer usually has not responded with price cuts to the entry of small generic companies. In other cases, major firms have entered with products at lower prices than that of the original producer, but it is too early to evaluate their effect. They still have a very small share of the market.

RESERPINE. Since reserpine is a natural product which has been known for many years, no product patent has covered it. Even as far back as 1963 many small generic firms manufactured the drug, and in that year generic prescriptions accounted for as much as 28 percent of all prescriptions.[11] By 1973 the share had grown to 57 percent. The growth took place at the expense of the share of the leading brand-name product, Serpasil (Ciba), which declined from more than half to about one-third over the same period.

Upjohn, Squibb, and SmithKline are the other firms manufacturing reserpine. Their sales, however, have been trivial. Total sales of reserpine alone do not exceed $5 million. Nor have firms been encouraged to increase their selling efforts by growth in total sales of reserpine. The growth has occured in the closely related rauwolfia diuretics, which are combination drugs and in non-rauwolfia hypotensives. The sales of the latter two groups are much larger, and many of the major firms are represented there.

It is not surprising, therefore, that the prices of Serpasil and Butiserpine show little change over the entire period (table 12-21). With no patent it is likely that prices have been too close to marginal cost to allow much room for downward price movement in the face of rising cost. As a matter of fact, the price of Butiserpine has increased over the 1964–72 period, although not as rapidly as the general level of prices of all goods.

MEPROBAMATE. The two major brands of meprobamate at the time that the patent expired in 1972 were Equanil (Wyeth) and Miltown (Wallace), and they continue to be the only brands of major firms which have significant sales. SmithKline and Parke Davis entered this market recently, but their sales remain

TABLE 12-21
Red Book and Effective Prices of Reserpines, 1960–72

	1960	1961	1962	1963	1964	1965	1966	1967	1968	1969	1970	1971	1972
					Red Book prices								
Serapsil (1000 tabs., .25 mg.) (Ciba)	$39.50	–	–	–	–	–	–	–	–	–	–	–	$39.50
Butiserpine (100 tabs) (McNeil)	2.94	–	–	–	–	2.94	3.25	–	–	–	3.25	3.60	3.60
					Effective prices (1964–72)								
Serapsil (1000 tabs., .25 mg.) (Ciba)					35.02	35.14	34.01	34.74	34.54	34.17	33.96	34.71	34.50
Butiserpine (100 tabs) (McNeil)					2.90	3.02	3.18	3.23	3.21	3.21	3.49	3.54	3.43

Sources: Drug Topics' Red Book, 1960–72; U.S. Pharmaceutical Market, Drug Stores, IMS America Ltd.
–No Change.

very small. No other major firms have attempted to enter. The reluctance to enter at the time that the patent expired may have been owing to the fact that Librium, which was introduced in 1960, and Valium, which was introduced in 1963, were highly successful new minor tranquilizers. Their influence can be seen in the decline in sales of meprobamate (table 12-22). A large number of small firms did enter the market upon the expiration of the patent, and by 1973, there were more than thirty firms selling meprobamate in the United States. [12]

Despite the absence of entry by a major firm over most of the period since the expiration of the patent, the number of generically written prescriptions increased enormously. Generically written prescriptions accounted for 10 percent of the total number of prescriptions in 1963 and 43 percent in 1973. As a result, Equanil's share of the number of prescriptions (not of dollar sales) declined from nearly 60 percent to about 40 percent, and that of Miltown went from one-third to one-fifth. The decline in the share of prescriptions written by brand name did not lead either Wyeth or Wallace to reduce their prices. Table 12-23 shows their effective prices from 1964 to 1973 and their list prices from 1960 to 1973. It is clear that the maintenance of prices by the two major firms in this market encouraged the increase in the number of generic prescriptions written. Despite the sharp decline in the share of the number of prescriptions written by brand name, the share of dollar sales of the two major firms did not decline appreciably during the period. Equanil's share remained about three fifths of the total, and Miltown's, which was about one-quarter of total sales at the beginning of the period, fell only slightly. However, the absolute dollar sales did decline as a result of the decline in the sales of meprobamate as a whole.

We can see that the original firms in the market behaved as we would expect them to. They did not cut their prices in an effort to retain their share of the total number of prescriptions in the face of entry by generic firms. Although this behavior did result in a loss of a large share of the total number of prescriptions,

TABLE 12-22
Sales of Meprobamates, 1963–73

	Sales ($000)		Sales ($000)
1963	52,497	1969	35,135
1964	53,366	1970	33,225
1965	44,525	1971	27,868
1966	38,287	1972	24,147
1967	40,450	1973	23,764
1968	40,084		

Source: U.S. Pharmaceutical Market, Drug Stores and Hospitals IMS America Ltd., 1963–73.

TABLE 12-23

Red Book and Effective Prices of Leading Meprobamates

	1960	1961	1962	1963	1964	1965	1966	1967	1968	1969	1970	1971	1972	1973
						Red Book Price								
Equanil	$3.25	–	$3.25	$2.90	–	$2.90	$3.25	–	–	$3.25	$3.65	–	–	$3.65
Miltown	3.25	–	–	–	–	–	–	3.12	–	–	–	–	–	$3.12
						Effective Price								
Equanil	NA	NA	NA	NA	2.95	–	–	2.99	3.03	3.33	NA	3.46	3.30	3.35
Miltown	NA	NA	NA	NA	3.26	3.16	3.20	3.24	3.24	2.91	3.26	3.22	3.17	3.19

Source: Drug Topics' Red Book, 1960–73; *U.S. Pharmaceutical Market, Drug Stores*, IMS America, Ltd., merica, Ltd., 1960–73.
N.A.: Not available.
–Unchanged.

the share of dollar sales was maintained. Price cuts would have resulted in a sharper decline in the total share of dollar sales.

We should observe that although the prices of the brand-name products were maintained, the average price paid did decline as a result of the increase in the share of total prescriptions written generically.

CHLORPROMAZINE. Chlorpromazine is a major tranquilizer which is used in the treatment of schizophrenia and other psychoses. The major market for this product is institutional. The patent, which was held by SmithKline, expired in 1970. In an apparent effort to discourage entry, the company cut its price in the same year by about 25 percent.

Only Parke Davis and USV, among the other major firms, has entered into the manufacture of the oral dosage form. One small firm sells another branded generic. Wyeth has entered with an injectable form. With the exception of Wyeth, which entered late in 1972, none of the other companies entered before 1973. In that year, their sales of chlorpromazine were very small.

It is too early as yet to see the full effect of the patent expiration and the entry of firms in the chlorpromazine market. Apparently the price cut by SmithKline on the expiration of its patent was effective in discouraging entry, for the firms that did enter did not do so for about three years. Even then, the number that entered was very small.

PROPOXYPHENE HCL. The patent on propoxyphene HCL expired in 1972. Lilly held the patent on this non-narcotic analgesic drug and has sold it under the brand name Darvon. In 1972 the sales of this product amounted to $17.4 million. Lilly has not been dependent on the single entity form of Darvon for the major part of its analgesic sales. For some time now it has been selling Darvon-Compound 65, which is a combination drug that contains aspirin, phenacetin, and caffeine as well as propoxyphene HCL. In addition, Lilly recently developed a new Darvon combination drug which it has given the brand name of Darvon-N. The active ingredient is propoxyphene napsylate and it is patent-protected. In recent years, the comparative effectiveness of Darvon as an analgesic has been challenged by studies which find it to be no more effective than aspirin. Nevertheless, the sales of Darvon have been well maintained.

In 1973 SmithKline entered the market, but so far its sales remain very small; sales by all other producers of propoxyphene HCL other than Lilly added up to less than $750 thousand in 1973. The prices of these other manufacturers' products to drug stores were set at about half that of Darvon. Lilly has not felt it necessary as yet to respond to these new competitors with reductions in its own price. One reason is that generic prescribing remains a very small fraction of the total number of prescriptions. It is too early to predict the course of the prices of the various propoxyphene HCL products. If other major companies enter the market and the entrants promote their products and sell them at much lower prices than that of Darvon, they are likely to take a larger share of the market. Lilly still may not choose to cut its prices, but the average price of propoxyphene should then come down.

NITROGLYCERINE. Nitroglycerine, which is a very old drug, is used in the treatment of angina pectoris. Generic prescriptions account for over three quarters of all prescriptions. The major brands are Nitrobid (Marion), Nitroglycerine (Lilly), and Nitrospan (USV). In this area, the small firm, Marion, has the leading position. Lilly, the only major firm with any significant share, had a much stronger position at the beginning of the 1960s than it currently has. Lilly's share of prescriptions has declined from about one-fifth to slightly more than 1 percent.

Prices have been generally stable. The manufacturers of different products did make small changes, but it cannot be said that there was any sharp price competition. One reason may be that the prices are low in relation to marginal cost. The price per 100 2.5-mg tablets is about $6.25, which is significantly lower than prices of most new drugs introduced since 1960.

DIGOXIN. Digoxin is a form of digitalis which is a drug used to treat heart failure. The market is not large, but it contains many sellers. Total sales do not exceed $7.1 million and are dominated by Lanoxin (Burroughs Wellcome), which had sales of $6.8 million in 1973. The price of Lanoxin seems to be unaffected by the generics; it fell from around $30.50 per 5000 .25-mg tablets in 1967 to around $26.00 in 1970, but then rose to around $28.00 in 1973. Due to its large share of the market, Burroughs Wellcome has been able to maintain price and not feel any pressure. Any price cut would only serve to decrease sales revenue.

CONSUMERS' BENEFITS FROM MANUFACTURERS' PRICE COMPETITION

Does price competition among manufacturers benefit consumers? As we have seen, when a large manufacturer reduces the price of a product, it will tend to increase its share of the market. This increase, however, may be the result of pharmacists taking all or most of the reduction in a larger retail margin. The pharmacist may substitute the low-price product for other products, and he may use it to fill generically written prescriptions. But the price that he charges customers may not be affected. To the extent that the retail market is competitive, price cuts at the wholesale level will be passed on to consumers. However, we do not know the extent of competition at the retail level. The R_xOTC, Inc., survey provides data which we can use to answer the question of how much the consumer saves as a result of manufacturers' price competition.

We will consider first the savings to consumers resulting from writing generic rather than brand-name prescriptions. The magnitude of the saving depends on whether a generic product or a brand product is used and on which brand product is used to fill such a prescription. Our comparisons will be among the arithmetic mean price of all generic prescriptions regardless of how filled, that of generically filled generic prescriptions, and the mean prices of prescriptions specifying brand name products which are filled as specified. For example, the arithmetic mean retail price for all generic prescriptions for ampicillin is $4.44, which is below the prices of prescriptions calling for the leading brand-name product, Polycillin, which are filled as specified (table 12-24). The mean price of such prescriptions is $5.05. It is also less than the prices of prescriptions of most of the other brand-name products filled as specified. But it is not below the average retail price of two brand-name products. These products are Pen-A and Totacillin; it is worth noting that the manufacturer's price for these products is relatively low, as we have seen.

TABLE 12-24
Comparison of Arithmetic Mean Retail Prices among
Prescriptions Filled for Ampicillin and Erythromycin
(20 tablets, 250 mg.)

	Average Retail Price
Ampicillin	
All generic	$4.44
Generic filled generically	4.31
Brand-name prescriptions filled as specified	
Polycillin	5.05
Amcill	5.08
Pen A	4.17
SK-Amp	4.65
Principen	4.69
Penbritin	4.94
Totacillin	4.30
Omnipen	5.11
Erythromycin	
All Generic	$4.58
Generic filled generically	4.21–4.31*
Brand-name prescriptions filled as specified	
Bristamycin	4.80
Erypar	4.46
Pfizer E	4.28
SK-Erythromycin	4.28
Ethril	4.32
Erythrocin	5.30
Ilosone	5.64
E-mycin	4.77

Source: R_xOTC, Inc., Philadelphia, Pa., 1973.
*Varies by type of generic product described by color of tablet.

The average price of all generic prescriptions for erythromycin is $4.58 compared to $5.30 for Erythrocin and $5.64 for Ilosone. The average savings to a consumer from a generic prescription compared to one specifying either of the leading brands is appreciable. Once again we see that there is no saving when the comparison is made among the retail prices of low price brands.

When generic prescriptions are filled with generic products, the savings to consumers are larger. Thus, the average retail price of a generic prescription for ampicillin which is filled generically is $4.31. Again, however, this price is not below that of brand products whose wholesale prices are low. In the case of erythromycin, savings to consumers result from generic prescriptions filled generically rather than by brand names. On the other hand, the average price of such prescriptions is only slightly below the price of some of the low-price brands.

Pharmacists have pressed for the right to substitute freely within the same generic class for drugs specified in a prescription on the ground that substitution will result in significant savings to consumers. According to this argument, the pharmacist can judge the quality of different drugs, and he will use low-price drugs when these are available and are of as good quality as the high-price drugs within the same class. The R_xOTC survey permits us to determine whether or not pharmacists do pass on to consumers savings resulting from substitution.

The average price of substitutes for Polycillin, Amcill, and Omnipen is lower than the prices of prescriptions which are filled as specified (table 12-25). It can be that the prices at the manufacturer's level of these three products are relatively high. On the other hand, when brand-name products whose manufacturers' prices are low are called for, substitution does not in general result in lower prices. In the case of Pen-A, for example, the price of the prescription is much higher when a substitute is used than when it is filled as specified. The same thing is true to a lesser degree for Penbritin and Totacillin.

The conclusion regarding the effect of substitution of erythromycin prescriptions is similar. Substitution results in savings to consumers only when the prescription calls for either Ilosone, Bristamycin, or Erypar.

The other question which we take up here is the effect of manufacturers' price cuts on retail prices. Table 12-26 shows the difference between the manufacturers' price and the retail price for each of the brand name products of ampicillin. We can see that the pharmacist obtains a large part of the difference in price between brand-name products. When a manufacturer offers a product at a lower price than that of the leading brand, the consumer does not receive the full benefit. Thus differences between manufacturers' and retail prices tend to vary inversely with manufacturers' prices. A similar pattern can be observed in the retail pricing of erythromycin product.

We can estimate the part of the reduction in price at the manufacturers' level which is passed on to consumers. The regression coefficient for ampicillin in equation 12.2 in Table 12-27 is 0.44. This means that when a manufacturers' price for a brand is $1.00 less than that of another manufacturers' brand, the

TABLE 12-25
Arithmetic Mean Prices of Prescriptions Written by Brand and Filled
As Specified and of Prescriptions Written by Indicated Brand but
Filled with a Substitute

	Average Price Filled as Specified	Average Price When Another Drug is Substituted
Ampicillin		
Polycillin	$5.05	$4.44
Amcill	5.08	4.78
Pen A	4.17	4.56
Sk Amp	4.65	4.46
Principen	4.69	4.69
Penbritin	4.94	5.14
Totacillin	4.30	5.03
Omnipen	5.11	4.56
Erythromycin		
Bristamycin	4.80	4.51
Erypar	4.46	4.37
Pfizer E	4.28	4.70
SK-Erythromycin	4.28	4.45
Ethril	4.32	4.44
Erythrocin	5.30	5.30
Ilosone	5.64	5.30
E-mycin	4.77	5.45

Source: R_xOTC, Inc. Philadelphia, Pa., 1973.

TABLE 12-26
Differences between Manufacturers' Average Effective Price
1973 and Average Retail Price of Prescriptions Filled by
Brand as Specified

	Manufacturer	Retail	Difference
Ampicillin			
Polycillin	$2.76	$5.05	$2.29
Amcill	1.77	5.08	3.31
Pen A	1.27	4.17	2.80
SK-Amp	2.32	4.65	2.23
Principen	2.26	4.69	2.43
Penbritin	1.81	4.94	3.13
Totacillin	1.66	4.30	2.64
Omnipen	2.02	5.11	3.07
Erythromycin			
Bristamycin	2.04	4.80	2.76
Erypar	1.63	4.46	2.83
Pfizer E	1.56	4.28	2.72
SK-Erythromycin	1.97	4.28	2.31
Ethril	1.53	4.32	2.79
Erythrocin	2.59	5.30	2.71
Ilosone	3.90	5.64	1.74
E-mycin	2.18	4.77	2.59

Source: R_xOTC, Inc. Philadelphia, Pa., 1973.

consumer's gain is only $.44 (the retail price is only $.44 lower). The difference, or $.56, is obtained by the pharmacist. The statistical nonsignificance of the regression coefficient indicates that the retail margins on different brands are not closely related to the manufacturers' prices. The nonsignificance is also due to the fact that the estimate is based on only eight observations.

A similar regression equation was run for erythromycin. In this case the results are highly significant, as can be seen in equation 12.3. The regression coefficient is equal to 0.60, which means that the consumer received $.60 out of a reduction of $1.00 in the price at the manufacturers' level, and the pharmacist received $.40.

It is also of interest to estimate the savings from manufacturers' price cuts realized by consumers who have generic prescriptions filled by brand-name products. In other words, when a pharmacist receives a generic prescription, does his price to the customer reflect the manufacturer's price for the brand which the pharmacist chooses? Equation 12.4 shows that in the case of ampicillin the consumer receives $.49 of each dollar difference between manufacturers' prices. This result is not very different from the one which we observed in the case of prescriptions filled as specified. However, among generic prescriptions, the relationship is much more significant. The corresponding equation for erythromycin shows no saving to consumers resulting from manufacturers' price cuts (eq. 12.5).

The third analysis is confined to prescriptions for which substitutes were used. In other words, the prescription called for a specified brand but another brand was in fact used. The regression equation for ampicillin (eq. 12.6) has a very large coefficient, 0.84, which indicates that in such prescriptions the consumer receives a large part of the manufacturers' price cut. The corresponding equation applied to erythromycin (eq. 12.7) indicates that the consumer receives about half of any price cut that a manufacturer makes. The high standard error relative to the regression coefficient indicates that retail pricing by pharmacists substituting one brand of erythromycin for another does not closely follow the indicated pattern.

We can conclude that drug retailing is sufficiently competitive for retailers to pass on to consumers part of the savings resulting from manufacturers' price competition. But, it is not sufficiently competitive for the consumers to receive the full benefit of such price competition among manufacturers.

CONCLUSIONS

The antibiotics market has seen a great deal of price competition among drug companies, both large and small, and price competition has set in even before the expiration of patents. The introductory argument emphasized the importance of the excess of average cost over marginal cost as a source of price competition. The discussion also stressed the importance of the distribution of

TABLE 12-27

Regression Equations Measuring Relationship between
Manufacturers' Prices' of Brands of Ampicillin and
Erythromycin and Average Retail Prices in 1973

A. For prescriptions specifying brand-name products and
filled as specified

Ampicillin $\quad R_{a_1} = 3.88 + .44W_a \quad$ (12.2)
$\qquad\qquad$ (t = 1.65) $\quad r^2 = .31$
$\qquad\qquad$ (SE = .27) $\quad F = 2.72$

Erythromycin $\quad R_{e_1} = 3.43 + .60W_e \quad$ (12.3)
$\qquad\qquad$ (t = 5.98) $\quad r^2 = .86$
$\qquad\qquad$ (SE = .10) $\quad F = 35.72$

B. For generic prescriptions filled by brand-name products

Ampicillin $\quad R_{a_2} = 3.54 + .49W_a \quad$ (12.4)
$\qquad\qquad$ (t = 2.50) $\quad r^2 = .51$
$\qquad\qquad$ (SE = .20) $\quad F = 6.24$

Erythromycin $\quad R_{e_2} = 4.92 - .05W_e \quad$ (12.5)
$\qquad\qquad$ (t = 1.41) $\quad r^2 = .03$
$\qquad\qquad$ (SE = .114) $\quad F = .167$

C. For prescriptions written for other brands but substituted by brands to which prices correspond

Ampicillin $\quad R_{a_3} = 2.83 + .84W_a \quad$ (12.6)
$\qquad\qquad$ (t = 2.91) $\quad r^2 = .59$
$\qquad\qquad$ (SE = .29) $\quad F = 8.48$

Erythromycin $\quad R_{e_3} = 3.66 + .50W_e \quad$ (12.7)
$\qquad\qquad$ (t = 1.94) $\quad r^2 = .38$
$\qquad\qquad$ (SE = .26) $\quad F = 3.74$

R = Mean retail price of brand-name product used to fill
prescription, as estimated by R_xOTC, Inc., on basis
of survey of June 1973.
W = Manufacturers' mean effective price of brand-name
product used to fill prescription based on IMS reports
of purchases by drug stores in 1973.
Subscripts: a = ampicillin; e = erythromycin; 1 = prescriptions specifying brand-name products and filled as specified; 2 = generic prescriptions filled by brand-name products; 3 = substituted prescriptions.

sales among many products within each company. Under these conditions firms which come into a market late are inclined to cut prices severely, and the original firms in any antibiotic market would be reluctant to do so. The price histories did not uniformly conform to the expected pattern of price competition. Thus, the two leading manufacturers of erythromycin cut their prices substantially well before the patent expired and prior to the entry of other firms. In the market for penicillin VK, it was again firms with established brands which began to cut prices sharply before entry occurred. The ampicillin market is the one which fulfills the prediction most closely. In this case, the new entrants continuously initiated the price cuts and the leading firm delayed its own price cuts for a long time. Similarly, in tetracycline the aggressive price competition came from firms with small market shares. Nevertheless, the model presents a roughly correct description of the price competition in antibiotic markets generally. In all of these markets, the firms with smaller shares were aggressive price cutters and those with larger shares tended to hold back. And in all of them the firms with the large shares eventually were forced to cut their prices due to losses in their shares of the market.

The markets other than antibiotics have not as yet seen a great deal of price competition among the major companies, and the leading brands have been able to maintain their prices. Entry by major companies is relatively recent; there has not yet been enough time for the major companies to have had a significant effect on the market shares of the original brands. On the other hand, in some cases—notably meprobamate—generic products have succeeded in capturing a large share of the market without precipitating price cuts by the manufacturers of the original brands. A critical factor in these markets may be that they are not sufficiently large to attract entry of major firms.

Price competition among the major companies results in some savings to consumers. Pharmacists pass on to consumers a part, but not all, of the initial price cuts by the manufacturers. The review of the material concerning pharmacists also reveals that they have acted as price agents for consumers. Their behavior has contributed to the sensitivity of manufacturers to price cuts by competitors within the same generic class. Even when doctors do not write generic prescriptions or choose a low-price brand, pharmacists shift sales to generic products and to low-price brands. They substitute generic products and low-price brands for more expensive products even when prescriptions specify the high-price products and doctors do not authorize substitution. In addition, they have also used low-priced brands and generic products to fill generically written prescriptions.

Prices of antibiotic products have not come all the way down to marginal cost. This is the reason the prices of some generic products manufactured by relatively small companies are lower than the prices of major companies' products. Apparently, despite the great decline in the prices of antibiotic products manufactured by major companies, they are still sufficiently high to permit some contribution to the cost of overhead, R & D, and promotion. The generic products of the smaller companies have not taken over the market. The reasons may include the possibility of poor quality and the fear of pharmacists to use the products of small and unknown manufacturers. In part, the inability of the low-price generics to take a major share of the antibiotic market may be the continued importance of brand prescribing by doctors and the reluctance of many druggists to substitute generics for brands specified in the prescriptions without specific authorization. Finally, the generic products may have been unable to capture a larger share of the market because of limits on their capacity.

Prices in these markets, including the antibiotics markets, are likely to decline further. The leading companies have in the last two or three years developed long generic lines of products and have committed themselves to promoting these products on the basis of price. In addition, public policy has moved in the direction of encouraging price competition in the industry. Very recently the HEW developed what is known as the Maximum Allowable Cost (MAC) regulation to govern the policy concerning the reimbursement of drugs under the Medicaid program. HEW will reimburse patients for drugs purchased up to a price which is not greater than MAC, plus a dispensing fee. The MAC will be set at the level of the lowest generally available price for any widely available drug in the same generic class. Firms which seek sales to Medicaid patients will be required to reduce their prices to *consumers generally* to that of the lowest price of any drug which is widely available and in the same generic class. This regulation promises to precipitate competition in the markets for multiple-source drugs. It is likely to force prices down to levels which are considerably lower than the present levels.

CHAPTER 13

REVIEW OF ECONOMIC LITERATURE

INTRODUCTION

The monopoly issue dominates the economic literature on the drug industry, while other issues, which may be more important in relation to the development of public policy towards the drug industry, are neglected. The focus on the monopoly issue is partly the result of congressional concern with the evidence of some high drug prices which are thought to imply exploitation of consumers by the industry. In addition, the field of industrial organization, within which the investigation of the drug industry has fallen, has been devoted to the study of the economics of competition and monopoly in all industries. Accordingly, practitioners in the field who have studied the drug industry have been primarily concerned with the same issues, and they have used the traditional approaches and tools of analysis. The drug industry is simply one of many industries. That some issues may be peculiar to it is not noticed, nor that some of these issues may be more important for public policy than the monopoly issue.

For example, the literature does not pay much attention to the particular conditions within the industry which influence the rate of drug innovation. Furthermore, whatever attention economists give to this question is incidental to the monopoly issue, with the result that the focus on the monopoly issue distorts the view of innovation. Thus, economists have viewed drug innovations by firms merely as the byproduct of oligopolistic avoidance of price competition. Drug firms' innovations, according to this line of reasoning, are not major advances in therapy but only new products which are sufficiently different from their predecessors to avoid infringement of patents. The important innovations, according to this view, come from outside the industry. The usual conclusion has been that the structure and the resulting competitive behavior of the industry have produced high, rigid prices and persistent high profits. The competitive behavior itself, which is characterized by product differentiation, is regarded as the product of a market structure, the most prominent elements of which are the protection provided to manufacturers by patents and resulting high concentration. The alternative view which has been advanced in this study is that past innovations in this industry stimulated the demand for more innovations and also the expectation of continuing success. Firms, according to the present study, have been induced to invest in R & D by the expectation of a high rate of return on their investment. This conclusion, of course, leads to policy conclusions very different from the conclusions of other studies.

Before we review the economic literature on the drug industry, it will be useful to outline the standard approach used in the study of industries. There are three parts to the standard approach: structure, behavior, and performance of an industry.[1]

The structure of an industry consists of the technological and other characteristics which determine the competitive behavior of firms. One of the problems which students have with this approach is that the important elements of the structure appear to vary among industries, so it is difficult to come to any general conclusions about their respective importance in all industries or, for that matter, in any single industry. Be that as it may, the list of structural elements invariably includes the condition of entry. In other words, one of the questions concerns the ease of entry. Ease of entry is a difficult concept which has given many writers trouble. We should regard it as a continuous rather than a dichotomous variable. Further, entry becomes more difficult as the height of the price required to attract an additional firm increases. More precisely, ease of entry varies inversely with the difference between the price which is required to attract the entry of an additional firm and the long-run competitive price. Ease of entry is determined by, among other things, the importance of patents in a particular industry. If patents prevent imitation of established products, entry may be difficult. Entry is also difficult if the economies of scale of production require a minimum size of firm which is large in relation to a given market, for then the entry of an additional firm may bring the price down to a level which is below the competitive level or the long-run average cost. When entry is difficult, we can expect the market to include only a few sellers. The number of sellers, which is the result of the condition of entry, is itself a structural element.

Usually economists use the concept of the concentration ratio rather than that of the number of sellers, since a market may contain many small sellers having only a small aggregate share of the market and, therefore, having little influence on price. The concentration ratio is the share of sales accounted for by some small number of the largest sellers. One of the major sets of questions posed by an examination of the structure of any market thus usually concerns the concentration ratio and its determinants. Indeed the structure of a market is seen as having its chief influence on competitive behavior through its effect on the concentration ratio. The prediction is that when there are only a few sellers each will be reluctant to provoke retaliation by cutting prices, and therefore, a high concentration ratio indicates monopoly power. Rivals in oligopolistic markets plausibly are expected to retaliate to price cuts because it would be suicidal for them not to do so, the effect of price differences on market shares being certain. They will prefer to compete by product differentiation. The effect of such differentiation is less certain and imitation which does not infringe on patent rights is more difficult.

Studies of the competitive behavior of firms examine the extent of the various types of competition, including price, product, and promotional competition. Thus, the studies look for evidence of collusion among sellers with respect to price or evidence of tacit understandings which limit price competition. These studies measure the frequency of price changes and their amplitude and attempt to assess the significance of the measurements against the background of an examination of the underlying changes in demand-and-supply conditions. They will also examine changes in products—quality changes, changes in the number of products—and they will try to assess the value of such changes to consumers. The discussion of promotional competition generally is from the standpoint that the less of it there is, the better. Promotional competition usually is viewed, at best, as an attempt by sellers to increase their sales without having to reduce prices and, at worst, as deception. The studies of promotional competition thus measure the proportion of sales which is spent on promotional activities, changes in the proportion, and evidence of interfirm rivalry in this area.

The appraisals of performances include assessments of the extent of the different types of competition. The literature approves of price competition, is ambivalent about product competition, and is hostile to promotional competition. Those industries, such as wheat growing, in which producers compete in price, produce a standard product, and spend nothing on promotion receive a high score for performance.

Economists have been skeptical of the value of product competition in general, since they see the important changes in product quality as emerging from scientific advances, which themselves are the product of the work of scientists in nonprofit laboratories rather than in industrial laboratories. Industrial efforts to alter products allegedly are intended only to differentiate them from those of their competitors at little cost and risk of failure, and they therefore allegedly usually consist of minor changes in appearance which do not add significantly to the utility of products to consumers but allow sellers to continue demanding high prices. This representation of the views of economists in the field of industrial organization with respect to quality competition may be a little unfair, but it is correct to say that the attitude has been ambivalent. Our own view is that product competition in some industries may be preferable to price competition. But discussions of performance in individual industries rarely attempt individual industry appraisals of the effects of product competition. To do so requires tedious attention to details of products and familiarity with the nuances of judgments of quality. More importantly we do not have a simple method of measuring the benefits of product improvements and translating them into price equivalents.

Studies of performance also assess the level of profits for evidence of exploitation of consumers. They generally take the position that if the average profit rate of firms in the industry persistently exceeds that in manufacturing as a whole, firms have been exploiting consumers. The same evidence is regarded as indicating monopoly power.

Finally, the studies look at the progressiveness and the efficiency of firms. These aspects of performance are difficult to appraise, owing to the absence of both standards and measurements. The main problem is that the studies must compare the cost of production with what the cost might be under some alternative market structure which does not exist. Despite the difficulties, attempts are made to pass judgment.

The chain of causation is traced from market structure, which is viewed as determined by conditions which are independent of the behavior of firms, including technology and characteristics of consumer demand, through competitive behavior, and finally to performance. The position is frequently taken, therefore, that it is necessary to alter the market structure in order to affect performance. This view runs into trouble if the market structure really is determined by technology, for then whatever may be done to correct the market structure may result in inefficiency and losses to consumers, and in any case the structure will revert to its original form. But the analysis becomes a little vague at this point, for the possibility is left open that what is regarded as part of the market structure, such as the degree of concentration, may be the result of actions of the firms, such as mergers, rather than of technologically inherent characteristics of the market.

The literature generally regards the model of perfect competition as representing an ideal market structure. The model specifies many sellers, homogeneous products, and quickly and readily available information concerning prices and quality. These conditions are seen to result in price competition and optimum performance, including maximum technical efficiency within a given technology and socially optimal outputs and prices. The analysis predicts with less confidence that competition defined in this narrow fashion will result in a high rate of innovation: the ideal environment for innovation is regarded as one in which many sellers compete for sales by introducing new techniques and products. This theory, which lacks empirical support, nevertheless has had enormous intuitive appeal.

STRUCTURE OF THE INDUSTRY

CONDITIONS OF DEMAND. The literature has selected the insensitivity of doctors to price differences between drugs as the most important characteristic of demand. This selection is partly owing to the influence of the approach, described in the introduction to this chapter, which gives primary importance to price competition, and also to the ambivalence of economists to product competition. Thus, according to Steele and Walker, doctors are less sensitive to price than consumers would be were they to make their own choices.[2] Frequently, doctors are not even aware of drug prices, for their principal source of information, *The Physicians' Desk Reference,* does not report prices. Steele and Walker believe that in the face of competition from other firms which sell good substitutes at lower prices, this insensitivity has the effect of permitting firms to maintain their sales without reducing prices.

One of the reasons offered for the insensitivity of doctors to prices is their susceptibility to the advertising appeals of drug companies.[3] Steele and Walker believe that identical generic titles indicate identical therapeutic properties. In addition, Steele believes that each therapeutic class includes several good substitutes, even though they may have different generic titles.[4]

According to Steele, in 1959 there were seven corticosteroids which were interchangeable in the treatment of many disorders, as demonstrated by the fact that these drugs were prescribed in every one of the seven disease groups requiring this type of drug therapy. He also suggests that any of the seven major tranquilizers can be used for any one of the five disease groups requiring such therapy. His evidence for the latter judgment is that the maximum usage of a drug in any disease group was only 41.3 percent, which he suggests is not much larger than the rate of usage would have been if the drugs were used at random. Random usage would have resulted in each drug being prescribed for one-seventh, or 14.3 percent, of all cases in each type of disorder. But the difference between 41.3 and 14.3 percent is highly significant statistically. The use of different drugs for treatment of the same indication is not evidence, moreover, of the substitutability of these drugs for every patient. Usually doctors prescribe a drug for a patient not only on the basis of a broadly defined indication, but they are also guided by other characteristics of the patient, such as susceptibility to various side effects. The major tranquilizers have different side-effects.

Steele also supports his assertion that physicians have been vulnerable to advertising with the observation that 88 percent of all prescriptions are written for brand-name products.[5] Obviously, however, one of the principal reasons doctors use brand names rather than generic products is that for most generic classes, only a single brand-name product is available. Since 1962, when Steele wrote his piece, the number of multiple-source drugs has increased, and generic prescribing has also increased. Furthermore, the assurance of quality which is provided by a brand-name product provides an inducement to prescribe such products rather than generic products, the sources of which are unknown.

As for substitutability of drugs within the same generic classes, it is not always certain that they have the same therapeutic properties and side effects. The products of small firms which may have no adequate system of quality control may be of inferior quality, and doctors may continue to prescribe brand-name drugs in order to protect their patients.

Moreover, it is not necessary for all doctors to prescribe generically or even for most of them to do so in order for the sales of a brand-name product to be sensitive to price differences. We have seen that a large percentage of the prescriptions for multiple-source drugs are written generically and that the low-price brand-name products and generic products tend to be used by druggists to fill generic prescriptions. We have even seen that druggists will substitute low-price brand-name products and generic products for high-price brand-name products in the same generic class when they are not authorized to do so by prescribers, despite the fact that they are legally required to obtain such authorization. Thus the fact that not all doctors prescribe generically has not prevented the demand for multiple-source drugs from being sensitive to prices.

It is true that doctors are more interested in quality differences among drugs than they are in price differences, and this has resulted in a great emphasis on product changes in the competitive strategy of pharmaceutical firms. This interest in differences in therapeutic properties has several sources other than the influence of advertising. One of these is simply that the doctor is more concerned professionally with the treatment and comfort of patients than with the prices of drugs. Another source is drug innovation. When new products come on the market, doctors are primarily interested in the qualities of the different products. Firms therefore seek to develop and market new drugs and inform doctors of their properties. The emphasis on product competition and on promotion thus has its roots in the high rate of innovation which has characterized the drug industry over much of its recent history. It is not surprising that price has failed to be the major focus of competition in this market. Product and promotional competition did not arise from an avoidance of price competition, but were the direct consequence of innovation. The competition in quality and advertising need not preclude price competition.

BARRIERS TO ENTRY. *Patents.* Obviously a firm cannot enter a market with a drug which is identical to one which is under patent; this is the intent of the patent law, and its effectiveness in this respect generally is not questioned. An important issue concerns the effectiveness of patents in preventing the entry of firms into therapeutic fields with new drugs which are not identical to established drugs but which are sufficiently similar to compete with them for sales. Another question is whether drug companies have excluded entry through the use of patents on products which are never marketed. Still another issue is whether drug companies have deliberately improved products in some minor aspect in order to extend the protection provided by a patent after it expired. Finally, leading drug companies are accused of excluding entry by restricting licenses to each other. The leading firms allegedly have created an exclusive club through cross-licensing to which smaller companies are not admitted and thereby have maintained their monopoly power.

Walker demonstrates that patents cover drugs accounting for a major part of total sales. He refers to the fact that between two-thirds and three-quarters of all prescriptions written in 1958 were for patented drugs. He also shows that a major part of sales were accounted for by single-source drugs covered by patents and produced by a single firm. In 1961, 54 percent of sales were accounted for by patented drugs, each of which was produced by only a single firm.[6] Walker's book, published in 1971, refers to the late 1950s and early 1960s. Although a major part of sales still is accounted for by single-source drugs, multi-source drugs are now much important than they were in 1958–61.

Steele finds it necessary to observe that a patent reduces the number of producers of a drug. He compares the number of producers of unpatented drugs with the number producing each of thirty-eight patented drugs. Not surprisingly, he finds that the patented drugs have fewer producers.[7] The surprise in these data is that in some instances the number of producers of a patented drug exceeded that of an unpatented drug.

Some authors suggest that patents are not effective barriers to entry because of the ease with which pharmacueitcal manufacturers can develop drugs similar to if not identical with those which are patented. Comanor cites testimony by George Frost, a patent attorney representing the industry before the Kefauver Committee, that the patents have not been effective. According to Frost, a drug patent usually is limited to a single compound or a small number of compounds when it represents a small advance in knowledge, because the applicant cannot anticipate all variants of the compound, and it is frequently possible to develop and patent new products which are based on the concept covered in the original patent.[8] Scientists in the research laboratories of pharmaceutical companies follow the patents filed by other manufacturers in order to keep abreast of critical developments. In addition, as Kemp has shown, manufacturers entered the diuretics field by introducing new drugs similar to the original ones.[9]

The comments by Comanor and Frost and the experience in diuretics, as described by Kemp, suggest that patents do not bar entry to a therapeutic field by an established drug manufacturer and that such entry is only moderately difficult. The condition of entry in fields other than diuretics, however, may be more difficult than Kemp's observations indicate. Considering the size of the market, there are not many generically different antibiotics; a similar observation holds for the minor tranquilizers. In any case, a patent does prevent duplication. A patent therefore is at least moderately effective in protecting a company which introduces a new drug against the competition of imitators.

Walker suggests that drug manufacturers have excluded firms from the industry through the accumulation of a large number of patents. They allegedly prevent the introduction of new drugs by threatening patent infringement suits. Walker depends on the general statement by Kaysen and Turner that this is a device frequently used by large firms in many industries to exclude entry.[10] Walker also refers to the fact that pharmaceutical manufacturers have persistently patented many more compounds than they have marketed. Thus, according to Walker, between 1950 and 1960, the mean number of single chemical entities introduced each year was 41.8, which is much less than the number of patents, 658, obtained for single chemical entities by the industry in 1961. Walker suggests that the industry deliberately patented 15.7 times as many products as were likely to be introduced in that year, in order to exclude entry. He infers that the companies' objectives were to monopolize the best products and also to prevent potential competitors from manufacturing similar, second-best products.

The comparison of the number of patented single chemical entities with the number of marketed new drugs does not prove intent to suppress competitive products. Patent applications, as we have seen, are made early in the process of research and development, prior to the determination of whether a particular compound will become a marketed drug or even whether it is marketable. The patent is applied for early so that if it turns out to be marketable, the company's interest is protected. In addition, an early patent permits discussion of the compound in journals without jeopardizing the rights of the company. The interpretation of the large number of patented chemical entities relative to the number which are actually marketed as evidence of deliberate suppression of new products is not supported.

Another way in which manufacturers are supposed to have extended patent protection beyond that which is granted legally is through improvements. Henry Steele contends that in the chemical industries, including the drug industry, patent grants are easily extended indefinitely by the deliberate timing of improvements.[11] But an important form of competition in the drug industry is product improvement, and the firm which introduced the original product is the one which is most likely to improve it. Furthermore, the high rate of turnover of leadership among companies in therapeutic fields suggests that companies do not usually maintain their positions by improving their products.

Finally, we come to Reekie's assertion that the leading firms limit competition by refusing to grant small firms licenses under their patents and by restricting the issuance of licenses to other leading firms.[12] Reekie offers no evidence to support this assertion. An analysis of de Haen's data on patents and licenses between 1941 and 1971 indicates that the distribution of patents is highly concentrated but also that the distribution of licenses is no more concentrated. Moreover, the leading companies did not license each other exclusively. The top fifteen companies by sales in 1960 obtained 65.8 percent of all of the patents granted during the period 1941–71 on marketed drugs, and they issued 71.1 percent of all licenses. It is true that they issued only 186 licenses on 354 patented products, and on more than half of the patents, no licenses were granted at all. But, more to the point concerning the number of licenses issued to small relative to large firms, the licenses issued by the fifteen leading firms were not limited to those which they issued to each other: only 40 percent of all licenses which they granted went to each other; thus 60 percent were granted to smaller firms.

The only evidence that Reekie presents to demonstrate that the leading firms used patents and licenses to limit competition is the contrast between the price behavior of penicillin, which was unpatented, and that of the prices of broad-spectrum antibiotics, which were patented. Reekie argues that the patents and cross-licenses permitted broad-spectrum prices to be stable over a long period in contrast to the decline of prices of penicillin products. The contrast suggests that patents have prevented entry and subsequent price declines, but it does not prove that large companies limited entry by refusing to license small firms.

To summarize the discussion of patents and entry, we can conclude that until patents expire, they prevent entry through the reproduction of existing drugs, except when licenses are granted. Since patent owners have not in general been generous with licenses, patents have limited the number of sellers in each therapeutic field.

Owners of patents usually have issued few licenses. A large pharmaceutical company will issue licenses to other manufacturers when these have through their own research efforts established patent positions which threaten infringement suits. In addition, licenses may be granted in exchange for technical information and cross licenses. In addition, large foreign firms, or small domestic firms which have lacked marketing organizations, have granted licenses.

To achieve entry prior to patent expiration, firms undertake R & D efforts. The large expenditures required for R & D and the associated risks have excluded small firms, but these requirements have not prevented firms which were already established in other fields of the industry from entering a particular field. Their laboratory scientists must have time to acquire familiarity with a field, but good profit prospects due to large potential sales and the likelihood of developing new products have encouraged R & D expenditures. In addition, the larger firms are engaged in R & D in a large number of fields, some of which have no drugs.

The Economies of Scale as Barriers to Entry.   The economies of scale in the production of drugs usually are small and therefore do not bar entry. The discussion by Steele is based on the FTC report of 1958 on antibiotics.[13] According to Steele, batch fermentation processes characterize the production of antibiotics and synthetic corticosteroids, which were the therapeutic fields with the largest sales at the time when Steele was writing. The large manufacturers of antibiotics each use from ten to fifty fermentation vessels, and they increase their output by increasing the number rather than the capacity of individual vats. The large firms thus gain no economies in production from their size.

In general, the economies of scale in production do not appear to have provided a barrier to entry. The significant economies, if there are any, are present only in the manufacture of active ingredients. In the case of the manufacture of active ingredients, frequently only a few manufacturers supply the bulk raw material. On the other hand, this has not prevented numerous plants from being established in the manufacture of finished products. The bulk materials are available for sale after the patent has expired, and sometimes before, to any manufacturer. The original patentee may supply other firms, despite the fact that these firms are competitors. They may do so because alternative sources of supply are available. Thus, bulk producers located in Italy supply active ingredients of a variety of drugs to final product manufacturers in the United States and elsewhere. Such producers have flourished in Italy because of its weak patent laws, but bulk producers which are independent of the major companies also are located in the U.S. These producers as well as the major companies realize whatever economies of scale are available in the production of active ingredient.

The economies of scale in the manufacturing processes in later stages of production have not set a minimum economic size of firm, which is a large fraction of the size of the market in most of the therapeutic markets or even of the sales of generic classes of drugs, which are much smaller. The output of a particular drug may be small, but even fairly small firms can produce several products using the same equipment and personnel.

The economies of scale in quality control, as we have seen in chapters 10 and 11, are sufficiently large to prevent small companies from being able to provide adequate assurance of efficacy and safety, but even this observation does not signify that a firm must account for the output of a large fraction of the sales in a generic class of drugs in order to provide adequate assurance of safety and efficacy.

Economies of Scale in Research. Chapter 5 showed that the economies of scale in R & D are large and require a large minimum size of firm. That chapter also reviewed the related literature. The economies are sufficiently large to prevent small firms from doing discovery research. Nevertheless, as Chapter 6 demonstrates, a large number of firms conduct research in the therapeutic fields with large sales.

Economies of Scale in Promotion. Comanor, Schifrin, and Steele[14] believe that the industry embarked on a policy of product differentiation following the experience of severe price cutting in the early 1950s in the penicillin and streptomycin markets. According to Comanor, the leading firms sought to avoid a similar experience later by developing and promoting special products. Both Comanor and Shifrin also say that product differentiation had the important effect of preventing entry by new firms into therapeutic fields. Comanor specifically suggests that an entrant now requires a technical advance and, therefore, must undertake the risk and cost of research. In other words, Comanor regards the expenditures for R & D as costs of product differentiation and further believes that these expenditures have the additional effect of blockading entry.

The other major barrier to entry created by product differentiation is the need for an entrant to undertake promotional activities. The height of this barrier increases with the economies of scale in selling.

As we have seen, detailing costs account for a major part of total selling costs, and direct mail and journal advertising account for most of the remainder. A pharmaceutical company requires large sales to carry the costs of detailing. According to Walker, a firm must spend approximately $2 million in order to visit every physician in the U.S. once.[15] This figure has probably risen considerably since Walker made his estimate.

Walker also points out that certain economies are available to firms operating nationally. The cost of advertising space per reader in national medical journals is lower than in regional journals. Firms which sell only regionally thus do not receive the full benefit of these journal advertising economies. Walker provides estimates which indicate the availability of large economies in selling to national companies.[16]

While Walker establishes a good case for the existence of economies of scale in selling, he overestimates the savings resulting from national operations by ignoring the fact that regional firms spend relatively more on direct mail advertising than on journal advertising. We also know that these economies have not been sufficiently large to prevent small regional sellers from flourishing. They have been able to sell their products to physicians and to retailers by using very simple direct-mail advertising.

In any case, the argument suggests only that economies of scale in selling increase the difficulty of small-scale entry. They do not block entry by large firms. Walker and others regard the therapeutic fields and even the generic classes as the true economic markets rather than the pharmaceutical industry as a whole. Pharmaceutical firms which have a marketing organization and which are not already established in a therapeutic field or in a generic class will not find the economies of scale in marketing a barrier to entry. Thus economies of scale in marketing do not limit competition in therapeutic markets.

CONCENTRATION. Despite the doubt concerning the validity of the concentration ratio as a measure of monopoly power, this ratio continues to be prominent in discussions of monopoly power in the drug industry.

Most of the studies accept the therapeutic field as the relevant market, and they conclude that in general the concentration ratio is high. Thus, Comanor maintains that the focus of competition is the therapeutic market, within which the number of firms usually is sufficiently small for each firm to consider the reactions of others to a price cut which it contemplates. Comanor cites data indicating that the leading five firms accounted for between 56 percent and 98 percent of sales in each therapeutic market.[17] Jadlow cites data for a later date which show that the five leading firms rarely have less than 50 percent of national sales in a therapeutic class and frequently more than 70 percent.[18] Both Comanor and Jadlow interpret the figures as signifying a high degree of concentration.

Jesse Markham suggests that the relevant market may be the entire industry.

He reports that in 1968 the four leading firms accounted for 27 percent of the total value of shipments of the entire industry (a figure which he considers to be low), but he fails to justify the use of industry concentration ratios.[19]

On the contrary, he prefers the use of individual therapeutic markets, which he agrees are highly concentrated. He also agrees that the degree of concentration is sufficiently high to induce firms to behave as a closely knit interdependent oligopoly and thus refrain from price competition. He accepts the common assumption that increases in concentration bring with them a decline in competition, but he provides no evidence. On the other hand, he makes the important qualification that the reluctance to compete is limited to price cuts. Markham also goes on to say that other elements in the structure of the market promote competition. He points to the instability of market positions in the therapeutic field as evidence of substantial competition. In sixteen of twenty therapeutic markets, Markham observes that at least two of the top five firms in 1951 had been displaced by 1960, and in eight markets at least three of the largest five firms had been displaced. Only in antibiotics was there no turnover. Markham attributes the generally high rate of turnover to the introduction of new products rather than to price competition.

Several observations can be made concerning this discussion. First, the discussion relates primarily to the experience of the 1950s rather than to the later period. During the 1960s, price competition did become much more vigorous in the antibiotics market, and new products displaced older products. At the same time, the concentration ratio remained high. Thus, the concentration ratio itself does not appear to provide a good index of the probability of price competition. It obviously depends on many other factors, which are difficult to identify. Nor does the evidence indicate that the high degree of product competition replaced price competition. During the 1960s a high rate of product turnover in antibiotics was associated with severe price cuts. We have seen that a major source of price competition in this segment of the market was the entry by major firms into antibiotics markets and their efforts to increase their market shares. In these efforts, they were not inhibited by the realization that previously established firms would retaliate with their own price cuts.

The implications of the acceptance of narrowly defined therapeutic markets as the relevant markets with respect to the condition of entry are not developed. If these are the markets, then many of the drug firms, including the large ones, are outside any one market. Thus many large firms have neither a major nor a minor tranquilizer. But they have the requisite technology, skills, capital, and marketing organizations to enter. The fact that more of them do not enter a market must be attributed to the effectiveness of patents in excluding entry, to the infrequency of new drug discoveries, or to low expected profit rates from investment in R & D. The arguments concerning the effectiveness of patents have been inconclusive, for as several authors have suggested, it is unusually easy for pharmaceutical manufacturers to invest close imitations of established products without infringing patents. They have also argued that much of the research in industry is intended for the development of minor product modifications. Thus, when firms do not enter a therapeutic market, it may very well be because of a low expected rate of return on investment in R & D rather than difficult entry.

Much of the discussion has been limited to the great successes. The patents on individual highly successful products such as Valium, Librium, the cephalosporins, and Darvon have effectively prevented entry through duplication, and competitors have found it difficult to capture a large share of the respective therapeutic market with similar, though not identical, drugs. Large investments by pharmaceutical firms have not yielded satisfactory substitutes, or, at any rate, doctors have not been persuaded of their adequacy. Thus, there appears to be some evidence of entrenched monopoly power resulting in high profits under the shelter of patents.

Nevertheless, it is a mistake to infer from these individual instances that entry is generally difficult to therapeutic markets. In most fields the sales of individual drugs have not been so large as to result in high realized rates of return on investment.

COMPETITIVE BEHAVIOR

PRICE COMPETITION. Comanor maintains that a deliberate policy of product development and product differentiation by industry leaders has prevented price competition. The industry structure is conducive to price competition, for the combination of a number of fairly large firms together with many smaller ones accounting for a substantial proportion of the total output usually results in price competition.[20]

He suggests that the leading firms have feared price competition because the lower limit to prices, the average variable cost, is well below average total cost. The average total cost includes expenditures on research and promotion, which are not included in variable costs, and these are major items. The leading firms, therefore, have competed in research and product differentiation primarily, with the consequence of price stability. The R & D expenditures have resulted in a large number of patented new drugs, which have accounted for a high proportion of total sales. The strategy thus has prevented price competition. Other consequences have been the importance of innovation for profits and more difficult entry, because entry requires a large investment in R & D.

We have suggested that the origins of the innovative focus of competition were preceding innovations and a high rate of return on investment in R & D rather than a deliberate policy of preventing price competition. Be that as it may, the public policy issue concerns the relative social merits of price and product competition. Comanor on the whole adheres to the usual economist's position that price competition is the more desirable form of competition, although he does express ambivalence.

The innovative strategy of the leading firms, however, may have been socially beneficial. This policy probably accelerated the rate of innovation. We have seen that the number of new single entities increases with expenditures on R & D. Some of the new entities may have been unimportant medical advances, but the number of important medical advances probably increased with the total number of new entities. Given the generally empirical methodology of pharmaceutical research, an increase in the amount of effort within any field will increase the probability of an important discovery as well as that of a lesser discovery.

Comanor's use of the expression "product differentiation" to describe the R & D effort has pejorative connotations. It suggests that firms deliberately seek products which are only slightly different from their predecessors. The suggestion that firms limited their efforts in this way is also conveyed by the use of the expressions "molecular modification" and "molecular manipulation" to describe the R & D activities. Molecular modification, as we have seen, is a standard research methodology of the chemists involved in drug research and is used because of the absence of theories for the prediction of effective drugs and the resultant dependence on empirical approaches. The confusion also arises from the fact that this approach to drug discovery resembles economists' representation of competition in oligopolistic industries in which competitors imitate highly successful products and refrain from price competition. Comanor's description of competition in the drug industry may contain some truth, but it is difficult to disentangle the part played by product differentiation as a motive from the part contributed by the standard approach to the discovery of drugs. In any case, the motivation matters little. The important consideration is that the business strategy of innovation probably accelerated the rate of innovation of important and useful drugs.

Moreover, Comanor gives too much credit to the companies' competitive policies for the high rate of innovation of the 1950s and early 1960s. He ignores completely the possibility that the strategy of product innovation was induced by a combination of factors independent of the decisions of individual firms. New fields were opened by important discoveries within a short period of time. The breakthroughs created the fields of antibiotics, hormonal products, contraceptives, tranquilizers, and diuretics, and opened the way for numerous developments which represented improvements of the quality of the original drugs. Comanor also ignores the great interest which physicians have in the potency of drugs, their efficacy, and their side effects. If drug manufacturers are to gain sales, they must pay particular attention to the quality of their products. Product competition in this market thus has a historical basis in the high rate of innovation of the age of discovery and strong support from doctors demands. There is little need, therefore, to attribute the product competition to an effort to evade price competition. In addition, there is no basis for the conclusion that consumers would have benefitted more from price cuts than from the product improvements which did take place.

Perhaps the emphasis on product quality was due in part to deliberate policy. We cannot be sure that the companies had no choice in the matter. If one or two of the major firms had been aggressive price cutters, the others might have been forced to follow. We see that in the 1960s Squibb did cut prices aggressively, and within the affected therapeutic fields the market leaders were forced to follow. It is not certain that in the 1950s price cuts would have been as effective as they were later, for in the earlier years, the products were still new and unfamiliar to doctors, who, therefore, would have been less inclined to prescribe generically and were more impressed with quality claims than they were later. Nevertheless, it is possible that the pattern of competition might have been different, and prices of antibiotics might have been reduced at the cost of a less rapid pace of product development. Society may be better off as a result of the preference for product competition as against price competition.

Much of the discussion concerning price competition focuses on the lack of flexibility of prices. Markham judges the prices of drugs to have been unusually inflexible. He shows that during the 1950s twelve out of the eighteen individual drugs in the vitamin class did not change in price. In cardiovascular agents, the number showing no change was fourteen out of twenty-three. Markham agrees with Comanor in his characterization of competition in the industry as consisting primarily of product changes. He points out that between 1951 and 1960 the industry introduced 432 new chemical entities, 1,064 new dosage forms, and 2,376 new combination products.[21] He quotes approvingly the industry's arguments that doctors are not guided by price considerations primarily in their choice of drugs but by their knowledge of the qualities of different drugs. He also refers to the argument that the large retail margin results in retail prices being insensitive to changes in manufacturers' prices. We have seen that retailers' prices are approximately double those of manufacturers. Markham does not offer any judgment on the performance of the industry. He does not suggest whether consumers would be better off were the industry more competitive in price.

Despite the apparent unanimity on the question of price stability, it is not certain that prices have in fact been stable. The method used in studies of price changes is to count the number of changes in list prices of each product over a period. The number of changes in drug prices then is compared with the number of changes in prices of products in other industries. A major deficiency of this method, which is generally recognized but then ignored, is that it depends on list prices. The effective prices, which reflect special deals by manufacturers, change frequently, while list prices remain the same. Another less generally recognized problem of the method is that it is based on the prices of a given set of products. Yet, as students have recognized, competition in this industry focuses on quality changes, and these quality changes are expressed by the introduction of new drugs. The quality changes are equivalent to price changes, but there is no way of expressing this form of competition in the count of price changes of given products. New drugs which offer the same therapy as old drugs but which are more effective or produce less discomfort are offered at the same price as their predecessors. In effect, the price has been cut, but it is difficult to identify such price cuts. Nevertheless to assess the extent of price competition without doing so is meaningless.

Further, to judge the degree of price flexibility, one must analyze the sources of price changes. Studies attempting to contrast industries with respect to their price flexibility must include an examination of the changes in demand and cost conditions. In the drug industry, some conditions which are not present elsewhere have contributed to price stability. One is the small part of total costs represented by variable costs and another is the growth of demand. Even large changes in raw material prices and in production-worker wages have a small percentage effect on the total costs of ethical drugs. In addition, there is little incentive to reduce prices as long as demand continues to grow.

The height of prices relative to production costs, which include the cost of materials and of direct labor, is also believed to demonstrate absence of price competition. Thus, Steele reports that the production cost of broad-spectrum antibiotics was low relative to price. In addition, he points out that during the 1950s the cost of production declined without accompanying price reductions.[22]

A related question concerns the prices of brands relative to those of generics. As Steele says, pharmacists can fill generic prescriptions with any available brand product or generic product within the same generic class. With price competition, the prices of name-brand products which are not under patent would be driven down to the same level as that of their generic competitors. Steele points out that this has not occurred. Ciba, for example, sold reserpine under the brand name of Serpasil at a wholesale price of $4.50 per hundred .25 milligram tablets. Some of the licensees sold the bulk powder to small companies who then undersold the advertised brands. Prices of bottled tablets varied greatly, the lowest price being Winsale's, at 45 cents, which was 10 percent of Ciba's price.[23]

These disparities in price were not limited to the period of the 1950s, but have persisted up to the present. We have seen that the prices of products in generic classes have frequently been far below those of the brand-name products. The latter have been able to maintain a large share of the market without cutting their prices. In addition, a recent study of antibiotic markets by the Council on Economic Priorities points to similar disparities.[24]

Such price differences have persisted despite the entry of large companies into various therapeutic markets with their own generic products. This entry usually forces price reduction on the manufacturers of the original brands, but the prices both of the original brands and of the generic products introduced by large companies do not come down to the level of the prices of the generic products of smaller manufacturers. Apparently the prices of the generic brands of large companies are not set as low as marginal costs but contain an allowance towards overhead, promotion, and R & D costs. The prices of generics produced by small companies do not include as much of an allowance for R & D and promotion, if any at all.

The critics suggest that the degree of price competition remains unsatisfactory despite the entry of large firms with generic products, and they support various measures, including reduction in patent life and the Maximum Allowable Cost regulation (MAC), both of which are expected to result in sharp price cuts. The MAC regulation requires HEW to reimburse patients under the Medicaid program for multiple-source drugs only up to the level of the lowest price of widely available drugs plus a professional dispensing fee. The combination of the reduction in patent life and the MAC regulation would have the effect of reducing prices over a large range of drugs. Under these conditions, the funds available for overhead, promotion, and R & D costs would be reduced sharply, unless the rate of innovation were to increase dramatically, which is unlikely. An institutional structure other than the private pharmaceutical industry would have to be developed to perform the functions of R & D and promotion.

PRODUCT DIFFERENTIATION. Critics of the industry, including Comanor, have maintained that the expenditures for R & D as well as for promotion are designed to differentiate products, and such expenditures have been excessive. Following the same argument, Steele also emphasizes the trivial nature of the changes represented by many of the new products.[25] We have already suggested that the choice of product competition as a business strategy was a fortunate decision from the standpoint of social welfare.

Other general issues related to promotional expenditures concern physicians' habits of prescription. The industry's critics insist that doctors should be required to prescribe generically, or, failing that, that pharmacists be allowed to substitute generically equivalent drugs for specific brands. In general, critics maintain that the differences in pharmaceutical properties among products within the same therapeutic class are frequently minor. The proposed regulations thus would not reduce the quality of medical care, and they would have the desired effect of encouraging entry and price competition. A related complaint concerns product proliferation. It is alleged that the available numerous brands represent unnecessary and wasteful duplication resulting from efforts to avoid price competition.

Therapeutic differences between drugs which are chemically different are frequently difficult to demonstrate in controlled trials on patients treated for an indication. But they may differ for subgroups of patients within the general population. Small differences in chemical formulas can be significant therapeutically; the potency and side effects may vary. Disagreements among doctors resulting from differences in direct clinical experience thus arise, and clinical studies which estimate the effects of drugs on patient populations do not reveal differences in effects between subgroups of patients. Within some fields, such as thiazide diuretics, the differences between drugs within a therapeutic class may be minor for most patients. But this field apparently is exceptional.

Concerning therapeutic differences between generically identical drugs, Walker and other critics maintain that generic products are as good as the corresponding brands, and doctors, therefore, should be required to prescribe generically. The standards of quality are specified by the U.S. Pharmacopeia and the National Formulary, and, according to Walker, there is little question concerning the adequacy of these standards, particularly in view of the fact that most doctors do not prescribe carefully but use standard prescriptions and disregard even the most elementary precautions, such as, in the case of respiratory infections, failing to discriminate between viral and bacterial infections.[26] According to Walker, doctors also use "shotgun" preparations in the treatment of anemia rather than discriminating between types of anemia. The assessment of hypertension, he also points out, is limited to the measurement of blood pressure. Moreover, doctors make no effort to guard against adverse drug reactions in the prescription of potentially dangerous drugs.[27]

The issue of the quality of different drugs should be separated from that of how well doctors prescribe. Concerning the adequacy of official standards, as embodied in the official pharmacopeias, they specify only the amount of active ingredients; not the quality or the amount of fillers and binders. Generic equivalence thus does not guarantee therapeutic equivalence.

Walker and others assume that the standards in the pharmacopeias are observed by all manufacturers. This assumption is not expressly made, but it is clear that they would be willing to accept only a very small risk of nonobservance of these standards for at least some drugs. Thus, the critics ultimately rely on the FDA to monitor the production of drugs by all companies in the U.S. As we have seen, however, the FDA has been unable and is unlikely to be able satisfactorily to perform this large task. Small establishments can be set up readily to supply local drug stores, and there are numerous small drug manufacturers in the U.S. The problem of surveillance is multiplied by the high rate of turnover of the small establishments.

Walker deals with the questions of good manufacturing practice by suggesting that the cost of quality control testing is small and therefore can be performed by any retail pharmacist. He suggests, therefore, that there is no reason for small manufacturers not to perform the tests or control the characteristics of drugs.[28]

Chapters 10 and 11 provide evidence that the costs of quality control are large. In addition, those chapters have shown that quality control procedures include not only the inspection performed by quality control laboratories in plants but also the procedures for control of manufacturing processes which are designed to minimize the risk of defective quality, and the cost of such procedures is not included in that of quality control but in the cost of manufacturing. Thus, small firms may very well not have sufficient resources to provide the assurance of good manufacturing practice. We have also seen evidence which indicates that the risk of defectives is significant in the purchase of drugs and that this risk is related to the size of the manufacturer.

Walker supports his argument with references to the experience of nonprofit hospitals which use formulary systems for dispensing drugs and purchase the products of small firms. He also points to purchases by military services from small firms. According to Walker, the military medical supply agency in 1959 awarded contracts to firms with an annual volume of business which was as low as $75,000.[29]

The nonprofit hospitals and the military supply agency, however, investigate their sources of supply. Retail pharmacists are in no position to conduct independent surveys of the quality of products of small manufacturers; they are more likely to depend on the assurances of the FDA. In any case, the doctor who relies on brand names rids himself of uncertainty of the possibility that the retailer has not checked the quality of the productions of his sources.

Walker also suggests that the promotional activities of the major drug companies have an undue influence on physicians. He refers to Lederle's heavy advertising campaigns for Achromycin, Pfizer's sponsorship of golf tournaments for physicians, Merrell's deceptive appeal to the ego of doctors in behalf of Kevadon, Pfizer's withholding of information regarding undesirable side effects of Diabinese, and Parke Davis's deliberate policy of ignoring chloramphenicol's undesirable side effects. He also quotes from the former medical director of Pfizer with respect to the excessive claims by companies for their drugs.[30]

Neither Walker nor the present author is in a position to evaluate the claims of drug companies. We have, however, seen that there is strong evidence to warrant the conclusion that the quality of drugs produced by large companies is superior to that produced by small generic companies. We can also say with some confidence that there are differences in therapeutic properties between brands of the different major companies, and the companies themselves inform doctors of these differences. Individual instances of excessive claims are not sufficient evidence to warrant the general conclusion that the promotional activities are uninformative or that the larger companies are not committed to the policy of ensuring that good manufacturing practices are followed.

Walker does examine data concerning legal actions by the FDA for violations of good manufacturing practices and the size of firm prosecuted. The period under investigation is that between 1950 and 1960. Table 13-1 reproduces his data. This table indicates that the number of legal actions per firm is small relative to sales for the largest size-class of firms.[31] It is also evident that among the small firms, the number of legal actions per million dollars of sales is largest for the smallest firms and varies inversely and markedly with the size of firm.

These observations signify that encouragement of entry through the reduction in the length of life of patents, the control of promotional expenditures, or the requirement that physicians prescribe generically, would increase the difficulty of the task of the FDA in controlling quality. If the FDA did not expand

TABLE 13-1

Legal Actions Initiated by F.D.A. according to Size of Firm

Size of Firms in terms of 1959 Sales ($ millions)	No. of Firms Engaged in Legal Actions	Total No. of Legal Actions	Mean No. of Legal Actions per Firm Engaged in Legal Action	No. of Firms Engaged in More than One Legal Action	Total No. of Legal Actions for Firms Engaged in More than One Action	Mean No. of Legal Actions per Firm for Firms Engaged in More than One Legal Action	Mean No. of Legal Actions per $ Million of 1959 Sales for All Firms Engaged in Legal Actions	Approx. No. of Firms in Category of Size	No. of Legal Actions per Firm
Less than 0.1	61	94	1.54	17	50	2.94	54.7	503	0.187
0.1–0.2	39	84	2.15	22	67	3.05	17.1	156	0.538
0.2–0.3	23	44	1.91	11	32	2.91	8.5	137	0.591
0.3–0.4	14	37	2.64	8	31	3.86	8.1		
0.4–0.6	16	38	2.38	8	30	3.75	5.0		
0.6–1.0	11	22	2.00	7	18	2.57	3.1	140	0.430
1.0–2.0	16	46	2.88	9	39	4.33	2.3	59	0.780
2.0–6.0	10	34	3.40	6	30	5.00	1.2	61	0.560
More than 6.0	10	18	1.80	2	10	5.00	0.06	58	0.310
Totals	200	417		90	307			1,114	

Source: Reproduced from Walker, Market Power and Price Levels in the Ethical Drug Industry (Bloomington: Indiana University Press, 1971), p. 77.

its resources for inspection very considerably, then the risk to consumers would be increased greatly.

Walker raises objections to the sampling procedure of the FDA. According to Walker, only forty-four of the firms against which actions were taken could be identified as small firms selling ethical drugs under generic names. In addition, Walker states that the FDA failed to provide estimates of the sales of thirty-seven firms which were referred to as "small," "dormant," "defunct," or "out of business." In addition, Walker points out that many of the firms for which sales estimates were provided were extremely small, and that these firms therefore were unlikely to be members of the industry.

Walker's objections do not destroy the validity of the general conclusion, which is that the incidence of legal actions in relation to sales among small firms exceeded that among firms in the top size group and considerably so.

Another objection which Walker makes to the validity of the FDA evidence is that the FDA samples small firms more intensively than large ones. According to Walker, the agency selected 8,376 samples from thirty large firms and based four legal actions on the samples. This is equivalent to 4.23 samples per million dollars of sales. From the remaining firms in the industry, the FDA selected 8,621 samples, which gave rise to 484 legal actions. The FDA took 29.13 samples per million dollars of sales. Small firms thus were inspected 6.89 times more intensively in relation to sales than large firms. Walker interprets these data to signify that the FDA does not allocate its samples to the different size groups of firms according to where quality checks would result in the greatest benefit. Walker claims that the larger firms have higher rates of violations relative to sales than the smaller firms, but he does not supply any data which show that the performance of larger firms is poorer.

Walker also believes that the FDA data are biased in favor of large firms' performance because the FDA prosecuted them less frequently than small firms. Walker says that eighty-four incidents of irregularities among large firms resulted in five legal actions and seventy-nine drug recalls. On the other hand, 690 irregularities among small firms resulted in as many as 206 legal actions, or relatively much more than for large firms. The ratio of legal actions against small firms to those against large firms was about forty to one, compared to a ratio of drug recalls issued against small firms to those against large firms of only five to two. Apparently, irregularities involving large firms were more frequently negotiated than those involving small firms. Walker interprets these data as signifying discrimination in favor of large firms by the FDA. An alternative interpretation is more plausible. The FDA probably could rely more on the assurances of the large firms that they would maintain quality control. They could not rely as much on the assurances provided by some small firms which were persistent violators.

Walker ignores an interesting feature about the data which he reports. The number of irregularities for small firms was much higher relative to their sales than the number of irregularities for large firms. He chooses only to comment on the possibility that the FDA favors large firms by not prosecuting them for violations as frequently as it does the small firms.

He emphasizes the possibility of discrimination in favor of large firms by saying that many of the employees of the FDA later are employed by the large firms in the industry.[32] In 1963 the FDA employed 1,150 persons in the classification of medical, scientific, and technical personnel. During the five preceding years, 813 employees in this classification left the FDA, and of these eighty-three were employed by industries (food, drug, and cosmetic) regulated by the FDA; twenty of these were employed by the major drug companies. Walker interprets these data as signifying that employees in the FDA are influenced in their decisions by the possibility of employment at high salaries in the regulated industries. They will tend to accept the large firms' viewpoint. The data which he reports, however, suggest that the probability of employment by a large company is small for FDA employees, and these data therefore suggest that the FDA is unlikely to be influenced by the interests of large firms.

Economists generally start from the premise that promotional activities are misleading to consumers and largely wasteful of resources. This view is expressed by the model of perfect competition which assumes that under competitive conditions consumers are well informed about the quality and prices of product, and therefore companies need not engage in activities intended to provide information on these aspects of products. In the model, then, competition is limited to price cuts. The assumption concerning information obviously simplifies the task of analysis of the competitive behavior of firms, and for many purposes it is a useful assumption. In relation to questions dealing explicitly with the role of promotion, however, it becomes excessively restrictive. The standard explanation of advertising and of promotion generally sees the assumption as a device used by oligopolistic firms to compete for sales without resorting to price cuts, which are avoided because of fear of retaliation. And, since customers supposedly find it difficult to evaluate the quality of advertised products and therefore are susceptible to false as well as to valid claims by sellers, oligopolistic avoidance of price rivalry is seen as the source of wasteful expenditures for deceptive promotional efforts. This analysis usually is supported by anecdotal illustrations of deceptive advertising. The argument also suggests that promotional activity which fixes brand names of products in the minds of customers provides a barrier to entry which protects monopolistic profits against potential competition from entrants. The cost of an advertising campaign to establish a new product in competition with previously established products may be so large as to block entry effectively.

A study by Comanor and Wilson of the relationship among industries between the ratio of advertising expenditures to sales with the after-tax profit rate supports the view that profits increase with advertising expenditures.[33] They find a positive relationship in a sample of forty-one consumer goods industries after controlling for the growth of demand, capital requirements, economy of scale, and the concentration ratio.

The procedure which Comanor and Wilson use leaves their results open to question. They follow the procedure of treating advertising expenditures as a current expense. Obviously, however, advertising expenditures represent an investment, and if these expenditures were capitalized, then the results might be quite different. The effect of capitalization on the rate of profit depends on the rates of growth of advertising expenditures and of sales and on the depreciation rate for advertising expenditures.

Concerning the effect of advertising on the condition of entry, Lester Telser suggests that rather than being a block to entry, advertising is a vehicle for entry. Were advertising to increase with the degree of monopoly power, then we would expect the ratio of advertising expenditures to sales—or, as it is frequently called, the "advertising intensity"—to increase with the concentration ratio. Telser finds no such relationship. On the contrary, he observes that the entry of new firms is frequently associated with large advertising expenditures. Telser grants the possibility that advertising in some cases may reduce competition, but he suggests that in other cases advertising serves to increase competition. His overall conclusion is that the effect of advertising is not monopolistic in view of the absence of the relationship between advertising intensity and the concentration ratio.[34]

Similar arguments have been made specifically about the role of advertising in the pharmaceutical industry. A study by W. Duncan Reekie examines advertising in the pharmaceutical industry from the same general standpoint as that which we have been discussing. He suggests that if advertising is largely the result of oligopolistic rivalry, then the amount of promotional effort will increase with the degree of concentration.[35] He also tests the hypothesis that advertising in the drug industry consists largely of misleading claims. If this hypothesis is true, then advertising would be heaviest in those areas where such claims are less readily validated. In other words, the companies would spend the largest amount for advertising in those fields in which doctors have relatively little knowledge of drugs. The third proposition which Reekie examines concerns the informational role of promotion. If promotional activities are intended to provide information, then advertising expenditures will be largest in those therapeutic fields in which the number of new products is relatively large.

His results do not support the hypothesis that advertising is largely due to seller rivalry. An analysis of differences among therapeutic fields in advertising expenditures in 1966 in the United Kingdom fails to indicate that concentration was a significant factor. The second hypothesis that firms use misleading claims receives support. He finds that the therapeutic fields in which the technology was relatively backward were associated with relatively large advertising effort. The third hypothesis concerning information also receives support. He finds that the relationship between advertising expenditures and the number of new products is very close.

Reekie's results thus are somewhat ambiguous, but on the whole they suggest that the oligopoly hypothesis is not valid and that information plays an important role. His results concerning the information hypothesis are the strongest. These findings agree with our own analysis of the relationship between advertising expenditures and a number of new products among firms (see Chapter 9).

John M. Vernon[36] has also examined the relationship among therapeutic fields between advertising expenditures and concentration. He examines 1968 data for the United States and does a regression analysis of concentration ratios in therapeutic markets on the ratio of promotional expenditures to sales. For 1968 he obtains nonsignificant results; the level of promotional expenditures has no effect on concentration. On the other hand, when he examines 1964 data, he obtains a statistically significant but negative regression coefficient. The results for 1964 are directly contradictory to the hypothesis in that high promotional expenditures apparently are associated with the low degree of concentration. Vernon does not attempt to explain these results.

The difference between the 1964 and 1968 results may have been caused by the decline in a number of new products over the intervening years.

GENERAL COMMENTS

This survey is not exhaustive, but it covers writings which are representative of the literature on the drug industry in books and articles by economists. This literature finds in general that the industry is monopolistic. The monopoly power is attributed to the effect of patents on the entry of new firms into therapeutic fields and to the prescribing habits of doctors who limit their prescribing to well-known brand-name products. These conditions have resulted in a high degree of concentration in therapeutic markets, which in turn has been reflected in oligopolistic interdependence and, therefore, a reluctance to compete in price. Instead, firms have competed in the development of new products and in promotion. The literature judges the performance of the industry to have been poor. The critics condemn the absence of price competition, the excessive promotional expenditures, excessive expenditures on R & D on trivial product changes, and high profits.

The alternative view developed in this book attributes the product rivalry among firms in the industry to important drug discoveries in the 1930s and 1940s which stimulated further search in the hope of discovering other new drugs. Further successes in the 1950s led to the expectation of a high rate of return from investment in R & D and, therefore, to large increases in such investment. Research in other fields contributed to the growth of pharmaceutical research by providing techniques of chemical analysis. The patent system also encouraged these developments by limiting the possibility of imitation of new drugs. Firms seeking increases in sales were required to discover and develop new products. This tendency also was encouraged by the emphasis by doctors on the quality of products rather than on price. The relatively high ratio of promotional expenditures to sales in this industry is attributed to the demand for product information by doctors and to the large number of firms, products, and doctors, rather than to oligopolistic rivalry.

The present study suggests that the product rivalry among firms resulted in a higher rate of innovation than would have come about were the competition to have been limited to price, as it would have been were new products less well protected by patents. The resulting new drugs included important advances as well as drugs which were of little therapeutic significance. The present study concludes also that the promotional effort was neither deceptive on the whole nor excessive. The drug companies have performed a valuable service in providing information to doctors. Finally, profits have not been excessive. The difference in average accounting rates of profit between the pharmaceutical and manufacturing industries as a whole has been due to the failure to capitalize R & D expenditures, the growth of demand for pharmaceutical products, and the relative riskiness of investment in this industry.

The important questions in relation to the drug industry concern sources of increases in the number of new drugs and the effects of public policy on the rate of innovation. The present study analyzes these sources and suggests that public policy has increased the rate of innovation by providing patent protection for new drugs. The decline in the rate of investment in the late 1960s is attributed partly to public policy and partly to problems of discovery which are independent of public policy. Increased demands by the FDA for evidence of efficacy and safety and more severe restrictions on human testing have reduced the number of innovations. These changes contributed to the decline in the expected rate of return from investment in R & D. If investment is to be maintained or increased, the expected rate must be allowed to rise from its present low level.

Discussion in the economic literature has been primarily concerned with the issue of monopoly power to the exclusion of these more important issues. The reason for the inappropriate emphasis is that this literature is part of the more general literature addressed to the monopoly issue. The monopoly issue is of more general interest both to economists and to others, and it embraces a large number of industries. We will not discuss whether or not the monopoly issue generally is important, but we will say that it is not the context within which to develop policy for the drug industry. The problem of appropriate policy for the encouragement of innovation is ignored, with the result that approaches to this problem remain undeveloped.

CHAPTER 14

GOVERNMENT PROPOSALS
FOR PUBLIC POLICY

INTRODUCTION

The pharmaceutical industry has been under almost continuous investigation by Congress since 1960 when the late Senator Kefauver charged the industry with monopolistic exploitation of consumers. In the past few years, Senator Nelson has been a particularly vigorous critic, and he has currently been supported by Senator Kennedy.[1] In addition, the FTC and the GAO have been investigating the industry. Recently, after much public debate, HEW adopted regulations for the reimbursement of payments for drugs used by Medicaid patients which will encourage generic prescribing. In all these discussions, the writings by some economists have been cited as pointing to the desirability of changes in public policy to encourage greater competition.

The continuing investigations may generate new proposals by government agencies for legislation and other measures. In the following pages, we shall briefly review the HEW Maximum Allowable Cost (MAC) regulation[2] and some of the major proposals for legislation, such as the Nelson Bill, for the compulsory licensing of drugs which are under patent.[3]

GENERIC DRUGS AND FORMULARY LEGISLATION

Legislative efforts to control drug prices have a long history and have generally been associated with the payment for drugs under programs for payments for medical care by the federal government. In 1966 Senator Long introduced a bill (S3614) which provided that drugs purchased under federally aided programs be prescribed under the generic rather than the brand names of drugs. Supporters of the bill maintained that the practice of brand-name prescribing prevented price competition among the large drug manufacturers, citing the findings of the Kefauver hearings on administered drug prices.[4] When he introduced his bill on July 13, 1966, Senator Long stated that brand-name prescribing was the basis of the monopoly power of the drug companies. According to Long, monopoly power prevented the substitution of cheaper drugs for those which were prescribed. He argued that in the absence of competition there was no safeguard against high prices. He suggested that brand-name prescribing was not essential for the protection of the quality of drugs used, since the FDA provided such protection. Subsequent legislative and administrative proposals designed to reduce the prices of drugs paid for by government programs have followed the lead provided by the Long Bill. In general, the proposals would require drugs to be generically prescribed in order to qualify for payment by the government. Although the proposal normally is limited to that part of the market covered by government programs for financing medical care, the effect of any legislation along these lines would be to encourage generic prescribing in general. Doctors would write generic prescriptions for patients who qualify for payments, and they would try to avoid errors in prescribing for these patients by prescribing generically for all patients. We defer our comments until later.

In 1967 Senator Joseph M. Montoya introduced a bill (S17) which provided for the reimbursement of the costs of "qualified drugs." A formulary committee would publish a list of qualified drugs together with the allowable costs for each drug. These costs would be based on the price paid by pharmacists plus a professional fee to the pharmacists. Reimbursement would be on the basis of the lowest drug cost provided the drug was of acceptable quality to the formulary committee. Although the bill would not compel physicians to prescribe generically, reimbursement under Medicare would encourage generic prescribing because it would provide only for what was considered a reasonable cost. Doctors who did not prescribe generically would have to take the time and trouble to know which drugs qualified for full reimbursement. In addition, a doctor would find it difficult to prescribe a brand-name product the price of which was above that of another drug of "acceptable" quality.

In the same year, Senator Long introduced S1303, which was a modification of his 1966 bill. Senator Long's bill adopted the proposal of the Montoya Bill to establish a formulary committee to determine the drugs for which the federal government would pay and to control the cost of these drugs. There was one important difference: this formulary would list drugs only under their generic name. A trade name was to be listed only if no generic-name product of acceptable quality was available. To reduce the risk of poor quality, the bill would require the FDA to expand its inspection and enforcement activities, and all manufacturers to place their name and FDA registration number on each package of drugs. Firms found to be producing substandard drugs would be barred from the sale of drugs eligible for reimbursement. The bill also contained a provision governing the cost of the drugs. Federal payments were to be limited to the "reasonable" cost of a drug which was generally available under its generic name. The reasonable cost was defined by reference to the drug as a generic class regardless of whether the prescription was written generically or by brand name.

It was to be a price within the range of prices charged by different manufacturers which sold the drug by its generic name.

The bill later was offered as an amendment to the administration's Social Security Bill (HR12080). On November 21, 1967, the Senate approved an amendment offered by Senator Long requiring that the government provide reimbursement under federal aid to medical-care programs for drugs prescribed and dispensed chiefly by their generic name rather than by brand name. The measure limited the amount of government reimbursement to a "reasonable charge" plus dispensing fee. The formulary committee would compile a list of drugs eligible for reimbursement and approve the range of acceptable charges for these drugs. The amendment provided that reimbursement was to be at a rate fixed on the basis of the prices of generic products, unless the physician specified a particular drug by designating its generic name together with the name of the manufacturer.

In 1972 Senator Long obtained the approval of the Finance Committee for an amendment to HR1, the Social Security and Welfare and Reform Act, which was reported out of the Finance Committee on September 22, 1972. The amendment was designed to provide for the payment for certain specified drugs used by out-patients in the treatment of common, crippling, or life-threatening chronic diseases of the aged. These diseases included arthritis, cancer, chronic cardiovascular disease, chronic kidney disease, chronic respiratory disease, diabetes, gout, glaucoma, high blood pressure, rheumatism, thyroid disease, and tuberculosis. Reimbursement was to be limited to certain drugs used in the treatment of these conditions. The amendment specified a method of reimbursement based on a reasonable charge and it incorporated a formulary apprach. It thus resembled Senator Long's earlier proposals. The Senate approved the amendment, but it was eliminated by the House-Senate Conference Committee.

MAXIMUM ALLOWABLE COST

Late in 1974 HEW announced that it was planning to change the rules governing the reimbursement to "providers" of drugs under the Medicare-Medicaid programs.[5] Providers include retail pharmacists, hospitals, and health maintenance organizations. The department stated that the purpose of the proposed change was to insure the most economical expenditures under the program. Despite this apparently limited purpose, the effects of the proposed change, which has been adopted in modified form, will be to reduce prices for multiple-source drugs.

The Department stated that drugs containing the same active ingredients were available from different producers at different prices and that its studies of prices in multiple-source markets estimated potential savings of 22 percent to 36 percent from the use of products at lower prices. The studies also estimated that such reductions in prices would result in prescription cost savings to the Medicaid program of between 5 percent and 8 percent.

HEW therefore proposed, under health financing and service programs which the department administers, to limit reimbursement for multiple-source drugs to the lowest cost at which chemically equivalent drugs are generally available, plus a reasonable fee for dispensing a drug. The department explained the phrase "generally available" to mean those drugs which are widely and consistently available to providers in the United States. This lowest cost, which it designated the "maximum allowable cost" or "MAC," would apply to a list of multiple-source drugs. In order to qualify for reimbursement under MAC, the pharmacist would have to substitute for any prescribed brand-name drug the chemically equivalent drug which was available at the lowest cost.

HEW recognized that the question about differences in quality among drugs had arisen in connection with the issue of price differences, but it maintained that such problems were dealt with through the FDA. The memorandum describing the proposal referred to the FDA's extensive drug surveillance program and more specifically to the batch certification of antibiotics, insulin, and other drugs which have been seen to vary significantly from official standards. The memorandum suggested that the FDA continue to develop improved laboratory methods and to revise standards as technology permits. It maintained that the present standards, the drug surveillance system, the batch testing requirements, and bioavailability requirements, where these are needed, will assure safe and effective drugs of consistently high quality.

In July 1975 HEW adopted the MAC regulations, modifying some of the original proposals. A Pharmaceutical Reimbursement Review Board consisting of members of the department and an outside advisory group, the Pharmaceutical Reimbursement Advisory Committee, is to set the MAC prices.

The board will first establish a list of drugs for which MAC prices will be set. This list will include multiple-source drugs, on which HEW spends significant sums under different programs and the prices of which differ significantly at the wholesale level. The FDA is to advise the board of any pending regulatory action to require bioequivalence certification for a drug. When there is no bioequivalence problem, the board will determine for each drug the lowest price at which the drug is widely and consistently available from any formulator or labeler. The advisory committee will review the proposed MAC price for each drug at meetings open to the public. In addition, public hearings may be held. The board will then determine the MAC price.

The pharmacist will receive in addition to reimbursement for the drug purchased a dispensing fee which is fixed by the states.

When doctors prescribe a specified drug for which the price exceeds the MAC price, then the pharmacist can obtain reimbursement only for the MAC price, unless the doctor certifies in writing that the drug is medically necessary. Such certification entitles the pharmacist to full reimbursement. Otherwise he must obtain the difference between the price of the drug and the MAC price from the patient.

The regulation can be expected to lead to severe price competition in the general market for multiple-source drugs, which currently account for about 40 percent of sales of ethical drugs. Since the marginal cost of a drug is well below the fully allocated average cost, manufacturers will cut prices of their generic products below average costs in order to increase their sales. A pharmaceutical manufacturer can deliberately not allocate overhead costs to individual products which account for a small proportion of its total sales. We have seen that these characteristics of costs in the industry have resulted in severe cuts in prices in those multiple-source drugs which have sufficient sales to have attracted the entry of several major manufacturers. These have included the markets for ampicillin, tetracycline, penicillin VK, and erythromycin.

The MAC regulation will intensify the downward pressures on the prices of multiple-source drugs. The provision that MAC will be at the lowest cost at which chemically equivalent drugs are generally available will induce the manufacturers seeking a share of the Medicaid market to reduce their prices in the market as a whole to marginal cost. Since MAC is based on the lowest price at which a chemically equivalent drug is *generally* available, the manufacturer must reduce the price to all buyers in order to obtain a share of the Medicaid market. The manufacturer cannot limit the price cut to Medicaid prescriptions.

The wisdom of the MAC regulation is questionable. Although price competition in multiple-source drug markets has already been severe, prices might have dropped further and price competition might have been more extensive than it actually has been. In those multiple-source drug markets where the prices of original brands have not come down, we may still see severe price cutting after major companies have entered and have established their own low-price brand-name product. It is not clear that prices should fall more than they have. Previous chapters have shown that the prices of many products are insufficient to cover the costs of their R & D, and the overall expected rate of return from investment in R & D is below the level required to maintain such investment.

The issues in this context are similar to those which arise in connection with pricing in other industries in which marginal costs are below average total costs. Discussion of the problems raised when average cost exceeds marginal cost has been limited in the literature to pricing in regulated industries, including telephone communications, electrical utilities, railroads, and airlines, where fixed costs are a large proportion of total costs. A contributing factor in these industries has been the regulatory requirement that firms provide to particular classes of customers service whose cost may be large and not fully covered by the prices to those customers. The discrepancy between average cost and marginal cost has induced firms in these markets to discriminate in price among different classes of customers. Companies have reduced prices to those customers who have access to alternative sources of equivalent service and for whom the price elasticity of demand therefore is large. In addition, firms have been attracted to those sectors of the market where the price-marginal cost difference is large, and in which they are exempt from the requirement of serving particular classes of customers at prices which do not cover average total cost. Thus, ICC regulation of prices for services by common carrier trucks has discriminated against freight having a high value-to-weight ratio and thus has encouraged contracting private carriers which are unregulated to serve this market. The regulation of airline prices has encouraged unregulated charter flights between certain major cities. Price competition in relatively profitable markets thus has contributed to the distressed condition of the railroads and the airlines. It has also been a factor in the elimination of railroad passenger service to many locations where the demand has been insufficient to permit continued service at fares which cover costs. The solutions which do not require the elimination of a service entail subsidies either by the government or by consumers of other related services. An alternative is to require consumers to pay a fixed fee for the availability of the service rather than for the units of the service which they actually consume. Such a system is represented by the flat basic charge for telephone service regardless of usage; usage charges are additional.

From the example of other industries, then, it can be seen that the problems of pricing in the drug industry and the solutions adopted by it are not peculiar. Present consumers of drugs subsidize future consumers by paying for current R & D, and both present and future consumers benefit from the subsidization of past R & D by past consumers. In addition, consumers of some types of drugs pay part of the cost of drugs used by others. More generally, consumers of drugs pay for related services including promotion as well as R & D from which they themselves may not directly benefit.

Political pressures to increase the severity of price competition through MAC and other devices threaten to reduce the quantity of service supplied by drug companies. The MAC regulation will encourage companies to price their multiple-source drugs at slightly above marginal cost in order to gain a large share of the Medicaid market and of other markets to which the same policy may be applied to the future.

The MAC regulation expresses the view that price competition in the multiple-source drug market is insufficient to prevent the accumulation of excess profits by the major drug manufacturers. This view is supported by comparisons of prices of brand-name products of major manufacturers with the prices of generic products in the same generic classes and by the apparently high level of reported profits. The comparisons are evaluated within the framework of the standard model of competitive price which suggests that the prices of identical products will be the same. This model ignores certain special conditions in the drug industry, including the excess of average cost over marginal cost and the difference in the dependence of individual firms on particular products for sales. The MAC regulation also is supported by the apparently high profits of pharmaceutical manufacturers. But the difference in profits between firms in the drug industry and firms in manufacturing industries as a whole is the result not of monopoly power but of the failure to capitalize R & D expenditures, the persistent growth in demand, and the difference in the riskiness of investment.

The MAC regulation creates problems for the control of quality over drugs. The regulation will encourage physicians to prescribe generically and thus not depend on the guarantees of quality provided by the large manufacturers of brand name products. HEW relies on the FDA to control the quality of drugs, but the FDA has not been successful thus far in enforcing good manufacuting practices among the many small firms in the industry. HEW has refused to accept the conclusions of various studies, most notably the Bioequivalence Panel report. Effective enforcement of the GMP regulations will require frequent inspection of individual plants. The FDA will have to specify the practices to be followed in individual plants much more closely than it has done in the past. The resources required both for the specification of GMP for each plant and for the continuous inspection of these plants will far exceed the resources which are presently used.

Finally, the MAC regulation assumes that competition in the drug industry within any particular generic class is limited to price competition. This again assumes that there is a standard of quality which must be maintained and the FDA can be depended upon to regulate practices in order to achieve that standard. It assumes that there is no possibility of improvement in quality, or else that such improvements are of trivial importance. Nevertheless, in some areas, such as insulin, the competition among firms has resulted in improvements despite the fact that these are multiple-source drugs. Firms continue to strive for greater stability of the products and greater assurance that the products are effective when administered to patients and also for greater assurance of safety through such devices as identicode. The MAC regulation, by emphasizing price, will create an incentive to reduce quality in order to cut costs and so reduce prices. It thus will have the effect of aggravating the present quality problem within the industry.

THE COMPULSORY LICENSING OF PATENTED DRUGS

In 1972 and again in 1973, Senator Gaylord Nelson proposed legislation to grant authority to the Federal Trade Commission to require compulsory licensing of drug patents. Senator Nelson's arguments are similar to those made by Senator Estes Kefauver during the investigation of the industry in the 1959–62 period by the Antitrust and Monopoly Subcommittee.

Senator Kefauver contended that the prices of ethical drugs were excessive in relation to the cost of manufacture and, in addition, the prices of the same drug varied among countries. He attributed the high cost of drugs to patents. He defended the proposal to reduce patent rights in the drug industry, on the grounds that, unlike other consumers, consumers of prescription drugs have no choice among products. He argued that the U.S. was the only industrialized country to issue drug patents with no provision for compulsory licensing or other protection of the public's interests. He also argued that excessive profits indicated the need for new policies. He pointed to data indicating a higher rate of profit on investment in the drug industry than any other industry.[6]

Accordingly, in April 1961, Senator Kefauver introduced S1552 to amend the patent laws as they apply to drugs by requiring compulsory licensing of drug patents.[7] The bill proposed to set a limit of three years from the effective date for patent exclusivity to be followed by an additional period of up to fourteen years in which the patent holder was to grant to qualified applicants an unrestricted license to make, use and sell the drug. The section further provided that if, during the additional period, the patentee failed to grant licenses within ninety days of a request, the Commissioner of Patents could cancel the patent.

The phrase "qualified applicant" was defined as any company holding a license to manufacture drugs under the Food, Drug, and Cosmetic Act. "Unrestricted license" was to include a grant of all technical information required for the manufacturer of the drug. "Effective date" was defined to be the date of filing the New Drug Application in the case of new drugs or date of application for the patent for other than new drugs. The maximum royalty was set at 8 percent of the selling price received by the licensee on the sale of the drug. The full Judiciary Committee approved a modified version of S1552, which eliminated the compulsory licensing provisions.

The Nelson Bill seeks to impose the licensing of drug patents through the rule-making power of the FTC. Under the bill, the FTC would act when the Surgeon General certifies that fewer than four manufacturers produce a drug or that the average price to the consumer is higher in the U.S. than either (1) five times direct cost of the producer or (2) the cost in any foreign country. The FTC would also be empowered to initiate its own investigation and determine whether the prices of drugs are above the levels indicated. If the FTC determines that the criteria had been met, then it will issue a rule requiring licensing of the drug. The Nelson Bill provides that the FTC will specify a reasonable royalty rate, balancing the public need for moderately priced drugs and the industry's need for a fair return. The bill provides that licenses will be made available to all applicants.

The Kefauver Bill's definition of the effective date of patent exclusivity would have reduced the exclusive commercial life to zero for some drugs. Thus, for new drugs, the effective date is defined as the date of filing an NDA. For these drugs, the period required by the FDA for approval might exceed the three-year limit under the bill. For other drugs, the date of application for the patent is defined as the effective date. In those cases, the patent office itself might require more than three years.

Senator Nelson retains the three-year period, but he defines the period as three years of marketing of the drug with sales of over one million dollars. Even this additional protection for patent holders is only apparent. The patent attorney, George E. Frost, in testimony on the Kefauver Bill;[8] stated that this protection would be useless. A patent attorney would advise a client proposing to market a drug copied from a competitor that the probability was small that a patent infringement suit would be decided before the end of the three-year period. In addition, the bill would prohibit suit for patent infringement after the FTC rule becomes effective. Further, it provides that no manufacturer shall be prosecuted for contempt of an injunction against patent infringement following the FTC rule. Thus, the bill provides no penalty for the instances where a patent infringement shall have been established within the three-year period and in fact encourages patent infringement during the three-year period by removing all penalties for infringement.

The Kefauver Bill would require the patentee to provide all of the technical data required for the safe manufacture and sale of the drug. The Nelson Bill would require the patentee to disclose such information in order to qualify for royalties. This type of provision, of course, reduces further the incentive for the development of technology.

The Kefauver Bill fixed 8 percent as the royalty payment, in contrast to the Nelson Bill, which would leave it up to the discretion of the FTC, which, it suggests, would be guided by the standard used by courts in assessing damages. The courts have been employing the standard of 6–8 percent of sales. This is not very different from Kefauver's maximum royalty. This level would probably not be sufficient to compensate the original firm for its investment in R & D, since patent infringers would select the most successful drugs for imitation. The number of failures by the major manufacturers result in the large costs of R & D undertaken and even the technical successes usually are not very great commercial successes.

The provision concerning the ratio of price to direct cost implies that a 5 to 1 ratio for the most successful drugs will be adequate to cover the indirect costs of the manufacture and sale of these drugs and also that there will be sources of revenue to pay for the costs, both direct and indirect, of other less popular drugs. Thus it assumes that the revenue from the sale of each drug will cover all of the costs associated with that drug and that the unallocated costs, such as research costs, which do not result in new marketed drugs will also be covered. In fact, the result of this provision would be to reduce the function of the drug industry to that of a manufacturer of standard commodities with the task of research and promotion being taken over by the government.

CONCLUSIONS

The proposals advanced both by members of the administration and of Congress for changes in public policy towards the drug industry see the principal problem as that of monopoly power based on the prescribing of brand-name drugs. These allegedly are no better than their generic equivalents which are available at much lower prices. The critics therefore call for restrictions on federal reimbursement of payments for drugs, which will have the effect of reducing the prices of brand-name products in multiple source generic drug classes to the level of prices of their generic equivalents. The Nelson Bill provides an alternative approach through compulsory licensing of drug patents.

The first approach is embodied in the MAC regulation. The regulation has a long legislative history and a good deal of support. The government can defend it on the ground that such a measure (it is hoped) would reduce the cost of drugs to the government.

Congressional approval for the Nelson Bill is unlikely in the near future, especially since the MAC regulation has been adopted. The regulation relieves some of the pressure for action in relation to the drug industry. But the Nelson bill cannot be considered a dead issue. The compulsory licensing of patents has precedents. In the UK and in Canada drug companies are required to license their patents to applicants after a short period of exclusivity In addition, compulsory licensing has been used in antitrust cases as a remedy against monopoly power. Indeed, in some cases, like the recent Xerox case, the defendant was required to give up its patent rights and agree to assist competitors in developing their manufacturing skills. Against this background, the compulsory licensing of drug patents after three years of exclusivity may not appear to be an extreme solution of the alleged monopoly problem. It is true that patents are more important for the drug industry than for other manufacturing industries, but this may appear to be a minor consideration to Congressional leaders.

Since the principal objective of public policy in relation to the industry should be to encourage R & D, the primary criterion should be the expected rate of return on R & D investment. We have seen that the expected rate is below the level required for the maintenance of the present level of investment. The enactment of the MAC proposal and of the Nelson bill would depress the expected rate still further.

In fact, government agencies and companies should consider proposals for *increasing* the expected rate of return from investment in R & D. The current low expected rate is at least partly the result of the administration of the regulations governing the introduction of new drugs since the enactment of the Drug Amendments in 1962. To the extent that the FDA can facilitate the introduction of new drugs without increasing risks to patients, the profitability of R & D investment will increase. In addition, Congress might consider an extension of the nominal patent life for drugs. We have seen that the effective patent life is considerably shorter than the nominal life, and an increase would encourage more investment in R & D. These are two obvious approaches.

A third, more questionable, policy proposal would be for the federal government to subsidize the industry's R & D activities. Limits might be placed on the subsidies so that they are designed to encourage research which would not take place without them. Companies are not inclined to investigate possible new drugs which promise small or no profits. Such possible drugs would treat relatively rare diseases, and the resulting sales would be small. The companies already do some of this type of research, but federal subsidies would promote such research. This would not be a novel experiment, for the government already has contracted with pharmaceutical manufacturers for research in the cancer area. We are only suggesting an expansion of such subsidies.

The government might also subsidize research which now is discouraged by poor prospects for patentable drugs. Promising compounds may be in the public domain because they are known, and therefore companies cannot obtain product patents for drugs based on such compounds. Patents covering medical uses or processes generally offer insufficient protection to the innovator to encourage substantial R & D expenditures.

The major conclusion of this discussion of public policy is that there is no obvious need for new legislation or for administrative regulations to reduce the level of profits in the industry. The proposals which Congress and HEW have been considering promise to do more harm than good

CHAPTER 15

ALTERNATIVE GOALS FOR PUBLIC POLICY

RESEARCH AND PUBLIC POLICY

From Kefauver to Nelson and Kennedy, a span of fifteen years, the main thrust of the many Congressional investigations of the industry has been negative. It has been directed at the alleged abuse of monopoly powers which supposedly results in higher than necessary prices, wasteful promotion, and research costs out of proportion to genuine new discoveries. We have seen in the preceding pages that these charges are unsubstantiated. There is much competition in the industry in products as well as in price. The price of a drug must be considered in relation to its benefits, and drugs are a low-cost method of therapy. Research has resulted in the introduction of new drugs which have virtually eliminated certain "killer" or disabling diseases (such as tuberculosis and diphtheria), have drastically reduced the morbidity rates of other infectious diseases, and have greatly reduced the rate of hospitalization and length of stay in hospital resulting from emotional and physical disorders. Such results are evidence of vigorous innovational competition. By focusing on alleged monopolistic abuses, Congress has neglected the really important problems of increasing the rate of new drug innovation and ensuring quality production of drugs.

The concern of Congress with alleged monopolistic abuses has resulted in proposals which conflict with the twin objectives of the development of a good medical care system and a reduction in the cost of medical care. The crucial point is that a sound public policy for the drug industry can be conceived only in the broader context of a general public policy for medical care. The drug industry is an integral part of the health care system and cannot, intelligently, be separated from it. Drugs are an economical medical technology. It is essential that maximum encouragement should be given to new drug innovation. The price paid is relatively very low. Yet Congress has failed to make the relevant cost/benefit analysis. There is need for Congress to concern itself with solving the important problems rather than being diverted from them into a witchhunt.

336

New drugs are still needed. They are needed even in the area which has seen the greatest advances—infectious diseases, which together still account for a significant fraction of all deaths and severe disabilities. The development of tranquilizers has not yet reduced the state hospital population to a small number. In addition, the decline in the death rate from cardiovascular diseases as a whole has been small.

Congress has recognized the importance of medical research for the reduction of morbidity and mortality rates by providing large appropriations for the support of medical research, chiefly through the National Institutes of Health. But one may wonder about the likelihood of practical success from the broadly based and largely academic program conducted by NIH. There has been little discussion of the process by which the knowledge acquired through biomedical research is applied to the development of new therapy. While the scientists in universities, hospitals, government laboratories, and nonprofit private laboratories perform research which adds to the basic knowledge of life processes, their work contributes to the discovery of new drugs only indirectly and in ways which are complex and not easy to discern. Some laboratories outside the industry conduct applied research, but by far the bulk of research explicitly seeking new drugs is carried on within the industry. It is the industry, and not academic or government institutions, which possesses the skills and resources required for applied research, and it is the industry which is society's chief instrument in the search for new drugs.

Drugs have become medicine's most important technology. The advances in drug therapy have led to much larger reductions in mortality and morbidity than advances in other medical technologies. Furthermore, most nonpharmaceutical modes of medical intervention are technically demanding and labor-intensive; the scarcity and costs of skilled manpower and facilities prevent their use on a massive scale. Drugs, by contrast, are mass-produced, generally simple to administer, and hence are relatively inexpensive. The cornerstone of modern medical treatment is drugs.

The source of new drugs is the pharmaceutical industry. The majority of new drugs have come from the industry, and its share has grown. Yet the discussion of medical research has neglected the industry's contribution. The neglect is due to the preoccupation with the alleged monopoly power of pharmaceutical firms. The attack on this aspect of the industry has distorted the understanding and discussion of important aspects of public policy towards the industry. It has resulted in a discussion about the pharmaceutical industry in which nothing can be looked at in straightforward, objective fashion. In particular, it has prevented us from investigating the important social question of how best to mobilize the skills and resources of the pharmaceutical industry against the human and economic costs of disease.

The concern over the monopoly issue, combined with a lack of understanding of the economics of the industry, has had other unfortunate effects. It has

produced legislative proposals for the reduction of drug prices through government controls or through a drastic reduction in the life of drug patents—
proposals which, if enacted, would have the disastrous consequence for society
of substantially reducing investment in pharmaceutical R & D and the rate of
innovation in therapeutics.

The rate of innovation, however, has declined, and more patents have expired
in recent years than have been granted. The emphasis therefore will tend to shift
from innovation to price. Yet the focus on innovation is to be preferred to that
on price in an industry where the output is a product for the treatment of
disease. It is not clear that public policy makers would be eager for a change,
despite their allegiance to the benefits of price competition. Nevertheless, the
emphasis on innovation is threatened not only by the expiration of patents and
the slowing down of the rate of innovation but also by proposed changes in
public policy designed to reduce profits in the industry.

The paramount issue in the development of public policy for the provision of
medical care thus is how to encourage the maintenance and perhaps even an
increase in the industry's traditional emphasis on new drug innovation as a
business strategy. A public policy aimed at this goal must recognize that R & D
expenditures are investments and that to undertake such expenditures, firms
must expect a rate of return at least equal to what they expect from alternative
investments.

The expected rate of return from investment in R & D has declined sharply
over the past decade in the pharmaceutical industry and is now quite low—lower
than from investment generally, and much less than it was in 1960. This decline
is caused by the drop in the number of new drug introductions in the market,
the increase in the costs of R & D, and the increase in the length of the required
development period. If this pattern continues, the inevitable effect of these
changes will be to reduce the R & D effort of the industry. If R & D expenditures are to increase, as they must if the rate of therapeutic innovation is to be
accelerated, the expected rate of return on R & D expenditures cannot persist
long at the current low level.

REPORTED PROFITS AND PRICING

Since public attention has focused on the reported profits, pricing, and promotion expenditures of drug companies, we have examined these aspects of the
industry's behavior. Our analysis has emphasized an outstanding yet often
neglected characteristic of the industry: profits have originated in the discovery
and development of a *few* highly successful new drugs reflecting a large random
component in the success of drug companies. Most of the marketed drugs do not
provide a satisfactory return on investment in R & D; it is the handful of very
successful drugs which companies must depend on to yield an acceptable rate of

return from all R & D. But public attention has focused on such drugs for the very reason that they are highly successful, and some proposed public policies threaten to prevent such individual great successes in the future. If these policies are adopted, the prospects for profits from investment in R & D become dismal indeed.

We have examined pricing from the same point of view. We have demonstrated that while the price of an individual product may seem very high when compared with its direct manufacturing cost, it is inappropriate to calculate the costs of individual products or even of individual firms to obtain economically relevant estimates of the expected rate or return on investment in R & D. The *industry as a whole* is the appropriate unit, and the individual firm's profits and prices are only relevant insofar as they influence the estimate of the expected return for the industry.

Many of the discussions feature the average reported rate of profit of the industry. Usually the estimate of this average is high because it refers to a group of leading companies rather than to a representative sample. The average reported rate even for a representative sample exceeds the average for all manufacturing companies, but the difference can be accounted for without resorting to the monopoly explanation. Thus, pharmaceutical companies' financial reports exaggerate their economic or true rate of profit by treating R & D expenditures as current expenses rather than capitalizing them. A second factor which generally has been ignored in analyzing the high profits has been the rapid growth in the demand for drugs. This oversight is probably due to the predisposition of economists to the belief that periods of market growth are short and therefore cannot produce high profits over a long period. But the demand for drugs has grown continuously over a long period owing to the introduction of new drugs, the growth in the general level of income, and the increase in the demand for medical service attributable to the increase in the share of payments for such service by third parties, including the government and private insurance companies. Another reason for the apparently high profits is the relatively high level of risk. The relative riskiness of investment in drug R & D inhibits new capital from entering and depressing the average rate of return. The evidence thus indicates that monopoly power is unlikely to have been an important source of the industry's profits. Other factors than monopoly power account for the differential between the industry's average reported rate of return and that of manufacturing as a whole.

The prices of individual drugs, even more than the overall profit rate of pharmaceutical companies, have drawn unfavorable public attention to the industry. Using various methods of estimating the costs of manufacturing individual drugs, critics have come to the conclusion that prices are excessive. Some of the measures are naïve, depending as they do entirely on the cost of ingredients with no allowance for manufacturing costs, administration, R & D, and promotion. But even some relatively careful estimates result in an unfavorable verdict. One practical result has been the British Monopolies Commission's order to Hoffman-LaRoche to reduce the price of Valium.

Analyzing the relationship between the costs and prices of individual drugs is a meaningless undertaking, simply because very few drugs have large enough sales to generate profits. The prices of the few successful drugs are the ones which come under attack, and naturally by the standards of hindsight, the costs of producing these individual big sellers may not appear to warrant their prices.

The price of a single drug may appear to be excessive even if a share of its manufacturer's total R & D expenditures is imputed to it on the basis of its share of total sales, and if other indirect costs are similarly imputed. The reason for this is that the appropriate unit of analysis is the industry as a whole and not the firm, but it is the firm, not the industry, that is the unit used to prepare these estimates of a drug's cost. If we do not permit individual firms to earn high profits, then the expected average rate of return for the industry will be too low to encourage continued investment. The appropriate economic criterion for public policy, therefore, is the expected rate of return from investment in R & D by the industry as a whole. Only if this is relatively high can a case be made for controlling prices or otherwise reducing profits.

The rarity of large-selling products also helps to explain observed differences in prices among different classes of buyers. Hospitals and other large institutional buyers pay less for drugs than do retail pharmacies. This is a form of price discrimination similar to that in other industries, including the publicly regulated utilities which sell power at lower prices to industrial consumers than to households. Lower costs of handling and distributing bulk orders account for only part of the difference in price; the main reason is the low marginal cost of production relative to the average total cost. In other words, producing an additional unit results in only a small incremental cost relative to the average cost per unit, including all overheads. A firm, therefore, can increase its profits by increasing sales even if the price for incremental units does not cover average costs, so long as it exceeds marginal cost. Over all of the units sold, however, the firm must cover average cost if it is to earn any profits. If a firm were to sell to retailers at the same low price as to a hospital, then total revenues would fall below total costs and losses would ensue. So long as a firm can restrict the low price to part of the market, a loss need not result. A firm would prefer to supply hospitals without having to reduce prices to below average cost, but it has to meet the competing bids of other sellers. These competitive pressures are great in relation to the large-selling drugs which attract the competition of other large manufacturers whose reputation for high quality products equal that of the original producer. Since the innovator has already met the costs of R & D and of promotion and doctors know the original product, these manufacturers can enter with little R & D and promotional expense and base their appeal on price.

These conditions of production and of the market also help to explain the observed international differences in prices. Prices of individual products have little relation to their costs of manufacturing.

In some countries, notably the U.K., the government has depressed drug prices to very low levels. Those countries do not carry their full share of the costs of research. This is the case even when, as in the U.K., the price negotiated with the government includes an allowance for such costs. This allowance is computed on the basis of the single firm, and we have already seen that the industry is the appropriate unit.

The absence of a cost basis for the prices of individual products raises the suspicion of monopoly power and provokes legislative proposals to encourage the early entry of generics. But the industry's inability to supply a cost justification of individual product prices is not the crucial economic issue; what matters is that the proposed legislation promises to reduce the rate of return from all investment in R & D and thus change the entire structure and behavior of the industry. The reduction of costs and the prices of existing drugs would become the focus of competition instead of R & D and innovation. Some other organization which does not as yet exist would have to perform the work that the industry now does in pharmaceutical research.

PROMOTIONAL EXPENDITURES

Many economists believe that promotional expenditures are the oligopolists' method of avoiding socially beneficial price competition. The promotional expenditures themselves apparently result in no direct and obvious utility to consumers but do add to the costs and, therefore, the prices of drugs. The critics suspect, moreover, that prescribers are unduly influenced by manufacturers' promotional efforts to encourage them to prescribe inappropriate or unnecessarily expensive drugs. And some physicians who appeared before the Nelson Subcommittee complained about the biased presentations of detailmen and journal advertisements and the large volume of promotional materials which they received and found difficult to go through.

Our study leads to the conclusion that promotional expenditures yield the service of providing information to doctors. This is not to suggest that companies are altruistic or that their main concern is something other than to increase sales. But to achieve this goal, firms must convey information to prescribers, and prescribers must be able to rely on it.

Even if doctors were far less busy than they are, they could not hope to keep up with the vast literature on drugs. And while the detailman is obviously an advocate, his claims have to be accurate if his company is to avoid contradiction by competitors, other detailmen, FDA action, liability suits, and the loss of its good reputation with doctors. What is more, effective selling of so complex a product as a drug to doctors, all of whom are highly trained, requires emphasis on its real therapeutic properties. An effective detailman cannot depend on his charm or the good will created by small gifts such as free prescription pads; he must show the physician that a product fills a need in that doctor's practice. To be sure, he will not emphasize the merits of rival products. But each company will promote its own drugs, and when a company knows that it can make strong claims for a drug, it can expect expenditures on promoting these claims to be far more productive than when a drug has no great advantage over competitive products. Doctors therefore can discover the advantages of different drugs. The influence of partisan sales claims on uninformed doctors should not be overestimated. Despite allegations to the contrary, there is no evidence of widespread misinformation of doctors by detailmen.

The informational service of manufacturers has been essential up to now, and it cannot be eliminated without the provision of some substitute. The only significant one which has been proposed suggests that either the FDA or some other federal agency rate drugs and advise doctors. Unless some such authority is created, doctors must continue to exercise their own judgment, and therefore they must be able to hear the rival claims of manufacturers. It should be noted, too, that this alternative of a federal agency is less simple than it appears to be, and the difficulties which it will create must be considered carefully. Doctors cannot unquestioningly accept the views of any expert, because experts are by no means unanimous concerning the efficacy and safety of individual drugs. Disagreements have been numerous. In addition, doctors, as well as patients, differ in their therapeutic objectives and their aversion to particular risks. Because the balance of therapeutic benefit and risk is always partly a subjective and personal decision, the general considerations of the expert cannot be decisive.

We must also consider the costs of promotion. Our estimate of the potential savings to consumers from the elimination of promotion is in the vicinity of 5 percent of their drug bill. Since any measures to reduce the cost of promotion will not eliminate it completely, the resulting savings would be less than 5 percent. Further, the elimination of promotion may raise the cost of medical care as a whole. Any saving is likely to be more than offset by the cost of the additional time required by doctors to keep informed of new drug developments, by a reduction in the quality of medical care, and by the greater use of alternative therapy (e.g., hospitalization) that results from the ignorance consequent to cutting back promotion.

There is also the question of whether the expenditures of individual companies are large enough to influence unduly doctors' prescribing choices. We have estimated that each of the eight leading firms spends an average of $138 annually per doctor on promotion; a high alternative estimate of these expenditures is $225. In 1973 the average promotional expenditures per drug among the fifty leading drugs per doctor was only approximately $10. We have also estimated that each of the eight leading companies calls on each doctor 3.4 times per year. These estimates do not warrant the impression of high-pressure selling. It appears that the impression of high pressure is created by the cumulative total effort of all firms (which include many more than the eight leaders). Doctors can feel overwhelmed even if each firm spends only a modest amount.

A less obvious but perhaps equally important consideration is that promotional efforts complement companies' innovative efforts. Promotional campaigns are built on the claims of superiority resulting from innovation. A successful innovator usually mounts a promotional campaign to accelerate the adoption and sales of its new product and to familiarize doctors with its properties. The innovator also protects its position against the possible entry of competitors with similar drugs. The first drug which is accepted and becomes widely used has an important advantage over new and unfamiliar drugs. Innovation thus increases the value of greater promotional effort by a company. This reasoning is supported by the finding that promotional expenditures increase among companies with the number of new entities introduced.

If companies shift away from a competitive strategy based on innovation, their promotional expenditures are likely to decline. Their new strategy will probably stress reductions in costs and in prices rather than improvements in the therapeutic properties of drugs and the resulting promotional claims. While some advertising will be needed to inform doctors of the existence of drugs and of new dosage forms, total expenditures on promotion probably will decline.

The shift may be taking place. The pharmaceutical industry, which has always contained small generic producers, has recently seen the larger firms enter the market with generic products. The result has been sharp price cuts. This trend toward more generic competition will probably accelerate with the expiration of the patents on many major drugs. Since many drugs were introduced in the later 1950s and early 1960s, their patents are now running out. In 1972 as much as 35 percent of sales were accounted for by drugs no longer protected by patents. On the assumption that new drugs have not appeared since 1972 among the leading 200 drugs, then the percentage will rise to 40 percent in 1975 and 69 percent in 1980 (see table 6-4).

New drugs have continued to appear, so the rise will not be as rapid as these estimates indicate, but a significant rise can be expected. We may be on the verge of a period of intense price competition, regardless of changes in public policy, and this whole discussion thus may be moot.

THE ECONOMICS OF PHARMACEUTICAL R & D

A strong economic case favors greater investment in R & D. Prices of medical services have risen, and society's medical bill continues to increase. Drugs would reduce the burden because they are less expensive than other types of treatment. Hospital care is very expensive, and the use of such treatment procedures as surgery and radiology requires highly trained skills and costly equipment. The economics of medical care thus adds an economic case to the humanitarian one for developing new drugs.

Contrary to popular belief, the pharmaceutical industry has been the major source of new drug discoveries. The industry discovered 91 percent of all new single entities introduced between 1960 and 1969. Despite this record, many people still believe that the important research leading to new drugs is performed in academic, government, and private nonprofit laboratories. They believe that these laboratories perform the necessary basic research while industrial laboratories merely apply the knowledge so obtained to prepare new drugs. The standard economic model of research gives a major role to the inventor, who is represented as familiar with the new basic knowledge and is the one to supply the insight to solve a practical problem. According to this model, large corporations are bureaucratic and therefore unable to make important discoveries but are proficient at the relatively routine and riskless but costly developmental work of designing products and production processes, where their risks are economic rather than technical. This model is supported by descriptions of individual inventions and innovations, which may be unrepresentative. Little systematic empirical work has been done to test this model; but, more to the point, this representation does not accurately describe contemporary research in pharmaceuticals.

Contrary to the model, corporate drug research is not bureaucratic: company laboratories have considerable independence. The model is also wrong about the risks. The firms take great technical as well as financial risks. Some have failed to discover a new single entity in particular fields after spending large funds over long periods. Contrary to the model, each pharmaceutical firm does its own discovery research; the work cannot be left to outside academic or other nonindustrial laboratories. Basic research is done in academic and governmental laboratories, but this research is not directed at the discovery of drugs; it is aimed at expanding the knowledge of particular disciplines. Furthermore, much of the basic knowledge and technique used in pharmaceutical research does not come from what is called basic research but rather is the product of applied research either within the general area of pharmaceutical research or of applied research in other fields based on chemistry. We have seen that some of the techniques of chemical analysis were developed in applied research seeking to solve practical problems connected with petroleum and with textile fibres.

The industry does most of the discovery research, which includes the synthesis of new compounds and their screening by animal tests to detect the desired activity. In the traditional model of invention a single inventor working alone combines the results of basic research in different disciplines. In actuality, discovery research in drugs requires the close cooperation of several different specialists. And, unlike much academic and basic research, it is not confined to a single discipline. Developmental research, moreover, must be closely linked with discovery research. Developmental research begins when a compound is submitted to animal toxicology testing. A clinical pharmacologist (physician), together with the chemists, pharmacologists, and toxicologists who were involved in the discovery research, then plans the clinical tests. In sum, the standard model of research draws a sharp line between discovery and developmental research and expects the inventor to transfer his patent to a developer after discovery research is complete. But drug research, as it is actually performed, draws no sharp line between discovery and developmental research. The interest and involvement of the chemists who synthesize a compound do not end with discovery. Their interest is maintained up to a late stage of what is called the development stage because of the great uncertainty of technical success. The probability of technical success after a proposed drug enters the development stage is estimated at 0.07. Despite the evidence of animal trials, it is only in phase II, after the proposed drug has passed some of the required clinical tests, that a research group can have confidence that technical success has been achieved. Indeed, it is only then that the drug is discovered, for many candidates reach this stage—and do not go beyond it.

Contrary to the model, industrial drug laboratories find it difficult to develop compounds from academic or from other industrial laboratories before a late stage of clinical testing. Pharmacological theory provides little guidance for the appraisal of a compound, and as a result the research is highly empirical. Few compounds demonstrating desirable biological activity eventually become safe, effective drugs, and clinicians who are responsible for the human tests are therefore very skeptical of the claims of chemists and pharmacologists.

It is thus clear that the high degree of uncertainty concerning the efficacy and safety of a drug which persists until late in the development stage, makes it difficult for compounds which are still being developed to be transferred from one firm to another. In addition, the chemists and pharmacologists who discover a proposed drug will work hard to overcome toxicological problems and other problems that come up later by modifying the compound and testing different analogs. The sale of patent rights prior to the completion of development thus is very difficult to negotiate, as evidenced by the high proportion of drugs discovered by the firms introducing them.

There are several other reasons for the concentration of pharmaceutical research in the industry. There are economies of scale in this type of research. Only large industrial firms have the required resources to organize large laboratories, with their large, multidisciplinary staffs. The employment of specialized skills is a source of economies of scale, and our study confirms their existence by demonstrating that innovative output increases more than proportionally with employment in industrial laboratories. Another reason is the need for large funds for R & D; our estimate of the average cost of research and development of a new drug is $24 million. While these funds are not needed in advance (the average period of research and development now is ten years), a firm will usually conduct several projects simultaneously, and consequently its annual R & D expenditures are large. In addition, academic scientists usually are interested in the advance of scientific knowledge rather than the discovery of new drugs. Their immediate preoccupations are with scientific problems, which fall *within* disciplines, and their work therefore is organized by discipline rather than as an interdisciplinary effort. Applied research utilizes the findings of research within disciplines, but it is usually not directly related to such research which is currently under way. Applied research also is unattractive to many academic scientists because it requires an excessive amount of tedious, repetitious trial-and-error experimentation. This characteristic of applied pharmaceutical research is duplicated in every field of technology which is based on chemistry, be it plastics, pesticides, or oil additives. The similarity is due to the fact that before a new product is invented, a chemist must create a large number of chemical compounds which must be systematically evaluated using techniques and end-use measures originating outside the discipline of chemistry.

These characteristics of drug research affect the productivity of different types of medical R & D expenditures. An investment in basic research is unlikely to generate practical discoveries at as fast a rate as the same investment in applied industrial research. For while the efforts of academic laboratories provide some basic knowledge for applied research, the transfer and utilization of this basic knowledge to the consumer is a complex and indirect process. This is due to the nature of drug research which, limited by the great complexity of biological organisms and our very incomplete knowledge of them, relies on empirical research rather than on the findings of basic research. To fund academic laboratories with the expectation of their providing knowledge of physiological processes which have a *direct* practical payoff in the form of drugs ignores the history of drug innovation. This is the reason why the vast investment in basic biological science funded by NIH since the 1950s has not resulted in rapid therapeutic progress, although it has added to the body of scientific knowledge. There is, on the other hand, much evidence to show that additional investment in R & D in the industry does lead to new drugs.

THE EXPECTED RATE OF RETURN ON PHARMACEUTICAL R & D

Investment in R & D will not be maintained at the current level if the expected rate of return is lower than that expected from alternative investments. We have estimated the expected rate of return on the R & D investment needed to obtain a new single chemical entity. Our formula estimated the expected rate of return from a stream of investment and the income which it generates. An equation was set up to determine the rate of return required to obtain a zero present value for a projected stream of investment and income. If this rate of return is high compared to that available from other investments, then the investment is undertaken.

Since the obvious goal of public policy is to encourage *significant* therapeutic discoveries, we estimated the expected rate of return on R & D investments directed only to the discovery and development of new single chemical entities (NCE's) rather than to new combination drugs or new dosage forms. In estimating the expected rate of return, we included the costs of failures as well as those of success. We assumed that in the future as much research effort will be required to obtain an NCE as in the period 1966–72 and that the R & D period is ten years. The resulting estimate of the R & D cost was $24.4 million. However, a company in fact invests only the after-tax cost, which is half, or $12.2 million. Assuming that the expenditures are equally spread over the whole R & D period of ten years, we obtain an annual after-tax R & D investment per NCE of $1.22 million. We also estimated the net income anticipated per NCE. We used the average domestic sales in 1972 of drugs introduced in 1962–68, $7.5 million, as the basis for estimating the net income. To estimate world sales we added 47 percent to the estimate of domestic sales, which brought the total to $11.0 million per NCE. The estimated profit margin, inclusive of R & D expenditures and after taxes, is 15.4 percent of sales. When we applied this margin after adjustment for other work to actual sales, we obtained $1.40 million in net profits per year. The commercial life was estimated at fifteen years. The expected rate of return on investment was estimated to be 3.3 percent. We also estimated the effect of extending the commercial life of the product from fifteen to twenty years, since the choice of a fifteen-year life is arbitrary, and that of increasing the gross margin to 17.5 percent and 20.0 percent.

Regardless of which estimate of the expected rate of return we use, it is *less* than the decision criterion used in other industries for determining new investment, which has been in the vicinity of 10 percent after taxes, and currently is probably much higher in most industries.

CONCLUSIONS

The case for product rather than price competition is especially appealing in the drug industry, since innovations have resulted in important new drugs. The minor product modifications which have also resulted should not obscure the significant advances. And while promotional competition may be less useful socially than price competition, the results of the combination of innovational and promotional competition may be difficult to surpass.

Since the pharmaceutical industry has been and remains the logical source of new drug development, we cannot count on existing nonindustrial organizations to invent these drugs. Nor could we easily develop an equally productive alternative system.

Current public policy threatens to hinder pharmaceutical R & D in several ways. First, it is likely to divert the limited scientific manpower to academic and other laboratories. Second, the MAC regulation promises to discourage new industrial R & D by reducing the expected rate of return from this type of investment.

The estimate of the expected rate of return from investment in pharmaceutical research has an ominous portent. If the profitability of R & D investment remains as low as is expected, such investment will decline and society will have to look to sources other than the industry for new drugs. Laboratories similar to those now operated by the industry will have to be organized and paid for. Criteria will have to be adopted for the selection of compounds to develop and produce, and new ways of transferring new technology to producers will have to be created. Results are not automatic; an enormous organized effort is required for the discovery and development of new drugs, and if profit incentives are absent, effective alternative incentives cannot be developed easily.

There is a tendency for those who find fault with private industry to seek the solution in government, and government institutions indeed may have to take over pharmaceutical research should the present level of the expected rate of return continue. Nevertheless, this is not a desirable development. The cost of R & D per drug developed in government laboratories is likely to be much higher than in private industrial laboratories. The incentives for economy are not as great. In addition, the selection of fields for research is likely to be based on political rather than on medical or economic considerations. Politically determined choices will result in the allocation of excessive resources to research seeking treatments of diseases which have caught public attention. The prospects for success may be minimal, and, in any case, the effort may require the abandonment of other research efforts which also are worthy but have less political appeal. The recent allocation of large funds for cancer research for example, reflects an essentially political view, and it has been criticized by scientists for diverting funds from other areas where success is more probable. The economic incentives of private pharmaceutical companies may not provide a fully satisfactory set of criteria for the selection of research objectives. These tend to result in the neglect of fatal diseases which are rare, such as certain types of cancer. The private companies do some research of this type, partly out of a sense of social obligation and partly in response to the interests of scientists in the laboratories who have some influence on the choice of projects. Nevertheless, the result may not be an adequate commitment of resources to the search for drugs to treat such rare diseases, and other funding institutions, including the government, probably should supply funds for this purpose. The cancer research financed by the federal government illustrates this recognition by policymakers, even if the result has been excessive appropriations in relation to what can be used well.

Though the proposals for reducing the profits of drug companies may very well entail a complex restructuring of the entire industry, the problems have not been thought through. The discussion has not even recognized that the central issue is the level of the expected rate of return from investment in R & D under the present system, to say nothing of the effects which the proposals would have. Once this point is recognized, it becomes clear that the expected rate of return under the existing system is already low and that there is a serious danger of a decline in the amount of resources devoted to research in this industry.

Public policy towards the industry should be formulated in the context of a broad program for the improvement of the medical care system. Drugs are the major medical technology, and the reduction of the suffering and cost of disease will require the developments of new drugs. These are the primary considerations which should guide the development of public policy.

THE EFFECT OF SUBSTITUTING SMALL VALUES FOR ZERO ON REGRESSION COEFFICIENTS CHAPTER 5

We used as a dependent variable the number of new single entities (N) either in the unweighted form or weighted by various indexes to measure either the importance or the novelty of new single entities. Since some companies introduced no new single entities over the period of the investigation, the value of N or any weighted version of N would be zero for these companies. Since logarithmic equations cannot handle zero values, we substituted an arbitrarily small value (.0001) for zero. We tested whether this procedure introduced a bias in the results which favored the conclusion that there are economies of scale in pharmaceutical research by substituting other values for zero to test the effect of the use of so small a number as .0001.

We reproduce here one of the equations (5.30) which utilized this value (.0001) instead of zero:

$$\ln N_s = -11.49 + 1.39 \ln S + .26 (\ln S)^2$$
$$(t = 7.10) \quad (t = 8.65) \qquad R^2 = .60$$
$$(SE = 0.184) \quad (SE = 0.030) \qquad F = 44.31$$

When we use .001 we obtain:

$$\ln N_s = -8.46 + .76 \ln S + .25 (\ln S)^2$$
$$(t = 4.97) \quad (t = 7.95) \qquad R^2 = .60$$
$$(SE = 0.152) \quad (SE = .032) \qquad F = 43.01$$

When we use .01 we obtain:

$$\ln N_s = -5.47 + .26 \ln S + .24 (\ln S)^2$$
$$(t = 1.65) \quad (t = 6.58) \qquad R^2 = .57$$
$$(SE = .158) \quad (SE = .036) \qquad F = 39.28$$

When we use .1 we obtain:

$$\ln N_s = -2.69 - .047 \ln S + .19 (\ln S)^2$$
$$(t = -.202) \quad (t = 4.024)$$
$$(SE = .23156) \quad (SE = .04726)$$

The substitution of .001 instead of .0001 has little effect on the final results. The use of .01 and .1 renders the linear coefficient nonsignificant (at the .05 critical level). On the other hand, the coefficient of the quadratic term remains positive and significant. Thus the hypothesis that large size of firm yields economies of scale in R & D remains confirmed even when we multiply the original proxy values for zero by a factor of 1000.

NOTES ON CONTROVERSIES
ON DRUG CHOICE

Experts do not agree on the best drugs to use for the treatment of diseases. The following sections discuss the drug use of different experts on problems in relation to the treatment of hypertension and schizophrenia and diabetes.

HYPERTENSION

The *Journal of Modern Medicine* (March 20, 1972) reported the proceedings of a symposium on the treatment of essential and malignant hypertension. At this symposium, Dr. Robert Wilkins took the position that the barbiturates are among the best blood-pressure lowering agents. He reported, however, that he did not prescribe them during the day because they produced somnolence. Dr. Edward D. Freis of Georgetown University disagreed. In his opinion controlled trials indicated that they were no more effective than a placebo. He said that there might be a great harm in temporizing by utilizing barbiturates instead of genuine antihypertensive drugs.

Dr. Freis also suggested that there was a good deal of uncertainty in the selection of a therapeutic program and suggested that before beginning drug treatment, it was worthwhile to tell the patient that there might be a good deal of trial and error required before finding the ideal treatment. He went on to say that there was no way of testing the equivalence of the various derivatives of rauwolfia. Alpha-methyldopa, for instance, produced somnolence which might become less severe as the drug is continued. On the other hand, perhaps 10 percent to 20 percent of hypertensive patients cannot take effective doses of the drug because of excessive sleepiness.

SCHIZOPHRENIA

According to Dr. Leo E. Hollister,[1] doctors use the more sedative phenothiazines, such as chlorpromazine and thioridazine, for patients with agitation and the less sedative drugs, such as trifluoperazine, for those patients exhibiting symptoms of withdrawal and retardation. But the approach has not been systematic, and the latest review of the entire subject of predicting responses to antipsychotic drugs concludes that the present evidence for the differential action of antipsychotic drugs is inconclusive. Dr. Hollister comments that studies showing differential action are based on retrospective analysis of group data which implicitly assume that doctors choose the correct drug for each patient, but the proper choice of drug for individual patients is very difficult.

A choice among the wide variety of antipsychotic drugs that are available should be based on learning the use of a few drugs well rather than on a superficial familiarity with all of them, maintains Dr. Hollister. The difference in treatment between the proper and improper use of the drug will probably exceed the effect of differences between drugs. He also says that the patient's past performance is a reliable guide. If the patient has done well previously on a drug, and especially if he has done less well on others, it would be foolhardy to change drugs or to reinstitute lapsed treatment with a different drug. According to Dr. Hollister the choice of drug for individual patients as much an art as a science.

Dr. Thomas A. Ban,[2] Associate Professor of Psychiatry and Director, Division of Pharmacology, at McGill University, agrees that the consensus concerning the best treatment for overactive behavior is not necessarily correct. Chlorpromazine is regarded as the drug of choice, but a study by J. Marks which Dr. Ban cites failed to confirm this consensus. Nor did Dr. Marks find that withdrawn patients responded better to the more activating phenothiazines. Dr. Ban also refers to the clinical observation that individual patients may be unaffected by a specific agent but may respond to some other drug.

DIABETES

In 1970 the FDA warned doctors against the possible dangers of oral antidiabetic drugs. It recommended that these drugs be given only to patients who cannot be controlled by diet or weight loss and for whom the use of insulin is unacceptable. The American Diabetes Association and the Council on Drugs of the American Medical Association have supported this view.

The recommendation is based on the study of the University Group Diabetes Program (UGDP) which began in 1961 in several universities. The study found that one of the oral antidiabetic drugs appeared to increase the death rate from cardiovascular disease. According to an editorial on the subject in *The British Medical Journal*,[3] the result is inconclusive, for the difference between the number of deaths from all causes in the control group and in the experimental group was not statistically significant. In addition, the study is subject to criticism on several grounds. The results in the different centers were not consistent. Although Cincinnati and Minneapolis contributed fewer than a quarter of the patients, these two centers accounted for more than half of the deaths in both the control and experimental groups. In addition, the reports of the causes of death are in doubt, since necropsies were done in only one third of the cases. There are other unusual features of the study. Women constituted 75 percent of the patients; excess mortality from cardiovascular disease in the experimental group was confined to women; half of all of the patients in the study were non-white; the excess of female cardiovascular deaths was largely among white women.

The result of the UGDP study disagreed with those recorded by H. Keene and R.J. Jarrett in Great Britain and by J. Paasikivi in Sweden. Both of these studies, according to the *British Medical Journal* editorial, suggested the opposite conclusion. They showed a decreased risk of cardiovascular disease in the experimental group.

The British Medical Journal expressed surprise at the recommendation of the FDA and more particularly at the decision of the American Diabetes Association to go along with the FDA. (A few months earlier the FDA had decided not to accept the UGDP study as evidence for the abandonment of oral agents as one of the methods of treatment. The reversal of this decision occurred without new evidence becoming available). The *Journal* pointed out that the UGDP study itself show that fewer than half the patients on a variable dose of insulin adhered strictly to their treatment, and that insulin treatment also has adverse effects, including hypoglycemia and weight gain.

A later article by A.M. Donkins and Arnold Bloom[4] points out that many of the subjects in the UGDP study were borderline cases which, in Great Britain at any rate, are usually treated by simple dietary restriction. The authors found in their study that when all therapy was discontinued, 31 percent of the patients remained as well controlled as when they had been taking tablets. Thus, even when poor initial response to simple dietary restrictions indicates a need for oral therapy, such therapy is not necessarily permanent. The dose can be reduced and then discontinued if control is maintained. They suggest that when hyperglycemia recurs it is reasonable to reintroduce oral therapy at the previous effective dose level. They also conclude that there is no firm evidence that insulin is more or less effective than oral therapy in preventing degenerative complications in diabetics that cannot be controlled on simple dietary restriction.

NOTES

CHAPTER 1

1. J. Fred Weston, "Implications of Recent Research for the Structural Approach to Oligopoly," *Antitrust Law Journal,* vol. 41, 1972; reprinted in *The Competitive Economy: Selected Readings,* ed. Yale Brozen (Morristown, N.J.: General Learning Press, 1975), pp. 86–93.

2. For example, W. Duncan Reekie, "Some Problems Associated with the Marketing of Ethical Pharmaceutical Products," *Journal of Industrial Economics* 1 (Nov. 1970):33–49.

3. See H. D. Walker, *Market Power and Price Levels in the Ethical Drug Industry* (Bloomington: Indiana University Press, 1971); William S. Comanor, "Research and Competitive Product Differentiation in the Pharmaceutical Industry in the United States," *Economica,* n. s. 31 (November 1964):372–84; Henry Steele, "Monopoly and Competition in the Ethical Market," *Journal of Law and Economics* 5 (October 1962): 131–63.

4. Textbooks in the field of industrial organization review this literature. See, for example: F. M. Scherer, *Industrial Market Structure and Economic Performance* (Chicago: Rand McNally and Co., 1970), pp. 351–52.

5. David Schwartzman, "The Burden of Monopoly," *Journal of Political Economy,* December 1960, 627–30.

6. See, for example, Edwin Mansfield, *The Economics of Technological Change* (N.Y.: W. W. Norton, 1968), chapters 2 and 3.

7. Pharmaceutical Manufacturers Association, *Prescription Industry Fact Book* (Washington, D.C.: PMA, 1972), pp. 41–42.

8. Comanor, "Research and Competitive Product Differentiation"; Walker, *Market Power and Price Levels.*

9. David Schwartzman, "The Expected-Profits Method of Locating Monopoly Power," *The Antitrust Bulletin* 17, no. 4 (Winter 1972).

10. Milton Silverman and Philip R. Lee, *Pills, Profits, and Politics* (Berkeley: University of California Press, 1974), chapter 3.

11. Joe S. Bain, *Industrial Organization,* 2d ed. (New York: Wiley, 1968), pp. 352–53.

12. Leonard W. Weiss, "The Concentration–Profits Relationship and Antitrust," in *Industrial Concentration: The New Learning,* ed. Harvey J. Goldschmid, H. Michael Mann, and J. Fred Weston (Boston: Little, Brown and Company, 1974) pp. 184–232.

13. James M. Ferguson, *Advertising: Theory, Measurement, Fact* (Cambridge, Mass.: Ballinger, 1974).

14. Stanley I. Ornstein, "Concentration and Profits," in *The Impact of Large Firms in the U.S. Economy,* ed. J. Fred Weston and Stanley Ornstein (Lexington, Mass.: Lexington Books, 1973), pp. 87–102.

15. Scherer, *Industrial Market Structure,* pp. 4–7.

16. Harold Demsetz, "Two Systems of Belief About Monopoly," in Goldschmid et al., *Industrial Concentration,* pp. 164–83; David Schwartzman, "Competition and Efficiency: Comment," *Journal of Political Economy* 81 (May/June 1973): 756–64.

17. Scherer, *Industrial Market Structure,* chapters 13, 14, 15, 17.

18. George J. Stigler, "The Kinky Oligopoly Demand Curve and Rigid Prices," *Journal of Political Economy,* October 1947, pp. 432–49.

19. Phillip Nelson, "Information and Consumer Behavior," *Journal of Political Economy* 78 (March/April 1970):311–29.

20. George von Haunalter, "Health Care Expenditures in the U.S. Through 1980," mimeographed (Menlo Park, Cal.: Stanford Research Institute, 1973), pp. 11–12.

21. See, for example, the discussions of the influence of drugs in reducing morbidity and mortality caused by tuberculosis and polio in Sam Peltzman, *The Regulation of Pharmaceutical Innovation* (Washington, D.C.: American Enterprise Institute for Public Policy Research, 1974), pp. 58–68.

22. Lewis Thomas, "The Future Impact of Science and Technology on Medicine," speech at Squibb Institute for Medical Research, Princeton, N.J., October 11, 1973.

23. David Schwartzman, *The Decline of Service in Retail Trade: An Analysis of the Growth of Sales Per Manhour* (Pullman, Wash.: Washington State University Press, 1970). The growth of the pharmaceutical manufacturing industry reflects two different types of substitution. The displacement of compounding in the retail establishment by a mass-production technology and the substitution of low-cost drug therapy for other more costly types of therapy.

24. U.S. Bureau of the Census, *Historical Statistics of the United States to 1957* (Washington, D.C.: Government Printing Office, 1960), and the *U.S. Statistical Abstract, 1972* (Washington, D.C.: Government Printing Office, 1972).

25. National Health Education Committee (NHEC), *Facts on the Major Killing and Crippling Diseases in the U.S. Today* (New York: National Health Education Committee, 1971), pp. 40–41.

26. There were over 84,000 reported cases of syphilis in fiscal 1974. Moreover, it is estimated that over 2,700,000 cases of syphilis and gonorrhea were unreported in fiscal 1974. Figures were compiled by the Center for Disease Control, Atlanta, Ga.

27. NHEC, *Facts on the Major Killing and Crippling Diseases.*

28. U.S. Bureau of the Census, *Statistic Abstract of the United States, 1973,* 93d ed. (Washington, D.C., 1973), p. 61.

29. Ibid.

30. NHEC, *Facts on the Major Killing and Crippling Diseases.*

31. Ibid.

32. *Alcohol and Health,* Second Special Report to the U.S. Congress from HEW (figures given to author over the phone from the National Council on Alcoholism, 2 Park Ave., N.Y., 212-889-3160).

33. But formidable difficulties stand in the way of utilizing this knowledge in the development of a drug. Interferon is difficult to extract and appears to be effective only in the species from which it is obtained. Rather than seeking a method of extraction, current efforts are directed toward the development of a drug that stimulates the production of interferon within the infected cells.

34. Jesse J. Friedman and Associates, *Economic Aspects of R & D Intensity in the Pharmaceutical Industry: A Composite Profile of Six Major Companies* (Washington, D.C., 1973), p. 2.

35. J. Spivak, *Wall Street Journal,* August 20, 1973.

36. See chapter 4. My estimate of the R & D cost of a new single entity in 1960 is $1.3 million; the corresponding estimate for 1973 is $24.4 million. The estimation procedures are described later; it should be noted that these estimates are in current dollars. Baily ("Research and Development Costs and Returns: The U.S. Pharmaceutical Industry," *Journal of Political Economy* 80, no. 1 [January/February 1972]: 78) estimates that the amendments increased the cost of R & D required for a given number of new single entities by 136 percent. Sam Peltzman estimates that the amendments doubled the constant-dollar cost of R & D required for an NCE; see "An Evaluation of Consumer Protection Legislation: The 1962 Drug Amendments," *Journal of Political Economy* 81, no. 5 (September/October 1973): 1049–91, esp. fn. 13, p. 1067.

37. These economists equate competition with price competition alone and are suspicious of other forms of competition, including innovation. See William S. Comanor, "Research and Competitive Product Differentiation"; reprinted in *Competitive Problems in*

the Drug Industry, U.S. Congress, Senate Select Committee on Small Business, Hearings Subcommittee on Monopoly, 90th Cong., part 5, p. 2070.

38. General Accounting Office, Comptroller General of the U.S., *Problems in Obtaining & Enforcing Compliance with Good Manufacturing Practices for Drugs,* Report to the Congress (Washington, D.C., 1973).

CHAPTER 2

1. John M. Blair, *Economic Concentration: Structure, Behavior, and Public Policy* (New York: Harcourt, Brace, Jovanovitch, Inc. 1972), pp. 216–19; Henry B. Steele, testimony, *Competitive Problems in the Drug Industry,* Hearings before the Subcommittee on Monopoly of the Select Committee on Small Business, U.S. Senate, 90th Cong., 1st and 2d sess. on Present Status of Competition in the Pharmaceutical Industry, part 5, December 1967 and January 1968, pp. 1911–13, 1938 (hereafter cited as *Competitive Problems in the Drug Industry*).

2. M. Tishler, "Drug Discovery–Background and Foreground," *Clinical Pharmaceutical Therapy,* 14, part 1 (1973):479.

3. Sir D. Dunlop, address before the American College of Clinical Pharmacology and Chemotherapy, Atlantic City, N.J., April 28, 1967.

4. J. Jennings, "Government Regulations and Drug Development: FDA," in Robert F. Gould, ed., *Drug Discovery: Science and Development in a Changing Society,* Advances in Chemistry series 108 (Washington, D.C.: American Chemical Society, 1971), p. 274.

5. J. Jewkes, D. Sawers, and R. Stillerman, *The Sources of Invention* (N.Y.: St. Martins Press, Inc., 1958), pp. 72–73, 98–99. Edwin Mansfield, *The Economics of Technological Change* (N.Y.: W.W. Norton & Co., 1968).

6. Mansfield, *Economics of Technological Change,* p. 93.

7. H. Feis, *Atomic Bomb and the End of World War II* (Princeton, N.J.: Princeton U. Press, 1966); R. G. Hewlett and O. E. Anderson, *A History of the United States Atomic Energy Commission,* vol. 1, *The New World, 1936–1946* (University Park: Pennsylvania State University Press, 1962).

8. A. M. Weinberg, "Prospects for Big Biology," from Conference on Research in the Service of Man: Biomedical Knowledge, Development, and Use, sponsored by the Senate Subcommittee on Government Research, Oklahoma City, Oklahoma, Oct. 24–27, 1966, Senate Document no. 55, 90th Congress, 1st Sess., November 2, 1967.

9. See chapter 3.

10. K. Sanow, "Development of Statistics Relating to Research and Development Activities in Private Industry," *Methodology of Statistics on R & D* (Washington, D.C.: National Science Foundation, 1951), p. 75.

11. Mansfield, *Economics of Technological Change,* pp. 45–46.

12. Ibid, pp. 56–61.

13. Jewkes, *et al., Sources of Invention.*

14. This description of the model of research and development as conceived by economists follows the discussions in Mansfield, *Economies of Technological Change,* pp. 50–52; F. M. Scherer, *Industrial Market Structure and Economic Performance* (Chicago: Rand McNally & Co., 1970), pp. 350–54; Daniel Hamberg, *R & D: Essays on the Economics of Research and Development* (N.Y.: Random House, 1966), pp. 16–20. The model is usually attributed to Abbott Usher, *The History of Mechanical Inventions* (Cambridge, Mass.: Harvard University Press), 1954.

15. Jacob Schmookler, *Invention and Economic Growth* (Cambridge, Mass.: Harvard University Press), 1966.

16. W. E. G. Salter, *Productivity and Technical Change* (Cambridge: At the University Press, 1960), pp. 133–34. For a similar idea, see Simon Kuznets, *Secular Movements in Production and Prices* (Boston: Houghton Mifflin Co., 1950), p. 11.

17. Cf. comments by Frederick M. Scherer and Leonard G. Schifrin in Joseph D. Cooper, *The Economics of Drug Innovation: The Proceedings of the First Seminar on*

Economics of Pharmaceutical Innovation, April 27–29, 1969 (Washington, D.C.: The American University, 1970), pp. 199–203, 208–13.

18. Cf. Scherer, *Industrial Market Structure*, pp. 350–54.

19. The role of patents is explained in chapter 9.

20. John H. Biel and Yvonne C. Martin, "Organic Synthesis as a Source of New Drugs," in Gould, *Drug Discovery*, pp. 81–111, esp. p. 85; and W. M. McLamore, "The Sulfa Drugs and Their Legacy," in Frank H. Clarke, ed., *How Modern Medicines are Discovered* (Mt. Kisco, N.Y.: Future Publishing Co., 1973), p. 42.

21. Harry F. Dowling, *Medicine for Man: The Development Regulation and Use of Prescription Drugs* (N.Y.: Alfred A. Knopf, 1973), p. 22.

22. John G. Topliss, "Diuretics," article no. 38 in *Medicinal Chemistry*, ed. A. Burger (N.Y.: Wiley-Interscience, 1970), part 2, pp. 976–1013, esp. pp. 984–85.

23. Biel and Martin, "Organic Synthesis," p. 84.

24. Windsor C. Cutting, *Handbook of Pharmacology: The Actions and Uses of Drugs*, 5th ed. (New York: Appelton-Century-Crofts, 1972), p. 1; C. H. Browning, "Emil Behring and Carl Ehrlich: Their Contributions to Science," *Nature* 175 (1955): 570–75, 616–19.

25. American Chemical Society, "Chemistry in Medicine," manuscript (Washington, D.C.: American Chemical Society), chap. 6.

26. Lloyd H. Conover, "Discovery of Drugs from Microbiological Sources," in Gould, *Drug Discovery*, pp. 34–38.

27. Biel and Martin, "Organic Synthesis," pp. 86–87.

28. Jack Peter Green, "Histamine," in Burger, *Medicinal Chemistry*, part 2, pp. 1623–41.

29. Charles L. Zirkle, "To Tranquilizers and Antidepressants from Antimalarials and Antihistamines," in Clarke, *How Modern Medicines Are Discovered*, p. 62.

30. Ibid. p. 66.

31. American Chemical Society, "Chemistry in Medicine," chapter 6.

32. Biel and Martin, "Organic Synthesis," p. 83.

33. F. Gilbert McMahon, "Sulfonyluneas, Science, and Serendipity," in *Molecular Modification in Drug Design*, ed. Robert F. Gould (Washington, D.C.: American Chemical Society, 1964), pp. 102–13.

34. Ibid.

35. E. G. Gale, *et al., The Molecular Basis of Antibiotic Action* (N.Y.: John Wiley, 1972).

36. J. A. Montgomery, T. P. Johnson, and Y. Fulmer Shealy, "Drugs for Neoplastic Diseases," in A. Burger, ed., *Medicinal Chemistry*, part 1.

CHAPTER 3

1. Nicholas C. Paulesco, *Archives of International Physiology*, August 1921; see also Ian Murray in the *Journal of the History of Medicines and Allied Sciences*, vol. 26.

2. G. T. Stewart, *The Penicillin Group of Drugs* (N.Y.: Elsevier Co., 1965).

3. Dr. Ira Ringler, "Splitting the Antipodes," Speech presented at PMA Science Writers Seminar, Rockefeller University, New York, May 24, 1972.

4. Lloyd H. Conover, "Discovery of Drugs from Microbiological Sources," in *Drug Discovery: Science and Development in a Changing Society*, ed. Robert F. Gould, Advances in Chemistry series 108 (Washington, D.C.: American Chemical Society, 1971), p. 54.

5. G. Bylinsky, "Upjohn Puts the Cells Own Messengers to Work," *Fortune*, June 1972, p. 96.

6. R. L. Rawls, "Prostaglandins: Chemical Foundation Is Laid," *Chemical Engineering News*, June 24, 1974, p. 18.

7. The following discussion of the research that led up to the Salk vaccine is based on the biography by Richard Carter, *Breakthrough: The Saga of Jonas Salk* (New York: Trident Press, 1966). See especially pp. 4, 19, 58, 69, 87, and 108.

8. H. L. Heroz, "Hormones and Control of Body Functions," in *How Modern Medicines Are Discovered*, ed. F. H. Clarke (Mount Kisco, N.Y.: Futura Publishing Co., 1973).

9. A. Q. Maisel, *The Hormone Quest* (N.Y.: Random House, 1965).

10. W. K. Pines, "A Primer on New Drug Development," *FDA Consumer,* February, 1974. p. 12.

11. The various estimates of the length of time funds are invested in the R & D program leading up to a new single entity are described later in this chapter.

12. Pharmaceutical Manufacturers Association, *Annual Survey Report,* 1970–71 (Washington, D.C.), p. 15.

13. See table 6-2 in chapter 6.

14. John Jewkes, David Sawers, and Richard Stillerman, *The Sources of Invention* (New York: St. Martins Press, 1959); F. M. Scherer, *Industrial Market Structure and Economic Performance* (Chicago: Rand McNally, 1970), pp. 351–54; Edwin Mansfield, *The Economics of Technological Change* (N.Y.: W. W. Norton, 1968), p. 98; Daniel Hamberg, *R & D: Essays on the Economics of Research and Development* (N.Y.: Random House, 1966).

15. R. H. Coase, "The Nature of the Firm," *Economica,* n. s. 5, no. 4 (1937): pp. 386–405.

16. In *New Product Survey* and *Nonproprietary Name Index* (New York, annual), Paul de Haen classifies new drugs into three groups: NCE's, new combination drugs, and new dosage forms. It is the first group that contains the new basic agents. A close inspection of even this group reveals derivatives of other more basic agents and other minor additions to the list of new drugs. The present study, therefore, removed from de Haen's, lists the following items as NCE's: diagnostic aids, hospitals solutions, nonabsorbed high-molecular weight compounds, impure extracts of natural origin, new uses and formulations of previously marketed drugs, new single components included in previously marketed mixtures, new salts and esters of previously marketed drugs, and drugs which were later withdrawn.

17. Based on an inspection of lists of innovations (in other industries), which contain many from small firms. Economists have inferred that small firms are more courageous and thus more prone to innovate. But, as I will demonstrate in chapter 6, the method is fallacious. The fallacy arises from looking only at those firms that do innovate and not at all firms.

18. Lewis H. Sarett, "FDA Regulations and Their Influence on Future R & D," *Research Management,* March 1974, pp. 18–20.

19. Harold Clymer in Joseph D. Cooper, *Economics of Drug Innovation* (Washington, D.C.: The American University, 1969), p. 109, and in M. Pernarowski and M. Darrach, eds., *The Development and Control of New Drug Products* (Vancouver, B.C.: Evergreen, 1972).

20. Prices of goods and personnel services used in academic research increased by 36.4 percent between 1964 and 1971. Between 1968 and 1971 the rate of increase of prices was about 6 percent per year and accelerating (cf. National Science Foundation, *A Price Index for the Deflation of Academic R & D Expenditures,* May 1972, NSF 72-310, p. 2, table 2). A conservative projection of the increase in prices to 1973 brings the estimate for the whole period up to 48 percent. A similar estimate is arrived at from the ratio of the index of nominal cost in 1973, as budgeted, on base 1963, to the index of laboratory employment. Both indexes are computed from PMA data. Laboratory employment is taken as the measure of total real input for this purpose. The estimate makes no allowance for the increase in costs due to the greater demands by the FDA for approval.

21. A rough estimate based on private inquiries to manufacturers. The percentage varies inversely with the number of compounds in the developmental stage of research and positively with the absolute size of the discovery program.

To my knowledge no estimate has previously been made of the share of total pharmaceutical R & D expenditures devoted to discovery research. The reason is that the expenditures per compound are only estimated by the research laboratories after the decision is made to perform clinical tests and toxicology testing begins, which in the industry's terminology marks the beginning of the development part of R & D. The discovery research will synthesize and test many compounds that never reach toxicology testing because they fail to show the desired biological reaction or because toxic effects are found in the early animal studies. The costs of such research are properly charged to the successful products, along with those costs that can be directly allocated to them. That discovery costs can constitute a large share of total R & D costs can be seen in the report by PMA that in 1970 its members "obtained, prepared, extracted, or isolated" 126,000 compounds, and tested pharmacologically 703,900 compounds. That actual developmental research was limited to a small number is shown by the fact that only 1,013 compounds were tested clinically (Pharmaceutical Manufacturers Association, *Annual Survey Report,* 1970–71), p. 15.

22. The share of total developmental cost accounted for by each product class is obtained by multiplying the number of new products in the class by the relative cost and expressing each product as a percentage of the sum of the products. On the basis of Jerome Schnee's estimates of costs of development the relative developmental costs are as follows: NCE 1.00; combination drug .30; dosage form .16.

The estimate of the number of drugs in each class is based on de Haen. His figure for NCE's corrected to exclude derivatives *et cetera* as described earlier, and the number so excluded are added to his number of new combination drugs. The final number in each class was: NCE's, 86; combination drugs, 280; dosage forms, 154. It should be noted that these numbers include drugs introduced by nonmembers of PMA, while the PMA research expenditure figures include only those of members. Nonmembers have accounted for a larger share of new combination drugs and of new dosage forms than of NCE's. The procedure thus results in an overestimate of the share of total R & D costs accounted for by combination drugs and dosage forms, and therefore, an underestimate of the cost per NCE. Hence, the resulting bias is to overstate the final estimate of the expected rate of return on investment in R & D. See Jerome Schnee, "Innovation and Discovery in the Drug Industry," in *Research and Innovation in the Modern Corporation,* ed. Edwin Mansfield, John Rapoport, Jerome Schnee, Samuel Wagner, and Michael Hamburger (New York: W. W. Norton, 1971).

23. The model assumes that the cost of R & D is reduced by the tax rate. It should be noted that a firm must have revenue in years 1 to 10 against which to offset the R & D expense. Otherwise the investment in R & D is larger than the estimated amount. The ability of the successful large drug firms to obtain this tax benefit from revenues resulting from drugs introduced in prior years has been a factor in their continued investment in R & D.

24. Martin Baily, "Research and Development Cost and Returns: The U.S. Pharmaceutical Industry," *Journal of Political Economy* 80 (Jan./Feb. 1972):78. Sam Peltzman "An Evaluation of Consumer Protection Legislation: The 1962 Drug Amendments," *Journal of Political Economy* 81 (Sept./Oct. 1973):1067, esp. fn. 13.

25. We have been told by people who were members of industrial research laboratories at the time that the R & D period was much shorter. Moreover, Schnee ("The Changing Pattern of Pharmaceutical Innovation and Discovery," mimeographed [New York: Graduate School of Business, Columbia University, 1973], p. 77) estimates the development period then to have been two years. Sarett's ("FDA Regulations and Their Influence on Future R & D") estimates for 1958–62 is the same. Our estimate, therefore, tends to understate the expected rate of return in that earlier period.

26. National Science Foundation, *Price Index for the Deflation of Academic R & D Expenditures,* p. 2.

27. "FDA Regulations and Their Influence on Future R & D." Dr. Sarett's estimate of the cost of developing a new drug in 1962 is much higher than my own for 1960. The costs at Merck, Sharp, and Dohme Laboratories on which he bases his estimate may have been higher than those in the rest of the industry. On the other hand, his estimate for 1973 is close to my own.

28. The rate of innovation has fallen, even though expenditures for R & D continue to increase as measured in constant as well as in current dollars. We are suggesting that the increase in R & D expenditures would have been larger were it not for the increased restrictiveness of FDA regulatory policy. There is no doubt *discovery* research spending would be larger.

CHAPTER 4

1. Jerome Schnee, "Innovation and Discovery in the Drug Industry," in *Research and Innovation in the Modern Corporation* ed. Edward Mansfield, John Rapoport, Jerome

Schnee, Samuel Wagner, and Michel Hamburger (New York: W. W. Norton, 1971), esp. p. 175, n. 35.

2. Ibid., p. 158.

3. Jerome Schnee, "The Changing Pattern of Pharmaceutical Innovation and Discovery," mimeographed (New York: Graduate School of Business, Columbia University, 1973). The survey covered the drugs introduced in 1963–1968. The selection for 1969–1970 consisted of the drugs reviewed in *The Medical Letter* in these years.

4. Schnee, "Innovation and Discovery in the Drug Industry," p. 178.

5. William McVicker, "New Drug Development Study," mimeographed (Washington, D.C.: Food and Drug Administration, 1972).

6. *Chemicals and Health,* Report of the Panel on Chemicals and Health of the President's Science Advisory Committee (Washington, D.C.: Science and Technology Policy Office, National Science Foundation, 1973), p. 48.

7. *Drug Safety,* Hearings Before a Subcommittee of the Committee on Governmental Operations, House of Representatives, 88th Cong., 2d sess., part 2, 1964, pp. 444–90; see especially the testimony of Dr. A. Burroughs Mider and of Dr. C. Gordon Zubrod.

8. Ibid., p. 421, testimony of Dr. Bernard B. Brodie, Chief, Laboratory of Chemical Pharmacology, National Heart Institute.

9. Ibid., p. 427, testimony of Dr. Sidney Udenfriend, Chief, Laboratory of Clinical Biochemistry, National Heart Institute.

10. Ibid., p. 314.

11. Hearings before Sub-committee of the Committee on Appropriations, House of Representatives, 93d Cong., 1st sess., part 4, 1973, pp. 132, 163, 718, 722–25.

CHAPTER 5

1. Joseph Schumpeter, *Capitalism, Socialism, and Democracy,* 3d ed. (New York, Harper, 1950), p. 106.

2. A good summary is provided by chapter 15 in F. M. Scherer, *Industrial Market Structure and Economic Performance* (Chicago: Rand McNally, 1970), esp. p. 353.

3. Edwin Mansfield, *Industrial Research and Technological Innovation* (New York: W. W. Norton, 1968), pp. 38–40; Henry G. Grabowski, "The Determinants of Industrial Research and Development: A Study of the Chemical, Drug, and Petroleum Industries," *Journal of Political Economy,* March/April 1968, pp. 292–305; William S. Comanor, "Research and Technical Change in the Pharmaceutical Industry," *Review of Economies and Statistics,* May 1965, pp. 182–90; Jerome Schnee, "Innovation and Discovery in the Ethical Pharmaceutical Industry," chapter 8 in *Research and Innovation in the Modern Corporation,* ed. Edwin Mansfield, John Rapaport, Jerome Schnee, Samuel Wagner, and Michael Hamburger (New York: W. W. Norton, 1971).

4. Pharmaceutical Manufacturer's Association, *Ethical Pharmaceutical Industry Operations and Research and Development Trends,* 1960–66 (Washington, D.C.: PMA, 1967), p. 49.

5. The list excluded other items as well, but these were the most important.

6. National Academy of Science–National Research Council, *Industrial Laboratories in the United States,* 1970.

7. Dr. J. G. Carpenter, unpublished material, Pfizer, Inc., Sandwich, England.

8. Prepared for the *Report for the National Economic Development Office on the Level of Innovative Activity in the Pharmaceutical Industry,* 1973.

9. *Industrial Research and Technological Innovation,* pp. 38–40.

10. Grabowski, "Determinants of Industrial Research and Development."

11. Ibid., p. 302, fn. 19.

12. "Research and Technical Change in the Pharmaceutical Industry."

13. Comanor multiplies both sides of his equation by S and expresses it as

$$Y = a + nR + cR^2, \text{ where } b = -4.671 - .000000128\, S^2.$$

Since $$2Y/2R = b + 2cR$$

then $$2Y/2R = -4.671 - .000000128\, S^2 + 2cR.$$

14. Schnee, "Innovation and Discovery in the Ethical Pharmaceutical Industry," p. 172.

15. John Jewkes, David Sawers, and Richard Stillerman, *The Sources of Invention* (New York: St. Martin's Press, 1959).

16. Daniel Hamberg, *R & D: Essays on the Economics of Research and Development* (New York: Random House, 1966), p. 71; Mansfield, *Industrial Research and Technological Innovation,* pp. 84–91.

17. See my comments on the importance of theoretically unspecified factors in the success of firms in "Competition and Efficiency: Comment," *Journal of Political Economy,* May/June 1973.

CHAPTER 6

1. Pharmaceutical Manufacturers Association, *Annual Survey Report, 1973–74.*

2. W. S. Peart, "Arterial Hypertension," in *A Textbook of Medicine,* ed. Russell Cecil and Robert Loeb, 13th ed. (Philadelphia: Saunders, 1971), pp. 1050–62.

3. See chapter 12, "Price Competition."

4. PMA, *Annual Survey Report, 1971–72,* p. 11; PMA, *Prescription Drug Industry Factbook,* 1972.

5. Laboratory employment from *Industrial Research Laboratories,* 13th ed. (N.Y.: R. Bowker Co., 1970).

6. Stanley I. Ornstein, "Concentration and Profits," in *The Impact of Large Firms on the U.S. Economy,* ed. J. Fred Weston and Stanley I. Ornstein (Lexington, Mass.: D. C. Heath, 1973), pp. 87–102.

7. William G. Shepherd, "The Elements of Market Structure," *Review of Economics and Statistics* 54 (February 1972): 25–27.

8. Harold Demsetz, "Two Systems of Belief about Monopoly," in *Industrial Concentrations: The New Learning,* ed. J. Harvey Goldschmid, H. Michael Mann, and J. Fred Weston (Boston: Little, Brown and Company, 1974), pp. 164–83.

CHAPTER 7

1. Martin Baily, "Research and Development Cost and Returns: The U.S. Pharmaceutical Industry," *Journal of Political Economy* 80 (January/February 1972): p. 78. Sam Peltzman, "An Evaluation of Consumer Protection Legislation: The 1962 Drug Amendments," *Journal of Political Economy* 81 (September/October 1973): 1054–56.

2. *U.S. Pharmaceutical Sales, Drug Stores and Hospitals,* IMS America, Ltd. 1972.

3. William E. Cox, "Product Life Cycles and Promotional Strategy in the Ethical Drug Industry" (Ph.D. diss., University of Michigan, 1963), chapter 4.

4. Harold Clymer "The Changing Costs and Risks of Pharmaceutical Innovation," in *Economics of Pharmaceutical Innovation,* ed. J. D. Cooper (Washington, D.C.: The American University, 1970).

5. Based on conversations with individuals associated with these industries.

6. Pharmaceutical Manufacturers Association, *Annual Survey Report, 1970–71* (Washington, D.C.), p. 15.

7. *Chemical Engineer News,* February 4, 1974. See also Harold Clymer of SmithKline Corporation, who has suggested that the return on investment in R & D will be low (Clymer, "The Changing Costs and Risks of Pharmaceutical Innovation," in Cooper, *Economics of Pharmaceutical Innovation*).

8. Lewis Sarett, "FDA Regulations and Their Influence on Future R & D," *Research Management,* March 1974, pp. 19–20.

9. Schnee, "The Changing Pattern of Pharmaceutical Innovation and Discovery," mimeographed (New York: Graduate School of Business, Columbia University, 1973), p. 77.

10. Cox, "Product Life Cycles and Promotional Strategy in the Ethical Drug Industry."

11. Sarrett, "FDA Regulations and Their Influence on Future R & D."

12. David Schwartzman, "The Expected-Profits Method of Locating Monopoly Power," *Antitrust Bulletin* 17, no. 4 (Winter 1972).

13. David Schwartzman, "Competition and Efficiency: Comment," *Journal of Political Economy,* 81 (May/June 1973).

14. Richard Mancke, "Causes of Interfirm Profitability Differences: A New Interpretation of the Evidence," *Quarterly Journal of Economics* 88 (May 1974): 181–93.

15. Recently the FTC has recognized that the rate of profit of companies that spend large sums on research may be overstated owing to the practice of expensing R & D.

16. Jesse J. Friedman and Associates, *Economic Aspects of R & D Intensity in the Pharmaceutical Industry* (Washington, D.C.: Jesse J. Friedman and Associates, 1973), p. 26. The "industry" average reported in table 8-5, a weighted average in which the leading companies have a large weight, refers to Friedman's estimate of the effect of the expensing procedure on the reported rate of profit for six of the leading companies; it is a good estimate of the required adjustment for this average.

17. Bloch estimates that Schering's reported rate of profit should be reduced by 6.0 percentage points in order to compensate for expensing of R & D. See Harry Bloch, "True Profitability Measures for Pharmaceutical and Economics," in *Regulation, Economics, and Pharmaceutical Innovation,* ed. Joseph D. Cooper (Washington, D.C.: American University, 1976), table 7, p. 155.

18. Gorden R. Conrad and Irving H. Plotkin, "Risk and Return in American Industry—an Economic Analysis," testimony for *Competitive Problems in the Drug Industry,* Hearings Before the Subcommittee on Monopoly, Select Committee on Small Business, U.S. Senate, 90th Cong. 1st and 2nd sess. part 5, December 14, 19, 1967; ibid., January 18, 19, 25, pp. 1746–84.

The ideal index of risk would be based on a dispersion of rates of return from investment projects in each industry. This is so because we are interested in decisions by firms to invest in R & D rather than by purchasers of securities to invest in a drug company. The dispersion of such rates of return would be much larger than that based on an estimate of the interfirm dispersion of profit rates. Further, the dispersion of rates of return from R & D projects in the drug industry would be much larger than the dispersion of rates of return from investment projects generally in other industries, and investment in R & D composes a large part of the total investment of the drug industry. On the whole, therefore, the Conrad-Plotkin Index provides a conservative estimate of the riskiness of investment in the drug industry. Since the dispersion of profit rates among drug firms is relatively large, the drug industry ranks high on this index, as the authors point out.

The FTC is scornful of this argument: firms have not suffered actual losses, and the profit rates of companies whose profit rate is low by industry standards have been higher than those of many companies in other industries. The FTC apparently is disregarding causes of high profits other than risk and monopoly power; no allowance is made for market growth, accounting methods, and overseas expansion (testimony of W. F. Mueller, *Competitive Problems in the Drug Industry,* pp. 1807–62).

19. Conrad and Plotkin's equation may provide a biased estimate of the effect of risk on the average rate of profit, because other variables affecting the rate of profit are not included. The estimate of the effect of risk may err either on the high or the low side as a result; there is no way of knowing. The error probably is small, because the equation explains a large part of the variance of the average profit rate. The coefficient of determination is .46.

20. Stanley J. Ornstein, "Concentration and Profits," *Journal of Business* 45 (October 1972): 519–41. W. G. Shepherd, "Elements of Market Structure," *Review of Economics and Statistics* 54 (February 1972): 25–37.

21. Charles L. Schultze et al., *Setting National Priorities: The 1973 Budget* (Washington, D.C.; Brookings Institution, 1972), p. 217.

22. Current-dollar foreign sales from PMA, *Prescription Industry Fact Book,* various years. The Firestone Price Index was the deflator.

23. Shepherd, "Elements of Market Structure." Between 1960 and 1969, Shepherd's period, U.S. pharmaceutical companies' world sales of ethical drugs increased by 120 percent. When we multiply this by Shepherd's coefficient for the growth of sales (.9), we obtain 1.1 as the contribution of the growth of demand to the profit rate.

Shepherd's equation refers to individual companies rather than to industries, and the present estimate is for the industry. The estimate is unlikely to err greatly, since the major part of interfirm variation of the change in sales over the long period 1960–69 that Shepherd examines consists of interindustry variation. Since the estimate itself is not large, errors are unlikely to affect the overall conclusion significantly.

24. PMA *Fact Book,* various years.

CHAPTER 8

1. U.S. Senate, *Congressional Record,* 87th Cong., 1st sess. April 12, 1961, p. 5638. Further discussion of Nelson's review is postponed to chapter 14.

2. See Sam Peltzman, *Regulation of Pharmaceutical Innovation* (Washington, D.C.: American Enterprise Institute for Public Policy Research, 1974), pp. 21–23.

3. Some drug manufacturers provide drugs free of charge to any low-income patient whose doctor requests free drugs for the patient.

4. C. T. Taylor and Z. A. Silberston, *The Economic Impact of the Patent System: A Study of the British Experience,* Cambridge University Department of Applied Economics, monograph 23 (Cambridge: At the University Press, 1973), p. 26.

5. In 1973, 30.7 percent of the total number of new prescriptions for the following drugs were written generically: thyroid, penicillin VK and V, oral penicillin G potassium, tetracycline HCL, erythromycin, oral ampicillin, barbiturates, nonbarbiturate sedatives, and digitalis preparations (see chapter 6 for details).

6. Edmund Kitch, "The Patent System and New Drug Application," in *Regulating New Drugs,* ed. Richard L. Landau (Chicago: University of Chicago Center for Policy Study, 1973), pp. 81–108.

7. Ibid., p. 85.

8. The following material is from William M. Wardell and Louis Lasagna, *Regulation and Drug Development* (Washington, D.C.: American Enterprise Institute for Public Policy, 1975), pp. 59–62.

9. T. Killip, "Ischemic Heart Disease," in *Cecil-Loeb Textbook of Medicine,* ed. P. Beeson and W. McDermott (Philadelphia: W. B. Saunders Co. 1971), pp. 1016–39; cited by Wardell and Lasagna, *Regulation and Drug Development,* p. 61.

10. Personal communication.

11. Harold Clymer, "The Changing Costs of Pharmaceutical Innovation," in *The Economics of Drug Innovation,* ed. Joseph D. Cooper (Washington, D.C.: The American University, 1970), p. 117, fig. 6.

12. *Federal Register* 35 no. 90 (May 8, 1970): 7250–53.

13. See Robert B. Helms, ed., *Drug Development and Marketing: A Conference Sponsored by the Center for Health Policy Research of the American Enterprise Institute* (Washington, D.C.: American Enterprise Institute for Public Policy Research, 1975), p. 196.

14. W. K. Pines, "A Primer on New Drug Development," *FDA Consumer,* February 1974, p. 12.

15. *Chemicals and Health,* report of the Panel on Chemicals and Health of the President's Science Advisory Committee, September 1973, Science and Technology Policy Office, National Science Foundation (Washington, D.C.: Government Printing Office, 1973) p. 125.

CHAPTER 9

1. George J. Stigler, "Economics of Information," *Journal of Political Economy* 69, no. 3 (June 1961): 213–25. Phillip Nelson, "Information and Consumer Behavior," *Journal of Political Economy* 78, no. 2 (March/April 1970): 311–29.

2. Count based on list provided by Ringdoc System, Derwent Publications, London, England.

3. Testimony of Dr. Harry L. Williams in *Competitive Problems in the Drug Industry,* Hearings Before the Subcommittee on Monopoly, Select Committee on Small Business, U.S. Senate, 90th Cong., 1st and 2d sess., part 2, May–June 1967, p. 457.

4. Richard Burach, *The Handbook of Prescription Drugs* (New York: Random House, 1967), p. 101.

5. *Competitive Problems in the Drug Industry,* part 18, August 1970, pp. 7453–60.

6. Discussion in parts 7 and 8, *Competitive Problems in the Drug Industry.*

7. *Report of the Committee of Enquiry into the Relationship of the Pharmaceutical Industry with the National Health Service, 1965–1967* (London: Her Majesty's Stationery Office, 1967); hereafter cited as Sainsbury Report.

8. Sainsbury Report, p. 139; the drugs were Ultralanum, Mogadon, Indocin, and Lasix.

9. Colinearity reduced the significance of the regression coefficient of sales, as can be seen in the following simple regression equation:

$$\ln \text{Pr} = 6.0628 + .2114 \ln \text{S}$$
$$(t = 2.3497) \quad R^2 = .29$$
$$(SE = .0900) \quad F = 5.521$$

Nevertheless, it explains very little of the interfirm variation in promotional expenditures, much less than sales-weighted NSCE's:

$$\ln \text{Pr} = 8.1968 + .1233 \ln \text{N}_S$$
$$(t = 4.7465) \quad R^2 = .29$$
$$(SE = .0260) \quad F = 22.529$$

Indeed, the firm-size variable adds little to the explanatory value of the equation.

10. That this is the true relationship is confirmed by a comparison of the results with those for an equation in which the age is represented by an arithmetic variable, as follows:

$$\ln \text{P}_p = 6.40996 + .21 \ln \text{N}_{rp} - .03_a$$
$$(t = 6.16) \quad (t = -2.39) \quad R^2 = .47$$
$$(SE = .034) \quad (SE = .012) \quad F = 20.877$$

11. W. Modell, ed., *Drugs of Choice, 1974–75* (St. Louis: C. V. Mosby Co., 1974), p. 84.

12. Sam Peltzman, "The Diffusion of Pharmaceutical Innovation," presented at the Conference on Drug Development and Marketing, American Enterprise Institute, Washington, D.C. July 25–26, 1974, p. 13.

13. The same kind of problem would arise in any case when a generic class contains many products. Many names are hard to remember and since each product would be used by a small number of doctors, the news of defects would not get around as rapidly. But the problem is much more severe when brand names are not used.

14. February 25, 1974.

15. H. E. Simmons and P. D. Stolley, "This Is Medical Progress?" *Journal of the American Medical Association* 227 (March 4, 1974): 1023–28.

16. The count is of certificates which show septicemia to be the primary cause of death. Either gram-positive or gram-negative septicemia was present in 24,504 cases in which death was attributed to other causes.

17. H. L. DuPont and W. W. Sprink, "Infections due to gram-negative organisms: An analysis of 860 patients with bacteremia at the University of Minnesota Medical Center, 1958–1966," *Medicine* 48 (1969): 307, 332.

18. R. L. Myerowitz, A. A. Medeiros, and T. F. O'Brien, "Recent experience with bacillemia due to gram-negative organisms," *The Journal of Infectious Disease* 124 (September 1971): 239–46.

19. W. A. Altemeier, J. W. Todd, and W. W. Ingre, "Gram-negative septicemia: A growing threat," *Annals of Surgery* 166 (October, 1967): 530–42.

20. M. Finland, "Changing ecology of bacterial infections as related to anti-bacterial therapy," *The Journal of Infectious Disease* 122 (November 1970): 419–31.

21. R. J. Bulger, E. Larson, and J. C. Sherris, "Decreased incidences of resistance to anti-microbial agents among Escherichia coli and Klebsiella-Enterobacter: A study in a university hospital over a 10-year period," *Annals of Internal Medicine* 72 (1970): 65–71; and R. J. Bulger and J. C. Sherris, "Decreased incidence of antibiotic resistance among

Staphylococcus aureus: A study in a university hospital over a 9-year period." *Annals of Internal Medicine* 69 (1968): 1099–1108.

22. *Quality of Health Care—The Pharmaceutical Industry, 1974,* Hearings before the Subcommittee on Health, May 20, 1974, p. 2 (chairman's opening statement). M. Silverman and P. R. Lee, *Pills, Profits, and Politics* (Berkeley: University of California Press, 1974), p. 264.

23. G. Caranasos, R. Steward, and L. Cluff, "Drug-induced illness leading to hospitalization," *Journal of American Medical Association* 228 (May 6, 1974): 713–16. S. Shapiro, D. Slone, G. Lewis, and H. Jick, "Fatal drug reactions among medical inpatients," *JAMA,* 216 (April 19, 1971): 467–72.

24. At least two other highly respected studies of this problem provide findings in sharp conflict with those presented in the Boston and Caranosos studies. See B. C. Hoddinott, C. W. Gowdy, W. K. Coulter, and J. M. Parker, "Drug reactions and errors in administration on medical ward," *Canadian Medical Association Journal* 97 (1967): 1001; N. Hurwitz, and O. L. Wade, "Intensive hospital monitoring of adverse reactions to drugs," *British Medical Journal* 1 (1969): 531; and N. Hurwitz, "Predisposing factors in adverse reactions to drugs," *British Medical Journal* 1 (1969): 536.

25. *Pills, Profits, and Politics,* p. 55. The authors cite the Task Force on Prescription Drugs, *Drug Makers and Drug Distributors* (Washington, D.C.: HEW, 1968), p. 27.

26. *U.S. Pharmaceutical Market, Drug Stores and Hospitals,* IMS America, Ltd., 1972.

27. Sainsbury Report, p. 64.

28. William S. Comanor and Thomas A. Wilson, "Advertising, Market Structure, and Performance," *Review of Economics and Statistics,* November 1967, pp. 423–40, app. 1. It should be noted that this estimate expressed the cost of advertising a ratio to manufacturers' sales.

29. PMA, *Prescription Drug Industry Fact Book,* Washington, D.C., p. 15.

30. Products ranked by sales as reported in *US Pharmaceutical Market, Drug Stores and Hospitals* 1973, IMS America, Ltd. Data on promotional expenditures per product from *National Detailing Audits,* 1973, *National Journal Audits,* 1973, and *National Mail Audits,* 1973, all IMS America, Ltd.

31. John Kenneth Galbraith, *Economics and the Public Purpose* (Boston: Houghton Mifflin, 1973), p. 158.

CHAPTER 10

1. This ceiling is known as the maximum allowable cost. It is calculated in various ways. The result is that all drugs priced below this level are fully reimbursed while those above it are reimbursed for only the ceiling price.

2. *Pharmacy Times,* April 1974, p. 35.

3. Estimate based on data for leading drugs. See table 6-5.

4. To capture a significant share of a market, a new drug must demonstrate some clear therapeutic advantage over established drugs or else sell at a lower price. The limit on doctors' time and effort probably is one of the factors in the concentration of sales among a few drugs in many therapeutic classes (chapters 6 and 9).

5. Drugs are an "experience" rather than a "search" good in Phillip Nelson's classification of goods: the quality cannot be judged from inspection of the product but must await experience. A prescriber need not, of course, depend on his own observations of the effects of a drug; usually he will depend greatly on reports of experience from many sources. See Phillip Nelson, "Information and Consumer Behavior," *Journal of Political Economy* 78, no. 2 (March/April 1970): 311–29.

6. *Code of Federal Regulations,* Title 21, "Food and Drugs," part 133.3, "Buildings," (Washington, D.C.: U.S. Government Printing Office, 1973), p. 119.

7. A. Kirshbaum, "Quality Control of Antibiotics," in Murray S. Cooper, *Quality Control in the Pharmaceutical Industry,* vol. 1 (New York: Academic Press, 1972), p. 40.

8. The data for SIC 283, "The Drug Industry," largely reflect those for SIC 2843, "The Pharmaceutical Preparations Industry," which is the major component. The data for

pharmaceutical preparations are shown in table 1-3. The other components of the Census Drug Industry are SIC 2831, "Biological Products," and SIC 2833, "Medicinals and Botanicals."

The census figure for the total number of plants in 1968 in the industry is much less than the GAO estimate of 6,400. The GAO is careful enough to indicate that the number refers to manufacturing establishments and not to distributors of warehousers. The discussion of the listing of establishments required by the FDA indicates that one source of the difference may be the number of establishments that produce drugs as a secondary product; the primary product may be foods, toilet preparations, or other products. Thus the census estimate of the number of establishments understates the FDA's inspection task, since the census only regards those whose primary product is drugs. Cf. General Accounting Office, *Problems in Obtaining and Enforcing Compliance with Good Manufacturing Practices for Drugs,* Report to Congress, 1973.

9. See chapter 11 for appraisal of FDA's enforcement activities.

CHAPTER 11

1. These results were reported by Commissioner James L. Goddard, Food and Drug Administration, on August 10, 1967, at Hearings before the Subcommittee on Monopoly of the Select Committee on Small Business, U.S. Senate, 90th Cong., 1st sess., *Competitive Problems in the Drug Industry,* part 2, p. 793.

2. Arthur W. Steers, "The Test Program of the National Center for Drug Analysis," in *Quality Control in the Pharmaceutical Industry,* ed. Murray S. Cooper (New York: Academic Press, 1972), vol. 2, pp. 55–75. Dr. Steers is a member of the National Center for Drug Analysis in St. Louis.

3. Detailed report provided in statement by Senator Robert Dole, *Congressional Record,* 91st Cong., 1st sess., July 30, 1969.

4. *Competitive Problems in the Drug Industry,* part 2, pp. 792–94. Testimony by Dr. Durward Hall quoted Commissioner Goddard as admitting that the study was sketchy and preliminary rather than final (ibid., part 1, p. 270).

5. Steers, "Test Program," p. 61.

6. Other members of the committee were Dr. M. W. Anders, Professor of Pharmacology, University of Minnesota; Dr. B. A. Cole, Deputy Associate Commissioner for Science, FDA (Staff Director); Dr. J. R. Crout, Professor of Pharmacology and Medicine, Michigan State University; Dr. W. A. Krehl, Professor of Preventive Medicine, Jefferson Medical College; Dr. L. A. Woods, Vice-President, Health Sciences, Virginia Commonwealth University.

7. "Report of the Ad Hoc Science Advisory Committee to the FDA," May 1971 (Ritts Report), mimeographed (Washington, D.C., 1971), p. 48.

8. *Agriculture-Environmental and Consumer Protection Appropriations for 1973.* Hearings before a Subcommittee of the Committee on Appropriations, House of Representatives, 92nd Cong., 2d sess., p. 149.

9. Testimony of Elmer B. Staats, Comptroller General of the United States, January 19, 1971, in *Competitive Problems in the Drug Industry,* pp. 8025–27. The specific reasons for disqualification cited under the headings of "Quality Control" and "Housekeeping" are as shown below (p. 8027):

Area of disqualification	Specific reasons cited
Quality control	Inadequate inspection program.
	Inadequate production records.
	Inadequate testing or testing program.
	Inadequacies in packaging.
	Inadequacies in written quality control procedures.
	Unauthorized people having access to label room.
	No program for maintenance and calibration of scales.
Housekeeping	Spillages not immediately removed from production area.
	Uncovered trash bins in bottle packaging area.

Trash barrel emptied too close to production line.
No program for periodic employee medical examinations.
Unsanitary raw material containers.

Since the time when this testimony was published, the Department of Defense has responded to pressure from the subcommittee and has agreed to permit the FDA to perform the inspection function for its own drug procurement.

10. "DPSC Interplay with FDA and the Pharmaceutical Industry," Conference, School of Pharmacy, University of North Carolina, February 14, 1972, mimeographed, p. 15.

11. Mr. Feinberg apparently estimated that, of the plants surveyed, 45 percent were found not to meet DPSC standards. The figure we quoted earlier in the text was based on the percentage of surveys resulting in disqualifications.

12. General Accounting Office, Comptroller General of the United States, *Problems in Obtaining and Enforcing Compliance with Good Manufacturing Practices for Drugs*. Report to the Congress, Washington, D.C., 1973.

13. *Drug Bioequivalence—A Report from the Drug Bioequivalence Study Panel to the Office of Technology Assessment*, U.S. Congress, July 1974. The chairman of the panel was Robert W. Berliner, M.D., Dean School of Medicine, Yale University. Senator Edward M. Kennedy had requested the Office of Technology Assessment to examine the problem of drug bioequivalence in order to settle the debate provoked by the Weinberger proposal. In response to this request, the OTA set up the Drug Bioequivalence Study Panel.

14. To limit the list of recalls to those affecting drugs which were the result of poor manufacturing practices, we eliminated from the list those which involved vitamins, those involving withdrawal of approval of the NDA, and those which were the result of class actions.

15. The formula for economic order quantity suggests that the average batch varies in proportion to the square root of average sales per product, or the average sales per product would have to be $(3.7)^2$, or 13.7 times larger. This is well within the range of actual variation in sales per product.

16. *Competitive Problems in the Drug Industry* part 20, p. 8026.

17. *Competitive Problems in the Drug Industry,* part 18, August 17, 1970, pp. 7569–7571.

18. Ibid., p. 7669.

19. Agricultural-Environmental and Consumer Protection Appropriations for 1973. Hearings before a Subcommittee of the Committee on Appropriations, House of Representatives, 92nd Cong., 2nd sess., p. 149.

20. "Drug Quality: Practicing Pharmacists' Viewpoints," *Medical Marketing and Media,* September 1973, pp. 24–31.

21. The results of these studies were reported by Dr. J. Fitelson, in *Competitive Problems in the Drug Industry,* part 2, June 28, 1967, pp. 550–558.

22. Testimony of Charles T. Silloway, *Competitive Problems in the Drug Industry,* part 3, September 14, 1967, p. 905.

23. The products which do not conform to USP specifications are mixtures of estrone and equilin and estrogenic substances from natural sources. These products do not contain appreciable amounts of 17-alpha-dihydroequilin, and others do not contain estrone or equilin within the specified limits. Statements on conjugated estrogen tablets supplied by Dr. Chester J. Cavallito, Executive Vice President, Ayerst Laboratories, to the Kennedy Subcommittee on Health, the *Committee of Labor and Public Health, Quality of Medical Care, the Pharmaceutical Industry,* February 1, 1974, 93d Cong., 2d sess., referred to on p. 84 of transcript.

24. Ibid., p. 87.

25. The study was one of those included in the Steers report, commented on earlier. The study of digoxin was included under the heading "cardiac glycosides." Steers did not analyze the results by brand-name and generic products.

26. Dr. Simmons goes on to say that even the major manufacturer experienced problems later in the production of digoxin in England. (Industry sources report that these were the results of changes in production methods.) Cf. Henry E. Simmons, Speech before the California Council of Hospital Pharmacists, San Diego, California, September 30, 1972.

27. Report by General Accounting Office on drug procurement system of federal agencies, January 19, 1971, *Competitive Problems in the Drug Industry,* part 20, p. 8050.

28. Since this was written, foreign purchasers have complained about the quality of wheat shipments despite certification by U.S. government inspectors. Apparently the standard example of product homogeneity is not all that homogeneous. Purchasers of wheat may also have to rely on brand names for quality assurance.

CHAPTER 12

1. Hugh D. Walker, *Market Power and Price Levels in the Ethical Drug Industry* (Bloomington: Indiana University Press, 1971), p. 31.

2. *National Prescription Audit,* IMS America Ltd., 1973.

3. Ibid., 1972.

4. *National Prescription Audits,* IMS America, Ltd., 1972.

5. The share of generic prescriptions filled by brand-name products equals 24/(100-31) × 100.

6. *National Prescription Audits,* IMS America Ltd., 1972.

7. Kentucky, Maryland, Illinois, and Massachusetts have repealed their antisubstitution laws. The district of Columbia has never had an antisubstitution law.

8. *U.S. Pharmaceutical Markets, Drugstores and Hospitals,* IMS America Ltd., 1972–73.

9. Process patents have not yet expired.

10. *U.S. Pharmaceutical Markets, Drugstores and Hospitals,* IMS America Ltd.

11. *National Prescription Audits,* IMS America, Ltd.

12. This estimate is based on a count of those firms for which sales were reported by IMS in *U.S. Pharmaceutical Market, Drugstores and Hospitals.* The estimate probably understates the number since the sales of some firms are too small to be picked up in the IMS audit.

CHAPTER 13

1. See F. M. Schemer, *Industrial Market, Structure and Economic Performance* (Chicago: Rand McNally, 1970).

2. Henry Steele, "Monopoly and Competition in the Ethical Drug Market," *Journal of Law and Economics* 5 (October 1962): 142–43; Hugh D. Walker, *Market Power and Price Levels in the Ethical Drug Industry* (Bloomington: Indiana University Press, 1971), p. 29–34.

3. Leonard G. Schifrin, "Ethical Drug Industry: The Case for Compulsory Patent Licensing," *Antitrust Bulletin,* Fall 1967, p. 900.

4. Steele, "Monopoly and Competition," pp. 151–53.

5. Ibid., p. 146.

6. Walker, *Market Power and Price Levels,* p. 48.

7. Steele, "Monopoly and Competition," p. 139.

8. William S. Comanor, "Research and Competitive Product Differentiation in the Pharmaceutical Industry in the United States," *Economica,* n. s. 31 (November 1964): 379. Comanor cites Frost at p. 2119, part 4, *Drug Industry Antitrust Act Hearings,* Senate Subcommittee on Antitrust and Monopoly, 87th Cong. 1st & 2d sess. 1961–62.

9. Bernard Kemp, "The RDTEM Process versus The Conventional Patent Protection Concept" (unpublished, 1971).

10. Walker, *Market Power and Price Levels,* p. 49; Carl Kaysen and Donald Turner, *Antitrust Policy: A Legal and Economic Analysis* (Cambridge, Mass. Harvard University Press, 1959).

11. "Monopoly and Competition," p. 137.

12. W. Duncan Reekie, *The Economics of Innovation with Special Reference to the Pharmaceutical Industry* (London: Association of British Pharmaceutical Industry, 1969).

13. Steele, "Monopoly and Competition," p. 134; Federal Trade Commission, *Economic Report on Antibiotics Manufacture* (Washington, D.C.: Government Printing Office, 1958), p. 118.

14. Comanor, "Research and Competitive Product Differentiation;" "The Drug Industry and Medical Research," *Journal of Business,* January 1966. Leonard G. Schifrin, "The Ethical Drug Industry," p. 899. Steele, "Monopoly and Competition," p. 141.

15. Walker, *Market Power and Price Levels,* p. 39.

16. Ibid., p. 43, table III-4.

17. Comanor, "Research and Competitive Product Differentiation," p. 380.

18. J. Jadlow, "Competition and Quality in the Drug Industry: The 1962 Kefauver-Harris Drug Amendments as Barriers to Entry," *Antitrust Law and Economics Review,* Winter 1971–72.

19. Markham, p. 170.

20. Comanor, "Research and Competitive Product Differentiation," pp. 374–375.

21. Markham, pp. 170–74.

22. Steele, "Ethical Drug Industry," *Journal of Industrial Economics,* July 1964, p. 217.

23. Steele, "Monopoly and Competition," p. 141. Steele cites the Kefauver *Hearings on Administered Prices,* part 18, pp. 105–95.

24. Paul A. Brooke, *Resistant Prices* (New York: The Council on Economic Priorities, 1975).

25. William S. Comanor, "Research and Competitive Product Differentiation," pp. 372–84, esp. pp. 373–74. Steele, "Monopoly and Competition," p. 148.

26. Walker, *Market Power and Price Levels,* p. 68.

27. Ibid., pp. 58–71.

28. Ibid., p. 64.

29. Ibid., pp. 65–66.

30. Ibid., pp. 74–75, 85–88.

31. Ibid., pp. 75–80. Walker cites references to the *1960 Administered Price Hearings,* Senate, 86th Cong., 2d sess., part 22, pp. 121–37 and p. 65.

32. Ibid., p. 80.

33. William S. Comanor and Thomas Wilson, "Advertising, Market Structure, and Performance," *Review of Economics and Statistics,* November 1967.

34. Lester G. Telser, "Another Look at Advertising and Concentration," *Journal of Industrial Economics,* November 1969.

35. W. Duncan Reekie, "Some Problems Associated with the Marketing of Ethical Pharmaceutical Products," *Journal of Industrial Economics* (November 1970): 33–49.

36. "Concentration, Promotion and Market Phase Statutory in the Pharmaceutical Industry," *Journal of Industrial Economics* (July 1971).

CHAPTER 14

1. United States Senate Subcommittee on Antitrust and Monopoly of the Committee on the Judiciary, *Hearings on Administered Prices,* 86th Cong., 1st sess., 2d sess., 1959, 1960. United States Senate Subcommittee on Antitrust and Monopoly of the Committee on the Judiciary, *Hearings on Drug Industry Antitrust Act,* 87th Cong., 1st sess., 2d sess., 1961, 1962. United States Senate Subcommittee on Antitrust and Monopoly of the Committee on the Judiciary, *Report, Administered Prices: Drugs,* 87th Cong., 1st sess., 1961, S. Rept. 448.

2. U.S. Senate Hearings before the Subcommittee on Monopoly of the Select Committee on Small Business, *Competitive Problems in the Drug Industry,* 90th Cong., 1st sess., part 1, May 1967. et seq. through part 23, 93d Cong., 1st sess., February and March 1973.

3. U.S. Senate Subcommittee on Health of the Senate Committee on Labor and Public Welfare, 93d Cong., 1st and 2d sess., 1973. *Examination of the Pharmaceutical Industry.* MAC proposal described in 39 Fed. Reg. 40302, Nov. 15, 1974.

4. See note 1, above.

5. 45 CFR Part 19, Dept. of Health, Education & Welfare, "Maximum Allowable Cost for drugs, Notice of Proposed Rule making."

6. *Congressional Record,* April 12, 1961, p. 5638.

7. The bill contained proposed amendments to the Food, Drug, and Cosmetic Act of 1938. This part of S1552 was modified and enacted into law in 1962 *(PL87–781)* and is cited as the "Drug Amendments of 1962."

8. *Hearings on S1552,* part 4, page 2130.

APPENDIX B

1. "Optimum Use of Antipsychotic Drugs," *Current Psychiatric Therapies,* vol. 12, 1972.

2. "Drug Treatment in Schizophrenia," *Canadian Psychiatric Association Journal,* vol. 16, 1971.

3. November 21, 1970, p. 444.

4. *British Medical Journal,* March 11, 1972, pp. 649–51.

INDEX

References to tables are printed in boldface type

LIBRARY OF CONGRESS
CATALOGING IN PUBLICATION DATA

Schwartzman, David.
  Innovation in the pharmaceutical industry.

  Includes bibliographical references and index.
  1. Drugs—Prices—United States. 2. Pharmaceutical re-
search—United States. I. Title.
HD9666.4.S38   338.4'3615'10973   76-7055
ISBN 0-8018-1844-3
ISBN 0-8018-1922-9 pbk.